A Radiological Atlas
of Diseases of the
Teeth and Jaws

A Radiological Atlas of Diseases of the Teeth and Jaws

R M Browne
BSc PhD DDS FDS RCS (Eng) FRCPath
Professor and Head of Department of Oral Pathology
University of Birmingham

H D Edmondson
MB ChB DDS FDS RCS (Eng) DA (Lond)
Professor and Head of Department of Oral Surgery and Oral Medicine
University of Birmingham

P G J Rout
BDS FDS RCS (Eng)
Lecturer in Oral Surgery and Oral Medicine
University of Birmingham

A Wiley Medical Publication

JOHN WILEY & SONS
Chichester · New York · Brisbane · Toronto · Singapore

Copyright © 1983 R. M. Browne   H. D. Edmondson   P. G. J. Rout

All Rights Reserved.
No part of this publication may be reproduced, stored in a
retrieval system, or transmitted, in any form or by any means,
electronic, mechanical, photocopying, recording or otherwise,
without the prior permission in writing of the copyright holder

Library of Congress Cataloging in Publication Data:

Browne, R. M. (Roger Michael)
  A radiological atlas of diseases of the teeth and
jaws.

  Includes index.
  1. Teeth—Diseases—Diagnosis—Atlases.   2. Jaws—
Diseases—Diagnosis—Atlases.   3. Diagnosis, Radioscopic
—Atlases.   I. Edmondson, H. D.   II. Rout, P. G. J.
III. Title.
RK309.B76   1983   617'.52207572   82–17349
ISBN 0 471 25616 1

British Library Cataloguing in Publication Data:

Browne, R. M.
  A radiological atlas of diseases of the teeth
  and jaws.
1 Teeth—Radiography   2. Teeth—Diseases
—Diagnosis   3. Jaws—Diseases—Diagnosis
  I. Title   II. Edmondson, H. D.
III. Rout, P. G. J.
  617.6'0757   RK309

ISBN 0 471 25616 1

Typeset in Linotron 202 Palatino by
Wyvern Typesetting Ltd, Bristol

Illustrations reproduced by
Wensum Graphics Ltd, Norwich

Printed and bound in Great Britain by
William Clowes (Beccles) Ltd, Beccles and London

To Eileen, Lilah, & Susan

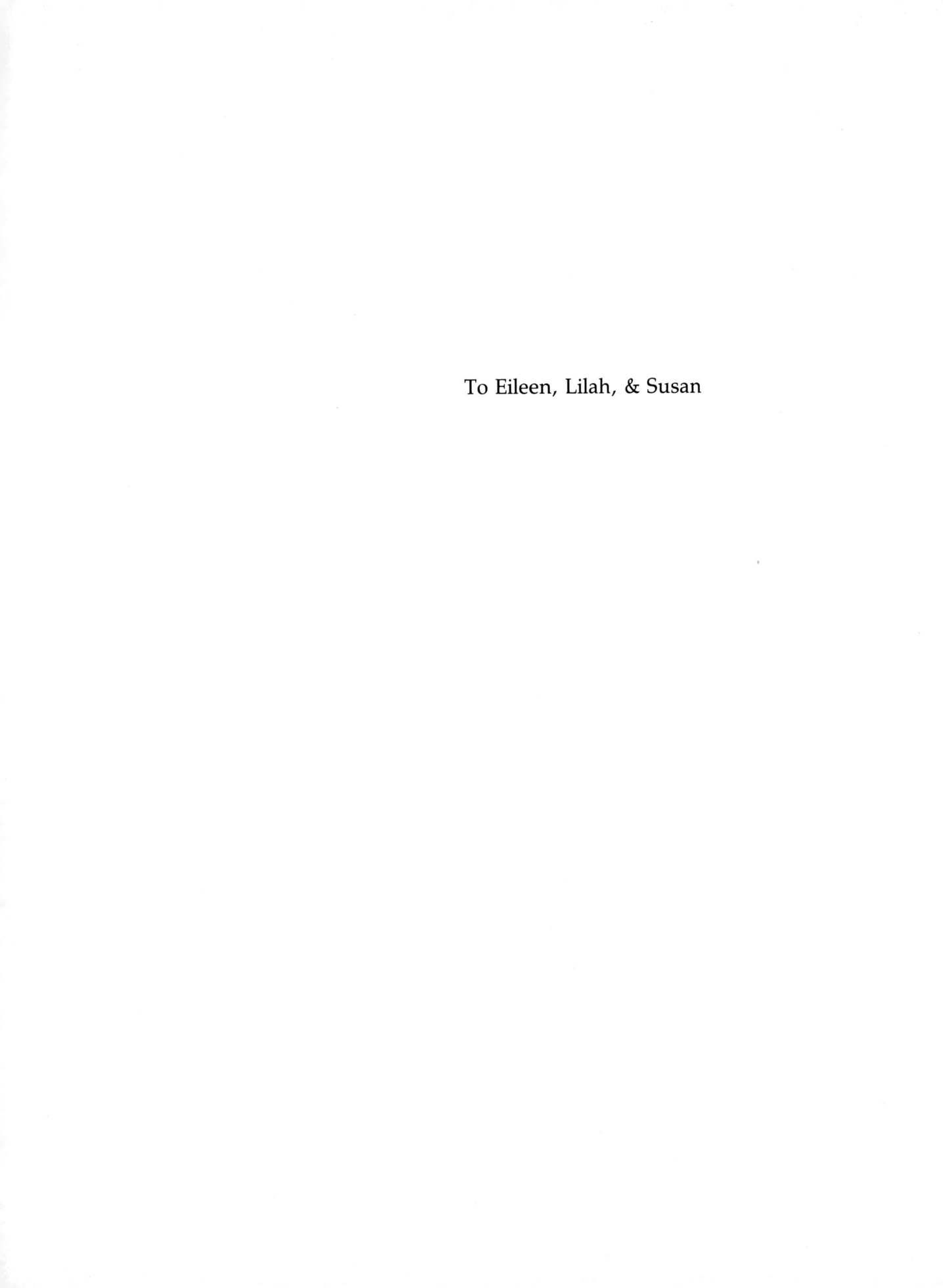

Contents

Preface		ix
Acknowledgements		xi
Abbreviations		xiii
Chapter 1	Introduction	1
Chapter 2	X-rays and Radiographic Technique	5
Chapter 3	Normal Radiographic Anatomy	15
Chapter 4	Technical Errors	47
Chapter 5	The Teeth	55
Chapter 6	The Periodontium	103
Chapter 7	The Facial Bones	117
Chapter 8	The Temporo-mandibular Joint	193
Chapter 9	The Soft Tissues including the Salivary Glands	207
Chapter 10	The Maxillary Antrum	227
Index		241

Preface

Investigation of the oral tissues by X-ray radiography is now an accepted everyday procedure in all aspects of dentistry. Whether a dental surgeon is working in general dental practice, in community dentistry or in hospital dentistry, the need for radiographic investigation of the patient is present. It is therefore essential for dental surgeons to be familiar with the variety of appearances, both normal and abnormal, of radiographs of the oral tissues.

As in many other aspects of dentistry, it takes many years to accumulate experience in the whole range of disease processes that can affect the jaws. It is the purpose in collecting together the radiographs contained within this Atlas, to help in reducing the time necessary to gain this experience. The authors appreciate that there is no real substitute for personal experience in acquiring diagnostic acumen, and that different examples of the same lesion frequently show variations in detail of the radiographic appearances. Nevertheless, it is hoped that this atlas will provide a reference for radiological diagnosis.

Since the majority of patients with disorders of the teeth and jaws are seen first by a general dental practitioner, radiographic appearances of these tissues on films commonly taken in dental practice are preferred. Although the diagnosis and treatment of the more unusual disorders may not be carried out by the practitioner, he or she should be aware of the diagnostic possibilities presented by each radiographic image. Where two or more diagnoses are likely, reference to the other commonly occurring disorders giving a similar radiographic appearance is often indicated in the text. The final diagnosis of many lesions is dependent, among other things, upon more extensive radiological investigation, and where necessary such radiographs have been included.

The radiographic appearance of a tissue is influenced firstly by its anatomical structure and secondly by the nature of the disease process which affects it. The first section of the atlas is concerned therefore with the variations in normal radiographic appearances occasioned by the different anatomical structures which may be present within or superimposed upon the structure under consideration. The remaining sections are concerned with changes in appearance brought about by different types of disease process. An understanding of the underlying pathology is essential for the correct interpretation of radiographs, and particular emphasis has been laid upon the correlation between different types of disease processes and radiological appearances in the text. Since the atlas is planned as an essentially practical book for use in the surgery, the disease processes have been presented as they may be considered at the chairside, in the form of a 'surgical sieve'. Further, where the radiological assessment is crucial to the proper management of a clinical problem (such as in the pre-operative assessment of impacted wisdom teeth), due emphasis has been paid to the necessary technical procedures.

It is anticipated, therefore, that this atlas will be of value not only to the general dental practitioner, but also, of course, to the dental undergraduate, most of whom are destined to become practitioners. Furthermore, it is hoped that those training for or pursuing a hospital career will find that the atlas provides a useful collection of radiographs for reference.

R. M. Browne
H. D. Edmondson
P. G. J. Rout

Acknowledgements

A collection of radiographs such as is presented in this Atlas can be achieved only as a consequence of the goodwill and collaboration of many people. The authors were very much aware of this when they set out on the task of compiling this Atlas, and wish to acknowledge the help and co-operation they have received from a great many people.

The majority of the radiographs presented have been selected from those contained within the Library of the Radiology Department of the Birmingham Dental Hospital. This collection has been accumulated over the past thirty years, and the authors are indebted to many of their predecessors who have so painstakingly documented and filed their radiographs in the past, as well as to their present day colleagues. In particular, they would like to thank Mr R. W. H. Tavenner, formerly Senior Lecturer in Dental Surgery, University of Birmingham and Consultant Dental Surgeon to the General Hospital, Birmingham; Mr J. W. Wheatcroft, formerly Tutor in Dental Radiology, University of Birmingham; and Mr C. L. Price, formerly Senior Lecturer in Oral Surgery, University of Birmingham. All three added many films to the Library and the authors have drawn heavily from their contributions.

Grateful thanks are due to all our present clinical colleagues working in the Hospitals of the Central Birmingham Health Authority, who have willingly agreed to our using films from their cases, and who have constantly borne our needs in mind. Grateful acknowledgement is also made to consultant colleagues from other authorities for contributing specific films, namely: Mr R. Bolton (Figs 7.148, 7.180, 7.181, 7.200, 9.50); Mr C. L. Brady (Figs 7.175, 7.190, 7.191); Mr D. Budd (Figs 5.177, 7.178); Mr J. G. Burland (Figs 7.53, 7.201, 7.202); Mr A. W. Grosart (Figs 7.75, 7.76); Mr A. Hamilton (Fig. 7.150); Mr G. S. Hoggins (Figs 5.98, 7.174); Dr P. Jacobs (Fig. 7.193);

Mr F. MacCauley (Fig. 5.86); Mr G. L. Manning (Figs 6.21, 7.179); Mr R. A. J. Mayhew (Figs 7.147, 7.170); Mr C. J. Meryon (Fig. 7.182); Mr K. Moos (Figs 7.54, 7.64, 7.167); Mr L. Oldham (Fig. 9.21); Mr. A. J. Sear (Fig. 7.152); and Mr C. Wishart (Figs 7.62, 7.151, 7.173).

We wish to thank particularly the entire staff of the Radiology Department, Birmingham Dental Hospital for their patience in putting up with our demands during the preparation of this book, and for their help, ever willingly given. In particular, we would thank Mr D. K. M. Toye, Consultant Radiologist, Miss D. Kelly, Superintendent Radiographer, and Mr C. Cook, Instructor in Dental Radiography, for their invaluable help and advice.

The diagrams were drawn and prepared partly by the staff of the Photographic Unit, Department of Oral Pathology, University of Birmingham, in particular by Mr G. O'Grady, and partly by Mrs C. A. Walker, to all of whom we extend our thanks. Similar thanks are extended to Mrs E. Merther and Miss H. Rupp, Department of Oral Pathology, and to Miss J. M. Preston, Department of Oral Surgery and Oral Medicine, for their assistance with the typing.

Finally, we would like to thank our publishers for their patience in awaiting this work.

Abbreviations

BW	Bitewing
CAT	Computerised axial tomogram
L	Lateral skull
LAO	Lower anterior occlusal
LC	Lateral skull cephalostat
LOO	Lower oblique occlusal
LTO	Lower true occlusal
OLM	Oblique lateral mandible
OM	Occipito-mental skull
OM30	Occipito-mental (30° angle) skull
P	Periapical
PA	Postero-anterior skull
PAC	Postero-anterior condyles
PR	Panoramic radiograph
RPA	Rotated postero-anterior skull
S	Soft tissue
SC	Scintiscan
SMV	Submento-vertex skull
T	Towne's view
TG	Tomogram
TMJ	Transcranial view of the temporo-mandibular joint
UOO	Upper oblique occlusal
USO	Upper standard occlusal (upper anterior occlusal)
UTO	Upper true occlusal
VO	Vertex occlusal

Chapter 1

Introduction

The successful practice of modern dentistry demands the use of X-rays under many circumstances, not only in arriving at a correct diagnosis, but also in monitoring and following up appropriate treatment programmes. Since the majority of dentistry is performed in the geographical isolation of general dental practice, the dental practitioner needs to be a competent radiographer in order to take the films which are necessary, and also an informed radiologist to be able to interpret them in the correct manner.

It was with the latter requirement in mind that we embarked upon the preparation of this collection of radiographs. As in any aspect of clinical dentistry, it takes a lifetime to accumulate experience of the whole range of disease processes that might affect the jaws. There is no substitute for personal experience, but it is hoped that a collection of this sort will accelerate the learning process and, to some extent provide a reference for some of the less common clinical conditions.

The ability to interpret radiographs correctly is dependent upon a correct understanding of four things: firstly, the physicochemical properties of X-rays and the factors involved in the production of a radiograph; secondly, the variety of angulations employed in the different radiographic techniques; thirdly, the full range of normal radiographic appearances that are a consequence of viewing the same anatomical structures by this variety of techniques; and finally, the variety of disease processes that might affect the jaws.

We have, therefore, presented a brief outline of the basic physics of X-rays, together with a simple explanation of the angulations involved in taking the radiographic views illustrated in this Atlas. We have made no attempt to describe in detail the procedures involved in taking the various types of radiograph, but have emphasised the direction of the X-ray beam relative to the structures of the head and neck in each example, so that a proper understanding of the anatomical structures displayed in each view can be obtained. Readers are referred to the appropriate texts on radiographic techniques for a detailed description of the procedures involved.

In addition, it is always advisable to emphasise the potential hazards of X-rays, not only to the patients being investigated, but also, and perhaps more importantly, to the staff carrying out the investigations. Brief reference is made to this.

The radiographic appearance of the normal anatomical features of the jaws and adjacent structures is presented for all the views illustrated in the main part of the Atlas.

It is our hope that besides being an invaluable teaching aid for both undergraduate and postgraduate students, this Atlas will also be of value at the chairside in helping with diagnostic problems. The main emphasis has, therefore, been in presenting radiographic views which can be readily taken in modern dental practices, although inevitably other views are also shown, since they are essential to the demonstration and interpretation of some of the diseases illustrated. In addition to conventional X-ray techniques, other forms of radiographic investigation have also been illustrated, including some of the more modern methods.

A collection of radiographs of the whole range of disease processes that can affect the jaws and adjacent tissues forms the main part of this Atlas. The different dento-facial structures are treated topographically so that the radiographic appearances of the whole range of diseases that can affect each anatomical area are presented together, thereby allowing them to be compared more readily. In presenting the examples for each anatomical area, they have been grouped according to disease processes as in the commonly used surgical sieve in the order: developmental, inflammatory, traumatic, neoplastic and metabolic.

The Atlas has been compiled with its main emphasis on the value of radiographs in aiding diagnosis. The examples chosen, therefore, illustrate predominantly diseases that have arisen *ab initio* and do not set out to demonstrate comprehensively the full range of radiographic appearances that may arise iatrogenically. In general, only when some iatrogenic procedure may be actiologic in a disease process, or provide a radiographic appearance that may be confused with some other disease, has it been illustrated.

The legends have been written bearing in mind how the disease process illustrated has contributed to the significant radiographic features. It is hoped that by the collaboration of an oral pathologist, an oral surgeon and a radiologist this objective may have been more satisfactorily achieved. Again, no attempt has been made to describe the histological features of the various diseases in detail, and it is suggested that in many instances an appropriate histopathology book may be studied concurrently to advantage.

It is probably true to say that each radiograph is unique and no two films are completely identical. The authors have been only too aware of this in seeking examples, and, as far as possible, films illustrating the most important changes have been chosen for the more common conditions. Clearly, for the more rare conditions, choice has not always been possible. In many instances, only one or at most two views of a lesion have been included. The views chosen are those considered to illustrate the radiographic features to the best advantage, and it cannot be emphasised too strongly that further views of the condition would often be desirable to obtain the maximum amount of information about many lesions. Routine radiographs provide a two dimensional image of a three dimensional object, and viewing a lesion from at least two different directions at right angles to each other is often necessary. It must also be emphasised that radiographs in themselves are not a means of making a diagnosis, but provide valuable information from which—together with a detailed clinical history and haematological, biochemical, immunological, microbiological and histopathological studies—a correct diagnosis may be reached. Indeed, in many instances the information to be gained from a radiograph, although bountiful, is limited in its diagnostic value and, as will be seen from the pages that follow, similar radiographic appearances may be given by a variety of lesions.

Finally, it is emphasised that the secret of successful radiographic interpretation is the ability to relate the changes displayed to the normal anatomy of the region being examined. In many unilateral lesions, opportunity is readily at hand, since the changes detected in the affected side can be compared with the appearance of the normal side. Fortunately, the human body is approximately symmetrical and thus provides an ideal basis upon which such comparisons can be made. Where bilateral comparison is not so readily available, either because of the systemic nature of the disease or because of limitation in the number of films taken, reference to the normal radiographic appearances presented early in this Atlas will be invaluable.

Cawson R. A. (1978) *Essentials of Dental Surgery and Pathology*, 3rd Edn, Edinburgh: Churchill Livingstone.

Lucas R. B. (1976) *Pathology of Tumours of the Oral Tissues*, 3rd Edn, Edinburgh: Churchill Livingstone.

Marsland E. A. & Browne R. M. (1975) *Colour Atlas of Oral Histopathology*, Aylesbury: HM + M Publishers.

Shafer W. G., Hine M. K. & Levy B. M. (1974) *A Textbook of Oral Pathology*, 3rd Edn, Philadelphia: W. B. Saunders.

Chapter 2

X-rays and Radiographic Technique

X-rays were discovered by W. Roentgen in November 1895 when, during experiments with a Crookes tube enclosed in black paper, he noticed a glow from a fluorescent screen close by. He attributed this phenomenon to an unknown ray, or X-ray, emitted from the tube. It is now known that X-rays are a form of energy which makes up part of the electromagnetic spectrum (Fig. 2.1) and have a very short wavelength. They have no mass, travel at the speed of light, cause certain salts to fluoresce, and darken photographic emulsions. X-rays can also exist as particles or quanta, referred to as photons.

X-ray Formation

In clinical usage, X-rays are produced in an evacuated glass tube (Fig. 2.2) with a copper anode containing a block of tungsten known as the target, or focal spot, and a cathode consisting of a spiral tungsten wire filament which, when heated by an electric current, liberates a cloud of electrons. A potential of many thousands of volts applied between the cathode and the anode causes the electrons to be propelled at high speed from the cathode and collide with the anode. Here their kinetic energy is converted mainly into heat which is conducted away by the copper anode, but about 1% is transformed into X-rays of various wavelengths and energy levels. The larger the filament current (measured in milliamps), the bigger the electron cloud and the greater the quantity of X-rays produced. The higher the voltage, the shorter the wavelength and the greater the energy of the X-rays and thus their ability to penetrate tissues. The X-rays emerge as a beam via a window in the otherwise shielded X-ray tube and pass through an aluminium filter of appropriate thickness to remove most of the low energy X-rays which would otherwise be absorbed by the soft tissue and not contribute to the formation of the image.

A lead diaphragm collimates the size of the beam to be no larger than 6 cm in diameter as it emerges from the end of the cone. The cone should be of such a length as to provide the necessary focus–skin distance.

X-ray Absorption

When X-rays penetrate tissue, their intensity is reduced by two processes, photoelectric absorption and Compton scatter (Fig. 2.3). In the former, high-energy photons displace an inner-orbiting or *k* electron from atoms within the tissue and, in the process, transfer their energy to the electrons, now referred to as photoelectrons. The atoms become ionised, but retain their stability by internal re-arrangement of the remaining electrons, a process which results in the emission of 'characteristic' radiation. Photoelectric absorption is more likely to occur with high atomic number elements such as the heavy metals. On the other hand, Compton scatter occurs when the X-ray photon displaces a relatively unbound or outer-orbiting electron from the atom. The X-ray photon loses only some of its energy to the electron, and is deflected from its original path and may subsequently react with other atoms. It is possible for an X-ray photon to be deflected by an atom without colliding with it, and this form of scattering is known as the Thompson effect.

Soon after Roentgen's discovery, it became evident that X-rays had harmful effects to both the patient and the operator, and that protective measures were needed. Continued improvements to X-ray equipment, and the establishment of safe radiographic techniques have resulted in dose levels acceptable to patient and operator. These improvements include X-ray sets incorporating the appropriate aluminium filtration and X-ray beam collimation, fast X-ray films, protective lead screens and aprons, intensifying screens and X-ray dose monitoring. Based on recommendations of the International Commission of Radiological Protection, most countries have a Code of Practice which sets out the principles of radiation control and provides guidance on the usage of X-radiation (United Kingdom Code of Practice 1972; Koren & Wuehrmann 1977).

The effects that X-rays have on the tissues depend on many factors, such as the dose received, the frequency of exposure, and the amount and type of tissue irradiated. Tissues whose cells divide frequently are more sensitive to X-rays than are tissues whose cells are less active. Cells may be injured by the production of radicals resulting from ionisation or from direct damage to their nuclear DNA. The biological effects that appear in the individual exposed to X-rays are known as the somatic effects and include radiation sickness, a reduction in blood cell counts, skin erythema, epilation, dermatitis, leukaemia and neoplasia. Following irradiation, there is a variable interval called the latent period (which may last many years) before any effects become apparent. The genetic effects are those that occur in the later generations of an irradiated person and result from the production of cellular mutations. It is possible that the genetic effects can occur from quite low doses of X-radiation.

X-ray Detection

Those X-rays that are not absorbed by the tissues will pass through them to reach the film. An X-ray film consists of a plastic base which is coated on either side with an emulsion of silver bromide crystals in gelatine, itself covered by a protective layer.

There are two types of film, non-screen and screen film. Non-screen film is used most frequently for intra-oral radiography and the image is formed on the emulsion by the direct action of X-rays. Since it is also sensitive to light, it is contained in a light-tight packet between two pieces of black paper, with a sheet of lead foil to absorb most of the X-rays which have passed through the film. Screen film, which is used mainly for extra-oral radiography, is placed within a cassette sandwiched between intensifying screens containing calcium tungstate crystals. The image is thus formed not only by the direct action of X-rays, but also by bluish light emitted from the intensifying screens when exposed to X-rays. The light emitted is multi-directional, its amount being a function of the crystal size. Thus, loss of definition of the image results when intensifying screens are used, being greatest with those screens which emit most light. However, considerably less radiation is required to produce an image. More efficient light emitters based on rare earths have recently been developed.

Since the atomic composition of tissues is variable, X-rays are absorbed to different degrees, and so an image of them can be recorded on X-ray film. A latent image is first formed due to alteration of those silver bromide crystals which have been irradiated, and is then made visible by reducing them to black metallic silver by a developer solution which contains hydroquinone and metol. In addition, the developer contains sodium carbonate to maintain the necessary alkalinity, potassium bromide to suppress reduction of the unexposed crystals, and sodium sulphite as a preservative.

For manual development, the manufacturer recommends a critical temperature and duration. After rinsing for a few seconds in water, the film is fixed in a sodium thiosulphate solution to remove the unexposed silver bromide so that the film becomes 'clear'. The solution also contains acetic acid for the necessary acidity, sodium sulphite as a preservative, and potassium alum, which hardens the emulsion. The temperature for fixing is less critical than that for development, but the duration is usually twice the time taken for the X-ray film to clear. After fixing, the film is washed in running water for about 20 minutes and dried in a warm, dust-free area. Because films are light sensitive, processing must be carried out in a darkened room illuminated by appropriate 'safe' lights.

Film processing may also be undertaken automatically, the majority of systems using rollers to transport the film through the various solutions, and subsequently produce a dry film ready for viewing. Other methods of processing include the monobath system, where the developer and alkaline fixer are present in one solution which is injected into the film packet, and subdued light processing, where the film emulsion contains a yellow dye which permits the processing to be undertaken by daylight.

No attempt has been made to describe the various radiographical techniques in detail, but a brief description is included below to assist the reader to interpret the whole range of radiographs presented. For a full account of these techniques, the reader is referred to an appropriate text (Mason 1982; Manson-Hing 1979; Smith 1980).

Intra-oral Radiographs

The majority of dental radiographs are taken with the film placed intra-orally, and consist of periapical, bitewing and occlusal radiographs. Periapical radiographs (P) record an image of the whole of the tooth and its surrounding tissues. There are two techniques commonly used to obtain this image, the bisecting angle technique and the paralleling technique.

The bisecting angle technique (Fig. 2.4) is based on the principle of isosceles triangles where AB is the length of the object, BC is the length of the image and BD is the bisector of the triangle ABC. The film is placed as close as possible to the lingual or palatal aspect of the teeth, in contact with their crowns, but inclined away from their roots, according to the shape of the investing tissues. The operator determines the plane of the bisector and directs the X-ray beam at right angles to it. The length of the tooth AB will thus equal the length of its image BC projected onto the film. The image will be elongated if the X-ray beam is directed at right angles to the teeth, and foreshortened if directed at right angles to the film. The film is placed as far as possible parallel in the horizontal plane to the crowns of the teeth, and the X-ray beam directed at right angles to the film in this plane (Fig. 2.5).

In the paralleling technique (Fig. 2.6), the film is placed parallel to the long axis of the teeth, which necessitates placing it away from them. To prevent magnification of the image, a nearly parallel beam of X-rays is used, which is obtained by increasing the anode–film distance. A relatively powerful dental X-ray set is required, since the intensity of the X-ray beam decreases as the distance from its source increases, as determined by the inverse square law. The film is held in position by a holder, some examples of which have devices to aid the correct alignment of the X-ray tube so that the beam is directed at right angles to the film.

Bitewing radiographs (BW)—so called because the patient stabilises the film by occluding onto an attached tab or wing (Fig. 2.7)—record the images of the crowns and the coronal portion of the roots of maxillary and mandibular posterior teeth and their investing tissues. The film is usually positioned with its long axis horizontal and parallel to the crowns of the teeth. The X-ray beam is directed with a downward angle of approximately 5° to the occlusal plane and at right angles to the film, passing between the contact points of the teeth being examined so that they do not overlap (Fig. 2.5).

In occlusal radiography, the film is larger than that used for periapical radiography and records an image of a greater area. The film is placed as far back into the mouth as is required and is gently held between the occlusal surfaces of the teeth. Occlusal radiographs fall into two groups: those that provide an image similar to that obtained in periapical radiographs and those in which a plan view of parts of the dental arches is obtained. The first group includes the upper standard (anterior) occlusal (USO), the upper oblique occlusal (UOO), the lower anterior occlusal (LAO) and the lower oblique occlusal (LOO). The upper views are frequently taken for the examination of unerupted teeth. The second group includes the upper true occlusal (UTO), which provides a plan view of the upper posterior teeth, the vertex occlusal (VO), which provides a plan view of the upper incisor teeth, and the lower true occlusal (LTO), which provides a plan view of the lower posterior teeth. These views are used in the localisation of foreign bodies and unerupted teeth, and the examination of expansile lesions of the alveolus. Since in upper views the beam is directed to the film from above, many structures in the maxillary skeleton may be superimposed upon the dento-alveolar image. In lower views, superimposition is little problem, since the beam is directed from below. Occlusal or periapical films (S) may also be used to detect foreign bodies in the lips, cheeks and submandibular salivary duct, in some instances necessitating positioning of the film extra-orally.

Parallax

A radiograph demonstrates a three dimensional object on a flat plane. Therefore, when superimposition of two or more structures occurs, it is not always possible to determine their spatial relationships. This information can be obtained by examining radiographs taken at right angles to each other, by tomography (see p. 9) or by employing the principle of parallax, the method of choice being determined by the particular circumstances. The parallax or tube shift technique involves taking two radiographic views of the same area with the film similarly positioned for both exposures, but with a different horizontal or vertical angulation of the X-ray tube. Structures lying in different planes will appear to move in relation to each other (Fig. 2.8). A structure positioned closer to the X-ray tube (Fig. 2.8b) moves in the opposite direction to that taken by the tube relative to a structure placed nearer to the film. Conversely, a structure lying closer to the film (Fig. 2.8c) moves in the same direction taken by the tube, relative to a structure positioned closer to it.

Extra-oral Radiographs

When an area larger than that of an intra-oral radiograph is to be examined, it becomes necessary to place the film outside the mouth so that a film of appropriate size can be used. To minimise the radiation exposure, screen film in a cassette with intensifying screens is required. Where the tissue density is not marked (as in an oblique lateral mandible view), a dental X-ray set may be used. However, for most examinations, the tissue thickness is such that a more powerful X-ray set with a variable current and voltage is required to allow for the appropriate exposure. The greater tissue thickness results in more scattered radiation, which impairs the image quality, but this problem can be minimised by the use of a specially designed grid system. The grid, which is placed between the object and the film, consists of a radiolucent plastic base containing a series of fine, linear, parallel, lead slats, which are so angled that the primary beam can pass between them, and the scattered radiation is absorbed by them (Fig. 2.9). Such grids may be either stationary or moveable (e.g. Potter–Bucky). The former cast a shadow of fine parallel lines on the film, but this problem is avoided with a moveable grid. The focus–film distance is much greater in extra-oral radiography in order to minimise magnification and blurring of the image. To aid accurate positioning of the head relative to the film and X-ray tube, certain base lines and planes (including the infra-orbital and orbito-meatal lines, and the sagittal plane) are used. The area of interest is placed closest to the film and the various radiographic views are usually described according to the direction of the X-ray beam.

Oblique Lateral Mandible (OLM) (Fig. 2.10)

This projection demonstrates one side of the mandible from its mid-point to the condyle, but may include part of the maxilla. The film is positioned against the upper and lower jaws, the head being turned to bring the area of interest parallel to the film, and the chin extended to draw the mandible away from the cervical vertebrae. The X-ray tube is centred just below and posterior to the angle of the mandible of the contralateral side, and is angled obliquely upwards so that the central ray passes between the ramus of the mandible and the cervical vertebrae to reach that part of the mandible of the side being examined.

Lateral Skull (L) (Fig. 2.11)

In this projection, the skull is viewed laterally, the patient being positioned with the sagittal plane parallel to, and the infra-orbital line perpendicular to, the film. The X-ray tube is directed at right angles to the film, so that there is superimposition of both sides of the skull, facial bones and mandible.

In orthodontic and oral surgery treatment planning,

accurate skull measurements and determination of skeletal growth are undertaken in a standardised form by cephalometric radiography (LC), whereby a reproducible relationship between X-ray tube, patient and film can be obtained. The patient's head is located in a specially designed holder, or craniostat, which incorporates an ear-plug fitting into each external auditory meatus. The film holder and X-ray tube are placed a set distance (approximately 1 foot and 6 feet, respectively) from the craniostat, at which separation the X-rays will be nearly parallel, and therefore magnification will be minimal. Such films should be taken with the teeth in occlusion. To demonstrate the soft tissues (S) of the front of the face, an appropriately positioned aluminium wedge may be used to attenuate the X-ray beam.

Occipito-mental (OM) (Fig. 2.12)

In this view, the patient faces the film with chin touching, so that the orbito-meatal line is at 45° to it. The sagittal plane is perpendicular to the film, the X-ray beam also being directed at right angles to the film. This view demonstrates well the middle third of the facial skeleton, including the maxillary antra, the orbits and the frontal sinuses, since these structures are projected away from the base of the skull and cervical spine. A modification to demonstrate the infra-orbital margins and zygomatic arches can be made by directing the X-ray beam downwards 30° to the horizontal (OM 30) so that it passes through the vertex to emerge at the infra-orbital margins.

Postero-anterior (PA) (Fig. 2.13)

In this view, the patient faces the film, the forehead touching it, with the sagittal plane, orbito-meatal line and X-ray beam at right angles to it. This view is used for demonstrating the posterior region of the mandible, the facial bones and nasal skeleton. There are several modifications to this technique, one of which is to expose the film with the patient's mouth open, which better demonstrates the condyles (PAC), and a second of which is taken with the patient's head rotated in the vertical axis so that the beam passes tangentially through the area of interest, thus avoiding superimposition upon deeper structures (RPA).

Submento-vertex (Base View) (SMV) (Fig. 2.14)

In this view, the vertex of the head touches the film so that the infra-orbital line is parallel to it. The X-ray beam is directed at right angles to the film, passing mid-way between the angles of the mandible. This projection demonstrates the base of the skull and, if the exposure is reduced, the zygomatic arches.

30° Fronto-occipital (Towne's View) (T) (Fig. 2.15)

In this view, the patient faces away from the film with the sagittal plane at right angles to it. The orbito-meatal line is perpendicular to the film and the X-ray tube is directed downwards at 30° to pass through the mandibular condyles. This projection demonstrates the condylar necks. The reverse Towne's view, in which the patient faces towards the film and the X-ray beam is angled upward at 30° to pass through the condyles, may also be used for this purpose.

Transcranial View of the Temporo-mandibular Joint (TMJ) (Fig. 2.16)

In this view, the patient is in a similar position as for a lateral skull radiograph, the X-ray tube being angled 25° downwards so that the central ray passes through the condyle under investigation, which is adjacent to the film. It provides an oblique view of the condylar head, articular surfaces and joint space, which may be examined with the mouth open and in the closed position.

Tomography (TG)

This technique demonstrates a selected plane within the head, whilst blurring out structures in other planes. It can be used to determine the extent of a lesion by taking a successive series of tomograms in parallel planes, or to examine a particular area which may be obscured by superimposition of other structures on conventional films.

Tomography (Fig. 2.17) involves movement of the X-ray tube and film, which are connected so as to rotate about a pivot. They move in opposite directions about a stationary object, so that there is a plane at which there is no relative movement between them (the pivot point). This plane is referred to as the tomographic cut, and structures in adjacent planes are blurred due to movement and so are not visualised. The thickness of the tomographic cut or plane is determined by the angle of travel taken by the X-ray tube, a small angle producing a thick, and a large angle a thin layer.

Panoramic Radiography (PR)

The principle of tomography is utilised in panoramic radiography, but instead of recording a flat plane, it focuses upon a curved layer corresponding to the upper and lower arches. The thickness of the tomographic cut varies, being narrow anteriorly, but much wider posteriorly. Originally this was achieved by rotating the X-ray apparatus about two, and subsequently three, pivots or centres of rotation, but recently eliptical paths of rotation have been used. The X-rays are collimated into a narrow slit beam. As the X-ray tube and film holder rotate around the patient, the film moves behind a slit guard in the front of the holder, so exposing it a bit at a time. In this way, a complete record is obtained of both jaws from front to back.

Computerised Axial Tomography (CAT)

Computed tomography is a technique able to demonstrate hard and soft tissues simultaneously in selected planes. A collimated beam of X-rays rotates around the patient, passing through the desired tissue layer. Crystal detectors measure the amount of attenuation of the X-ray beam and convey this information to a computer, which reconstructs the image on a cathode ray tube. This image may be recorded photographically or stored for future reference on an electromagnetic disc, either in its original form or as a digital scattergram in which the figures correspond to the absorption values of the tissues.

Sialography

In this technique, a radiopaque, fluid contrast medium is used to demonstrate the duct system of the parotid and submandibular salivary glands. Plain radiographs are usually taken prior to sialography, although they do not demonstrate the salivary glands themselves, but may reveal a ductal calculus provided it is sufficiently mineralised. There are two types of contrast media, one of which is water-soluble (e.g. Hypaque) and the other oil-based (e.g. Lipiodol). Water-soluble media are miscible with saliva and of lower viscosity than oil-based media, which are in general more radiopaque.

The duct orifice is located and dilated with a blunt probe to allow the introduction of a suitable cannula, through which sufficient contrast medium is slowly injected to slightly distend the gland. Radiographs are taken immediately after injection with the cannula still in place, and again, if an oil-based medium is used, 30–60 minutes after the cannula has been removed, to demonstrate the amount of contrast medium retained within the duct system, as an indication of gland function.

Scintiscanning (SC)

Scintiscanning involves the adminstration of a labelled radionuclide tracer, the emitted γ radiation of which is recorded and thus located by scintillation counters placed outside the body. The most commonly used radionuclide is technetium because it emits radiation of the appropriate energy level, has a short half-life (approximately six hours) and is almost completely excreted from the body within 24 hours. The uptake of radionuclide is an indication of the metabolic activity of a tissue, and by choosing an appropriate tracer, the metabolism of selected tissues can be studied. Scintiscanning can thus be used to investigate the activity of suspected benign and malignant neoplams particularly those affecting the deeper tissues, fibro-osseous disorders of the jaws, and the secretory activity of salivary glands.

Code of practice for the protection of persons against ionising radiations arising from medical and dental use (1972). London: HMSO.

Koren K. & Wuehrmann A. H. (1977) Radiation protection in dentistry. *Manual on Radiation Protection in Hospitals and General Practice*, Vol. 4. Geneva: WHO.

Manson-Hing L. R. (1979) *Fundamentals of Dental Radiography*. Philadelphia: Lea & Febiger.

Mason R. A. (1982) *A Guide to Dental Radiography*. Bristol: John Wright & Sons.

Smith N. J. D. (1980) *Dental Radiography*. Oxford: Blackwell Scientific Publications.

X-rays and Radiographic Technique   11

	ANGSTROM UNITS
Cosmic Rays	0.0001 Å
Gamma Rays	0.001 Å
X-Rays	0.1 - 10.0 Å
Ultra Violet Light	100 Å
Visible Light	5000 Å
Infra Red	50,000 Å
	METERS
Microwaves & Radar	0.01 M
Television	1.0 M
Radio	10M - 100M

2.1 A diagram illustrating the relative position of X-rays in the electromagnetic spectrum.

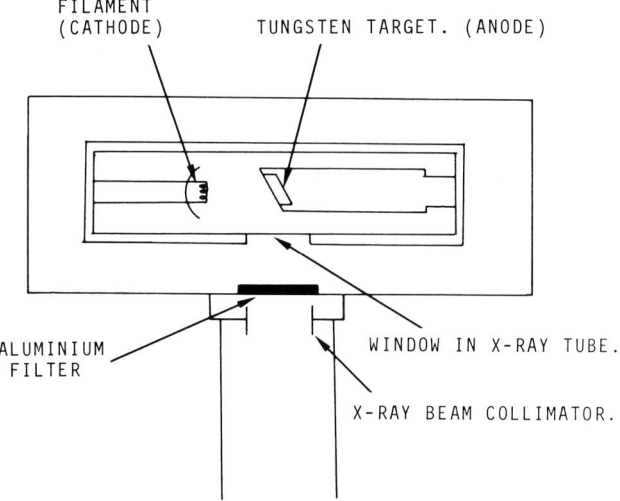

2.2 The basic components of an X-ray tube.

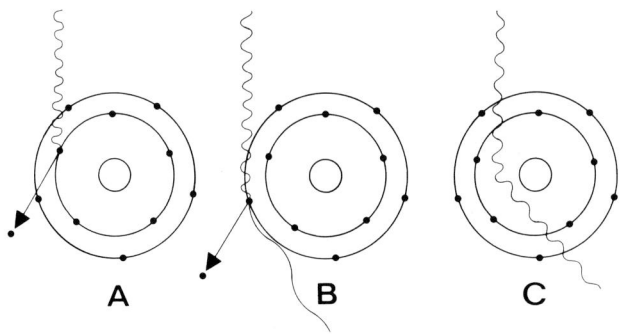

2.3 The interaction of X-rays with matter: A, photoelectric absorption; B, Compton scatter; C, the Thompson effect.

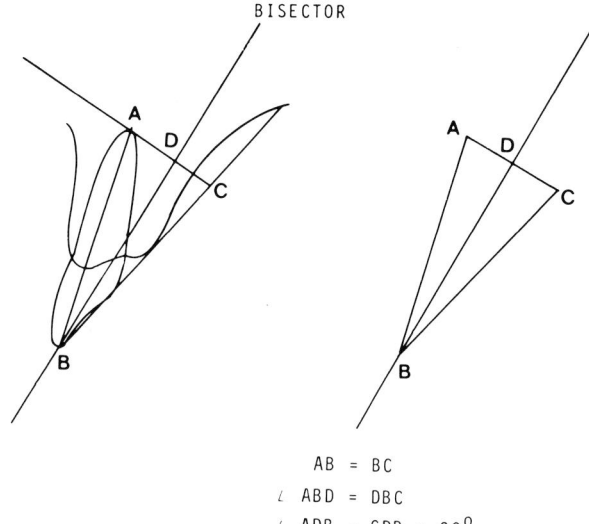

$AB = BC$
$\angle ABD = DBC$
$\angle ADB = CDB = 90°$

2.4 The bisecting angle technique for taking intra-oral radiographs (see text).

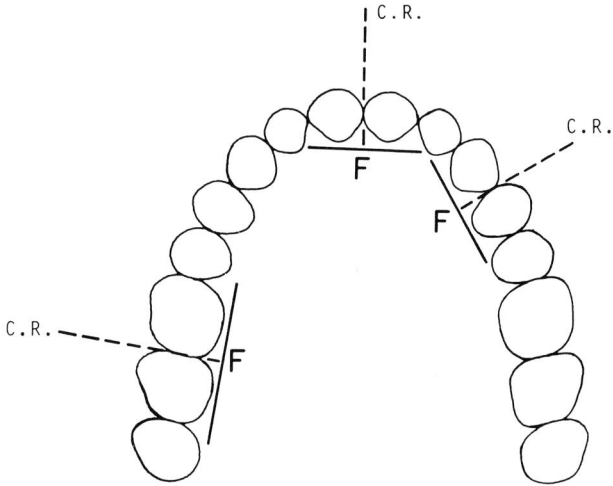

2.5 The alignment of the X-ray beam relative to the teeth in intra-oral radiographs: CR, centre ray of the X-ray beam; F, film.

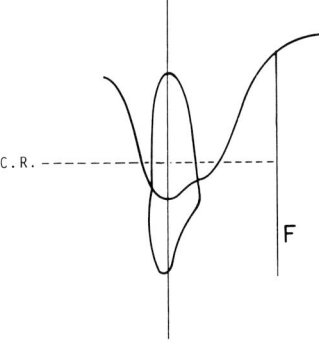

2.6 The paralleling technique for taking intra-oral radiographs: CR, centre ray of the X-ray beam; F, film.

12 *A Radiological Atlas of Diseases of the Teeth and Jaws*

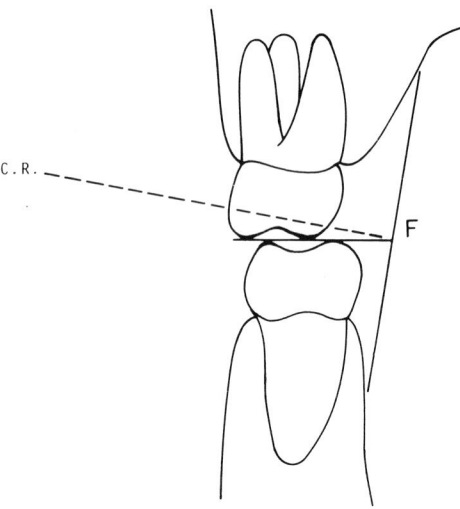

2.7 The bitewing technique in which the film (F) is held in place by occluding on a tab: CR, centre ray of the X-ray beam.

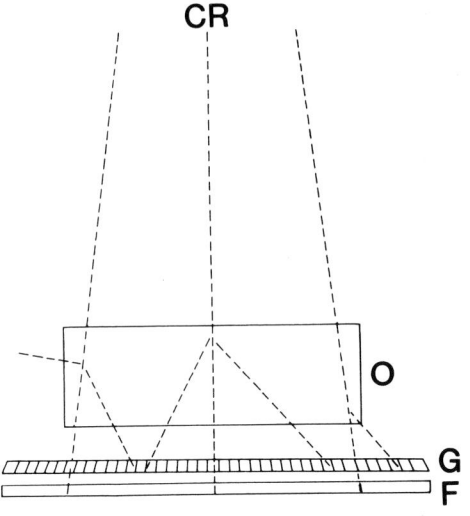

2.9 The Potter–Bucky grid. Scattered rays emerging from the object (O) are absorbed by the grid (G) and thus prevented from reaching the film (F). Only undeviated rays reach the film. CR, centre ray of X-ray beam.

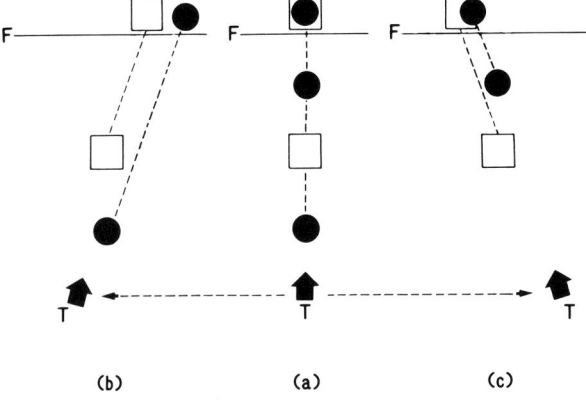

2.8 The principle of parallax. When two objects are superimposed (a) it is not possible to be certain if the reference object (open square) is nearer or further from the film (F) than the object of interest (full circle). If the object of interest is closer to the tube (T) it moves in the opposite direction (b) relative to the reference object, whereas if it is further away, it moves in the same direction (c).

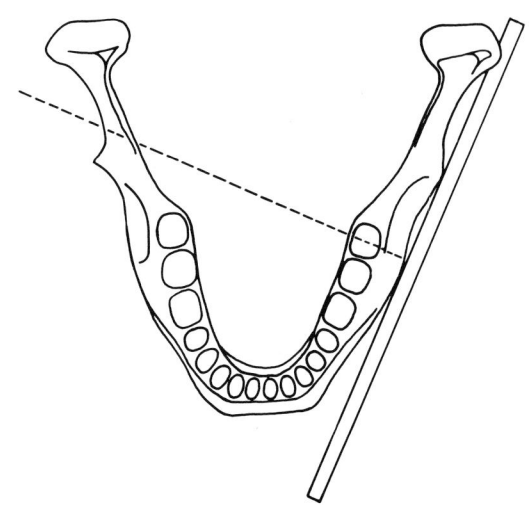

2.10 Oblique lateral mandible view.

X-rays and Radiographic Technique 13

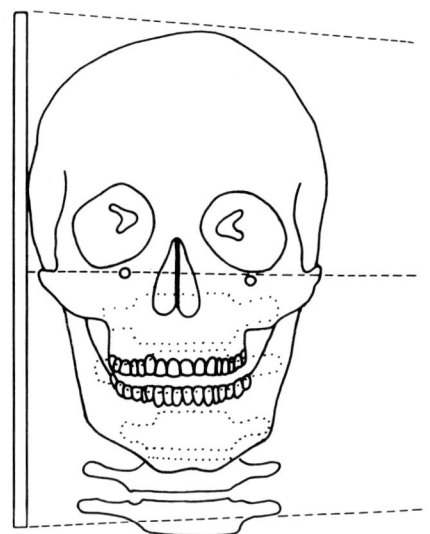

2.11 Lateral skull view.

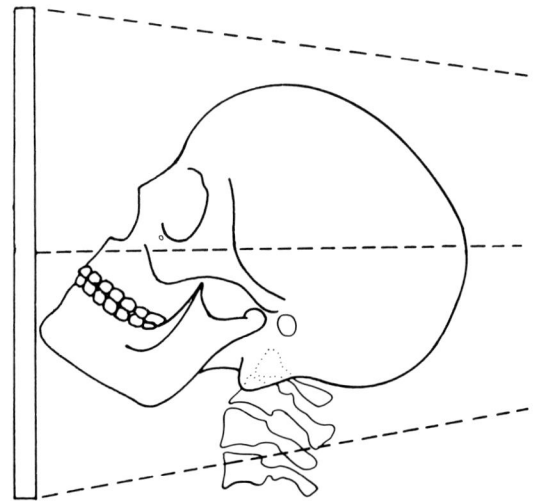

2.12 Occipito-mental view.

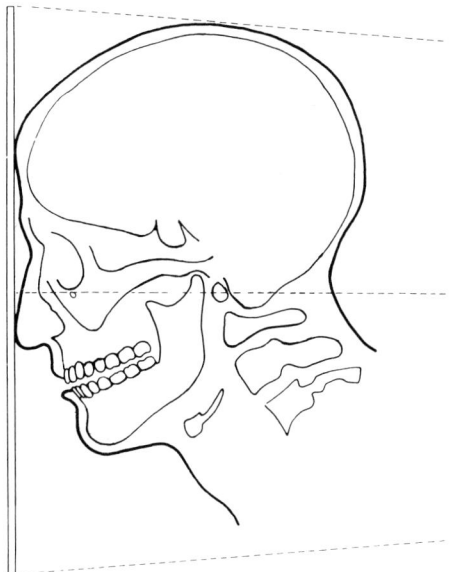

2.13 Postero-anterior view.

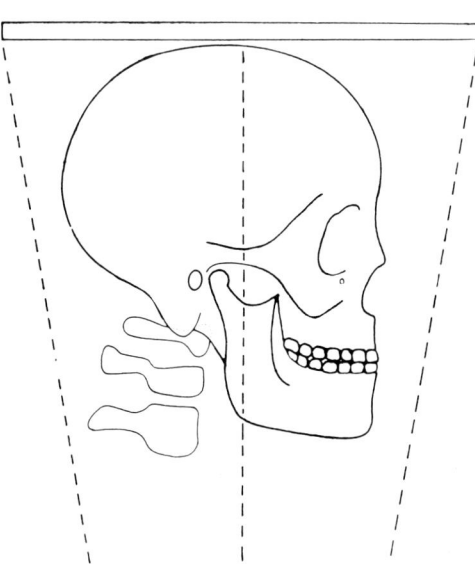

2.14 Submento-vertex (base) view.

14   A Radiological Atlas of Diseases of the Teeth and Jaws

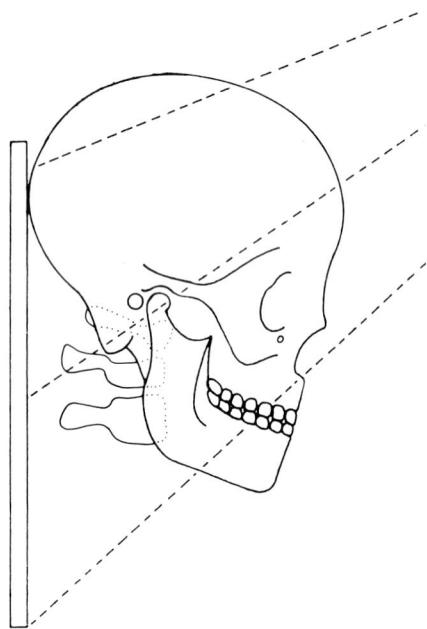

2.15   30° Fronto-occipital (Towne's) view.

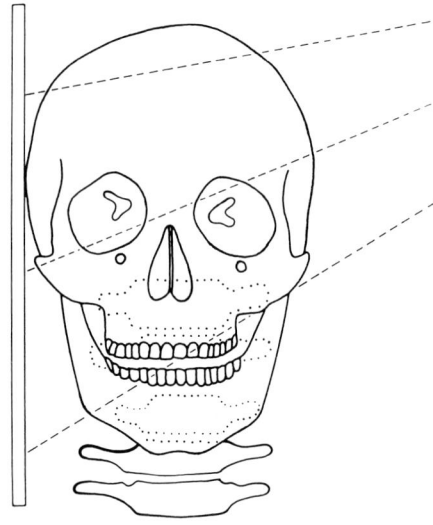

2.16   Transcranial view of the temporo-mandibular joint.

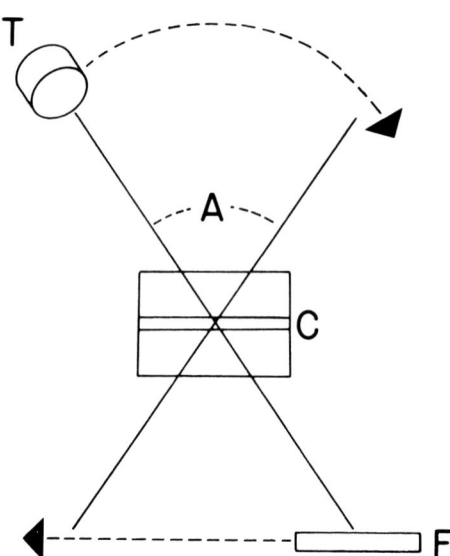

2.17   The principle of tomography. The X-ray tube (T) and film (F) rotate in opposite directions around a fixed plane (C), which remains in focus. The thickness of the plane visualised is determined by the angle of travel (A) of the tube.

Chapter 3

Normal Radiographic Anatomy

Normal Radiographic Anatomy 17

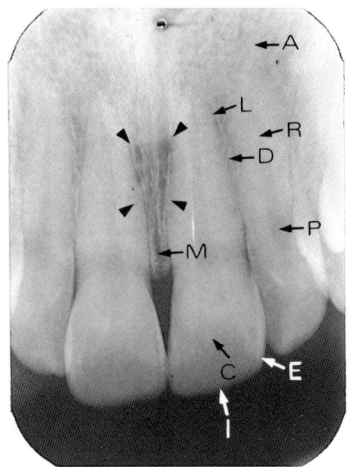

3.1 Periapical (P), incisor teeth:
- E enamel
- P pulp chamber
- R root canal
- A root apex
- D lamina dura
- L periodontal ligament space
- M anterior midline suture
- C cingulum
- I incisal edge

small arrows indicate incisive fossa

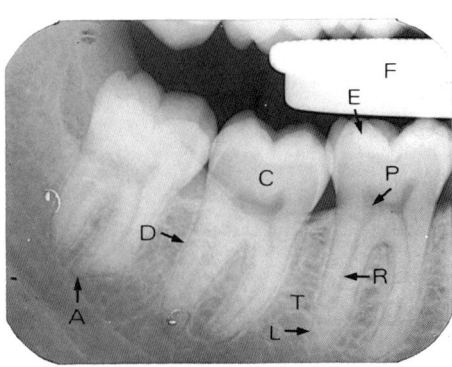

3.2 Periapical (P), molar teeth:
- E enamel
- P pulp chamber
- R root canal
- T bony trabeculae in the interdental septum
- L periodontal ligament space
- D lamina dura
- A root apex
- C coronal dentine
- F film holder

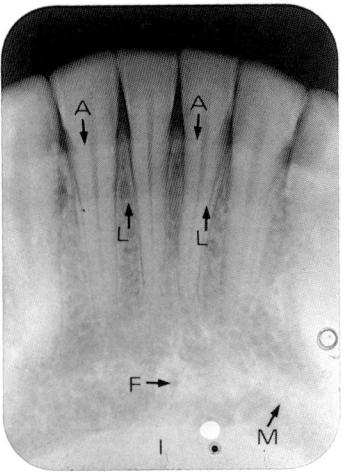

3.3 Periapical (P) $\overline{321\,|\,123}$ region, bisecting angle technique, demonstrating the spiny interdental crests and the trabecular pattern of the bone:
- M mental ridge
- F lingual foramen
- L lip line
- A alveolar crest line
- I inferior cortical plate

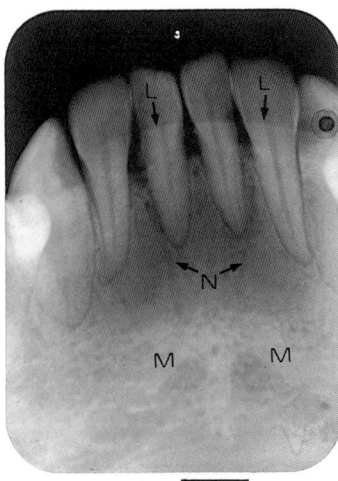

3.4 Periapical (P) $\overline{321\,|\,123}$ region, bisecting angle technique:
- N Hirschfeld's nutrient canals
- L lip line
- M mental ridge

18 A Radiological Atlas of Diseases of the Teeth and Jaws

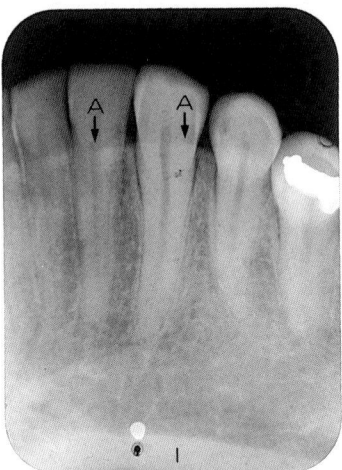

3.5 Periapical (P) $\overline{12345}$ region, bisecting angle technique, demonstrating the trabecular pattern of the bone:
- A alveolar crest line
- I inferior cortical plate

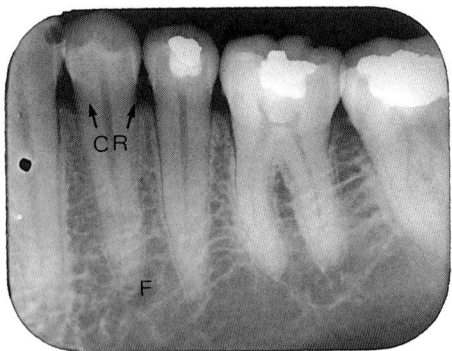

3.6 Periapical (P) $\overline{34567}$ region, bisecting angle technique, demonstrating the plateau form of the interdental crests and the horizontal distribution of the trabeculae in the alveolar bone, both interdentally and inter-radicularly:
- F mental foramen
- CR cervical radiolucency, due to the relative contrast between the enamel-covered crown superiorly and the bone-invested part of the root inferiorly, and the cervical part of the root which is covered by neither.

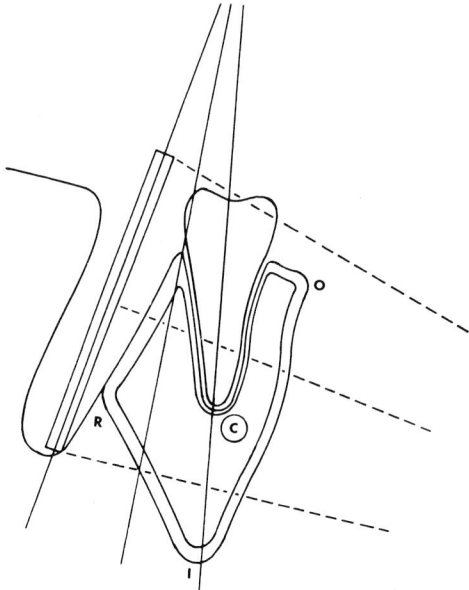

3.7 A line drawing illustrating the anatomical features that commonly appear on a mandibular molar periapical film, taken by the bisecting angle technique:
- C inferior alveolar canal
- O oblique ridge
- R mylohyoid ridge
- I inferior cortical plate

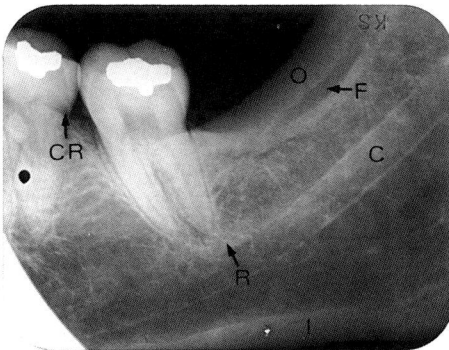

3.8 Periapical (P) $\overline{78}$ region, bisecting angle technique:
- C inferior alveolar canal
- O oblique ridge
- R mylohyoid ridge
- F retromolar fossa
- I inferior cortical plate
- CR cervical radiolucency

Normal Radiographic Anatomy 19

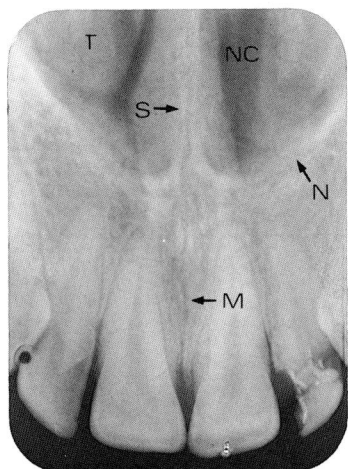

3.9 Periapical (P) 21|12 region, bisecting angle technique, demonstrating the trabecular pattern of the alveolar bone:
N lateral margin of floor of nose
S nasal septum
NC nasal cavity
T inferior turbinates, covered with soft tissue
M anterior midline suture

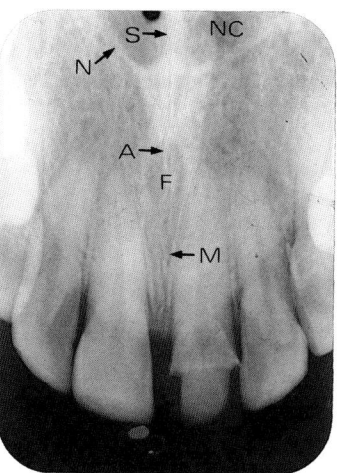

3.11 Periapical (P) 21|12 region, bisecting angle technique:
N lateral margin of floor of nose
S nasal septum
NC nasal cavity
F incisive foramen
A anterior nasal spine
M anterior midline suture

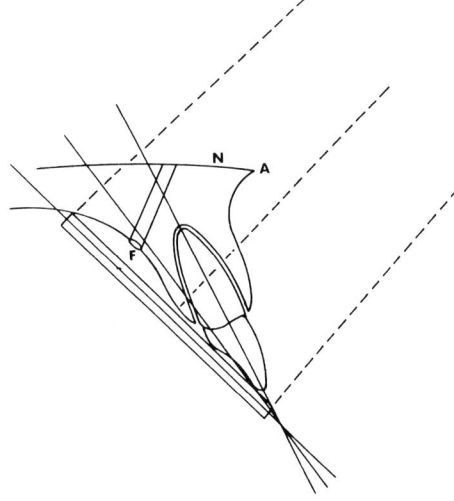

3.10 A line drawing illustrating the anatomical features that commonly appear on a maxillary incisor periapical film taken by the bisecting angle technique:
N floor of nose
A anterior nasal spine
F incisive foramen

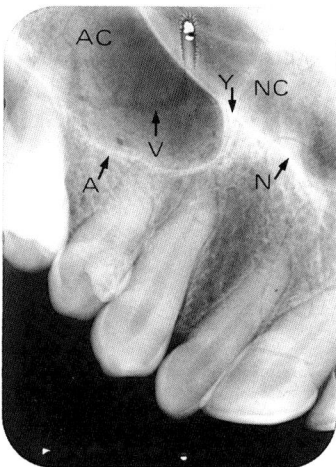

3.12 Periapical (P) 54321| region, bisecting angle technique:
A floor of antrum
AC antral cavity
V vascular canals in antral wall
N floor of nose
NC nasal cavity
Y point of confluence of the structures making up the Y formation of Ennis, i.e. lateral margin of the floor of the nose and anterior part of the floor of the maxillary antrum

20 *A Radiological Atlas of Diseases of the Teeth and Jaws*

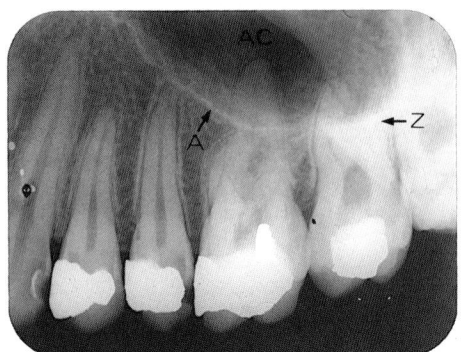

3.13 Periapical (P) |345678 region, bisecting angle technique:
- A floor of antrum
- AC antral cavity
- Z root of zygoma

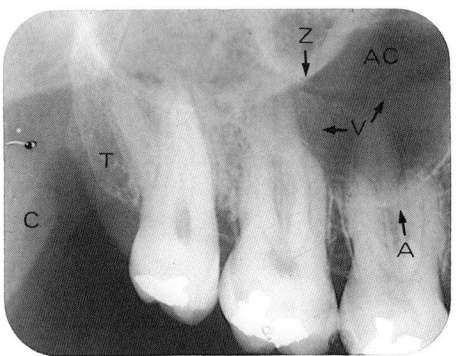

3.14 Periapical (P) 876| region, bisecting angle technique:
- A floor of antrum
- AC antral cavity
- Z root of zygoma
- C coronoid process of mandible
- T maxillary tuberosity with mucosal covering
- V vascular canals in antral wall

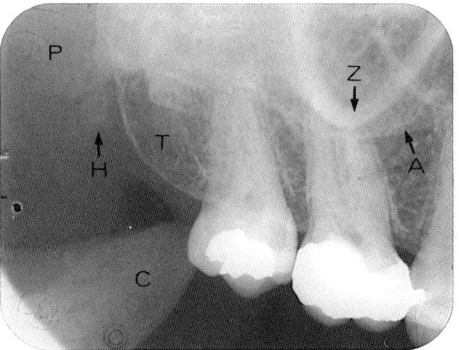

3.15 Periapical (P) 87| region, bisecting angle technique:
- A floor of antrum
- Z root of zygoma
- T maxillary tuberosity with mucosal covering
- H pterygoid hamulus
- P pterygoid plates
- C coronoid process of mandible

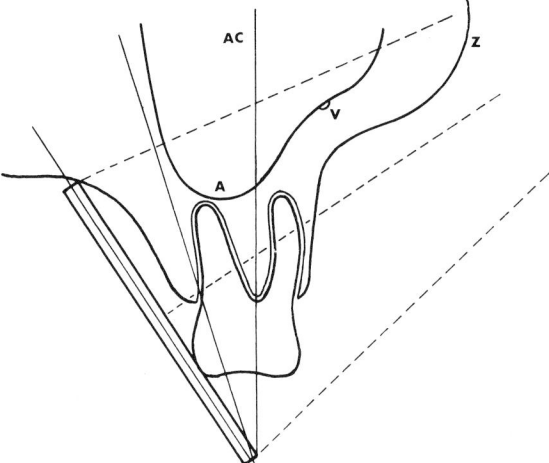

3.16 A line drawing illustrating the anatomical features that commonly appear on a maxillary molar periapical film taken by the bisecting angle technique:
- AC antral cavity
- A floor of antrum
- V vascular canal in antral wall
- Z root of zygoma

Normal Radiographic Anatomy   21

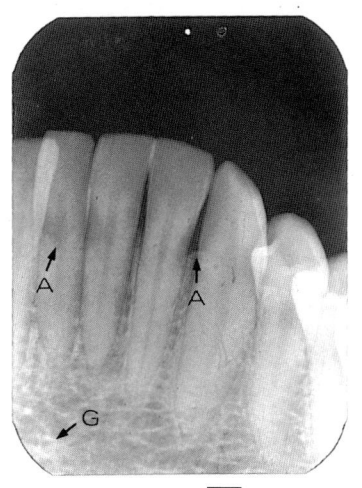

3.17 Periapical (P) |123 region, paralleling technique:
   A   alveolar crest line
   G   genial tubercles

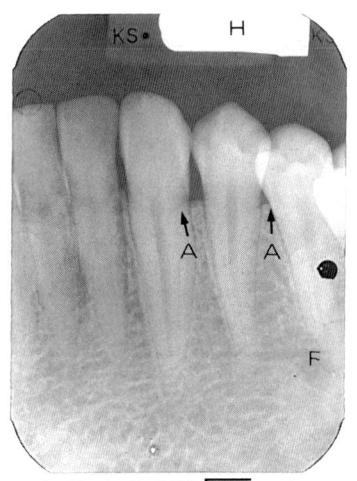

3.18 Periapical (P) |2345 region, paralleling technique:
   A   alveolar crest line
   F   mental foramen
   H   film holder

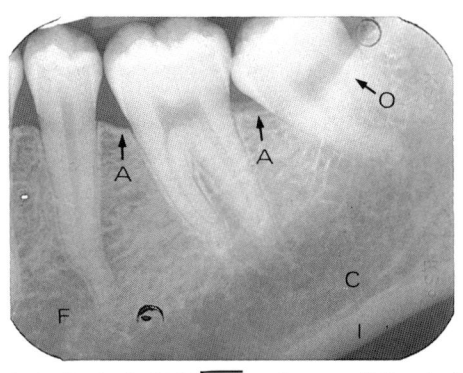

3.19 Periapical (P) |5 78 region, paralleling technique:
   O   oblique ridge
   I   inferior cortical plate
   C   inferior alveolar canal
   F   mental foramen
   A   alveolar crest line
Note that |6 is absent

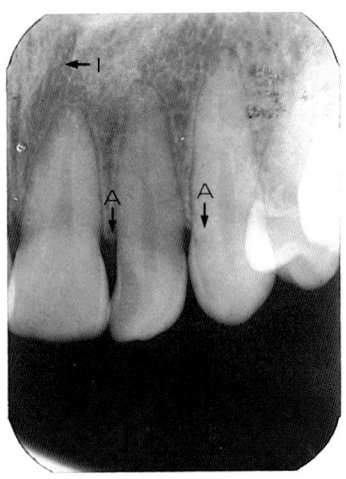

3.20 Periapical (P) |123 region, paralleling technique:
- I incisive canal
- A alveolar crest line

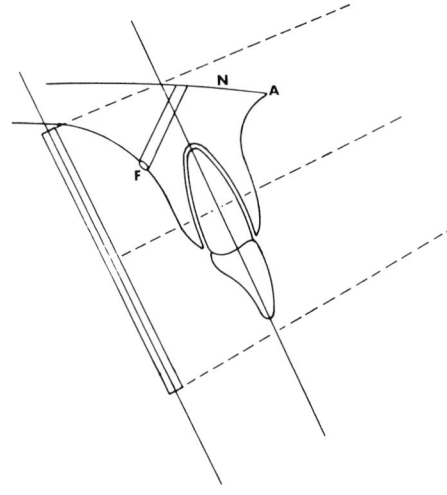

3.21 A line diagram illustrating the anatomical features that commonly appear on a maxillary incisor periapical film taken by the paralleling technique:
- N floor of nose
- A anterior nasal spine
- F incisive foramen

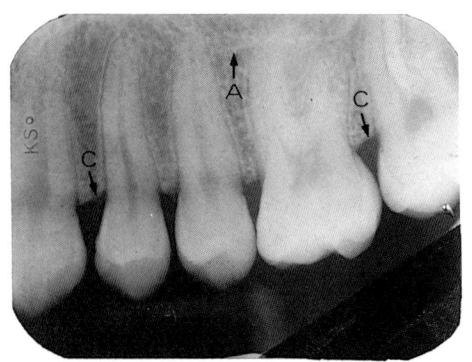

3.22 Periapical (P) |456 region, paralleling technique:
- C alveolar crest line
- A floor of antrum

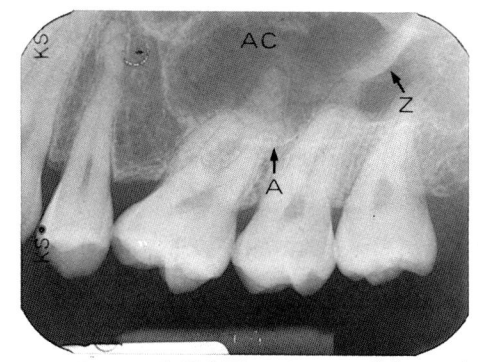

3.23 Periapical (P) |678 region, paralleling technique:
- A floor of antrum
- AC antral cavity
- Z root of zygoma

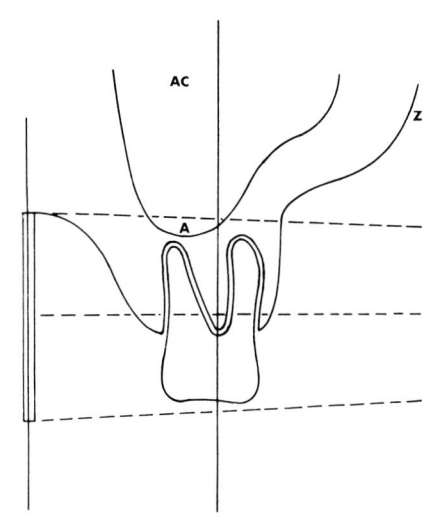

Normal Radiographic Anatomy 23

3.24 A line diagram illustrating the anatomical features that commonly appear on a maxillary molar periapical film taken by the paralleling technique:

AC antral cavity
A   floor of antrum
Z   root of zygoma

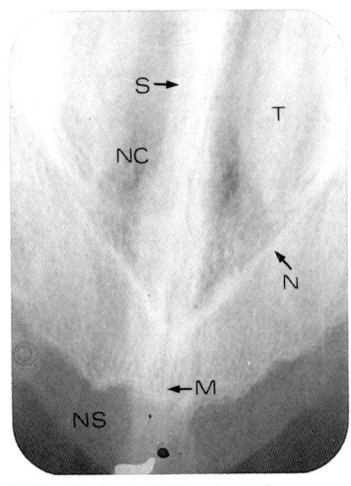

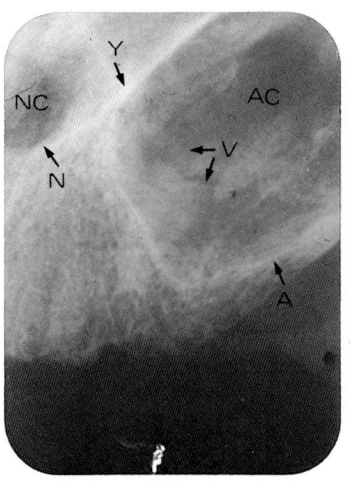

3.26 Periapical (P) edentulous maxillary premolar region:

N   floor of nose
NC nasal cavity
A   floor of antrum
AC antral cavity
Y   Y formation of Ennis
V   vascular canals in lateral wall of antrum

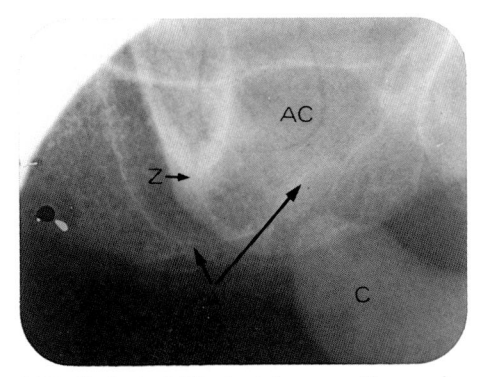

3.25 Periapical (P) edentulous maxillary anterior region:

N   floor of nose
S   nasal septum, bony and cartilaginous
T   inferior turbinate bones covered with soft tissue
NC nasal cavity
M   anterior midline suture
NS soft tissue of nose

3.27 Periapical (P) edentulous maxillary molar region:

A   floor of antrum
AC antral cavity
Z   root of zygoma
C   coronoid process

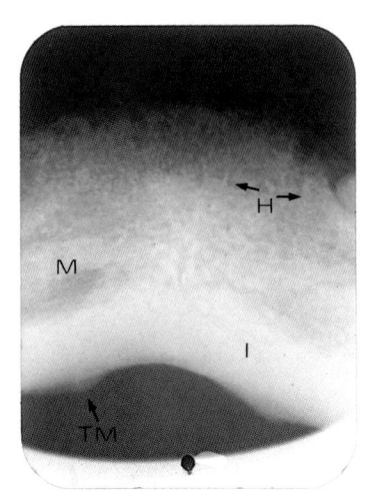

24 A Radiological Atlas of Diseases of the Teeth and Jaws

3.28 Periapical (P) edentulous mandibular incisor region:
- H nutrient canals (Hirschfeld's canals)
- I   inferior cortical plate of mandible
- TM torus mandibularis
- M mental ridge

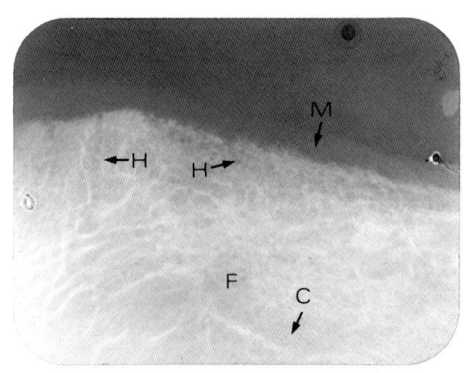

3.29 Periapical (P) edentulous mandibular premolar region:
- H nutrient canals (Hirschfeld's canals)
- F mental foramen
- C inferior alveolar canal
- M mucosal covering

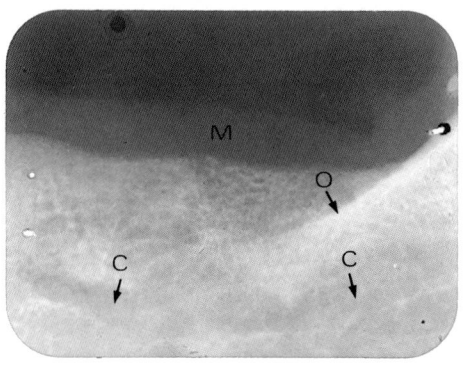

3.30 Periapical (P) edentulous mandibular molar region:
- C inferior alveolar canal
- O oblique ridge
- M mucosal covering

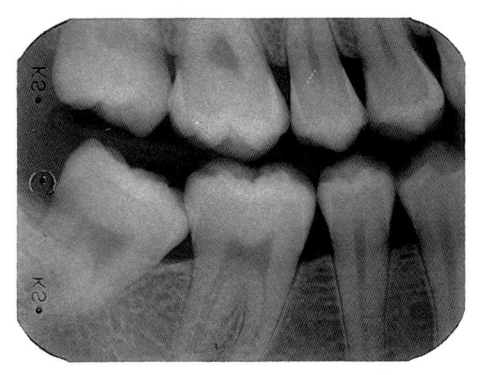

3.31 Bitewing (BW) demonstrating the lack of overlapping of the enamel of contiguous teeth, the normal relationship between the alveolar crest and the amelo-cemental junctions of the adjacent teeth, and the horizontal arrangement of the trabeculae in the interdental septa.

Normal Radiographic Anatomy 25

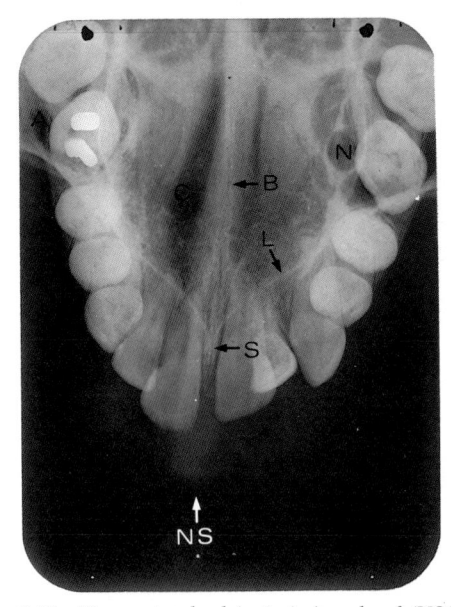

3.32 Upper standard (anterior) occlusal (USO):
- N nasolacrimal canal
- A maxillary antrum
- L lateral margin of floor of nose
- C nasal cavity
- S anterior nasal spine
- B nasal septum
- NS soft tissue of nose

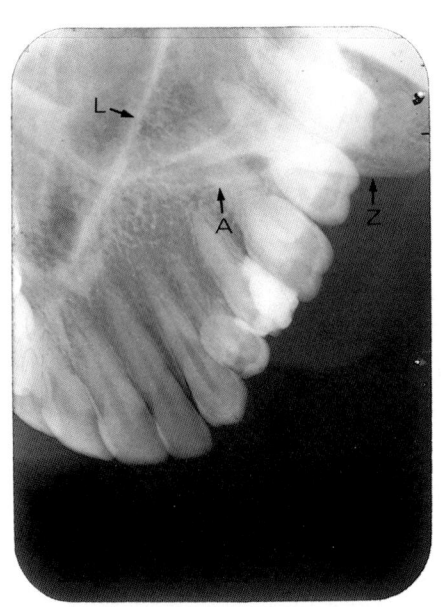

3.33 Upper oblique occlusal (UOO):
- L lateral margin of floor of nose
- Z root of zygoma
- A floor of maxillary antrum

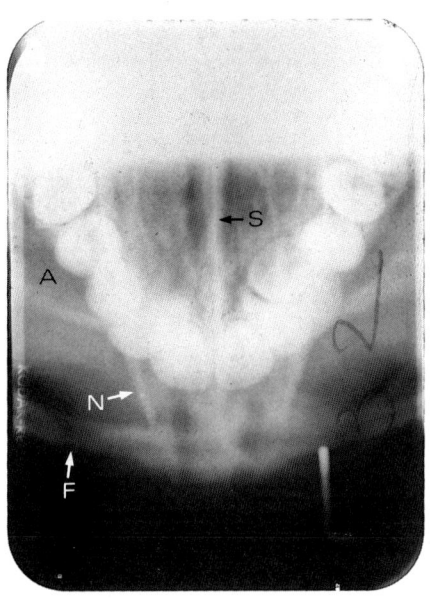

3.34 Upper vertex occlusal (VO):
- F frontal bone
- N nasal bones
- A maxillary antrum
- S nasal septum

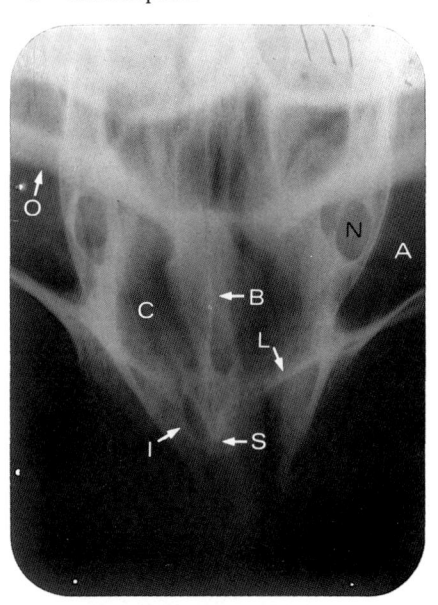

3.35 Upper true occlusal (UTO):
- N nasolacrimal canal
- A maxillary antrum
- L lateral margin of floor of nose
- S anterior nasal spine
- I incisive foramen
- C nasal cavity
- B nasal septum
- O infra-orbital margin

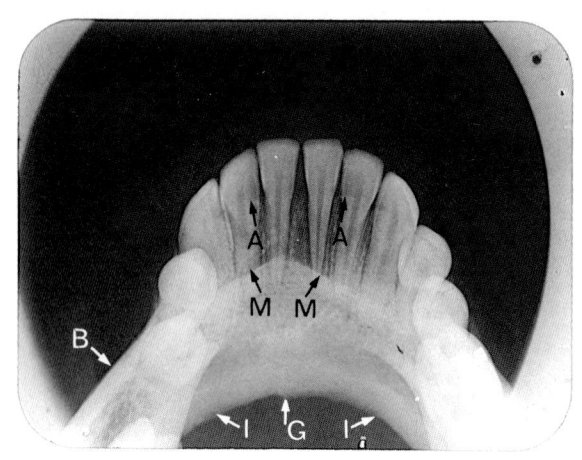

3.36 Lower anterior occlusal (LAO):
 M mental ridge
 G genial tubercle
 A alveolar crest line
 I inferior cortical plate
 B buccal cortical plate

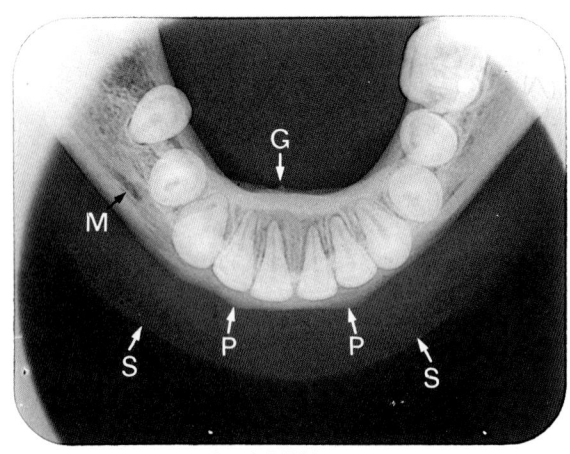

3.37 Lower true occlusal (LTO):
 M mental foramen
 S outline of soft tissues of lip and chin
 G genial tubercle
 P mental protruberance

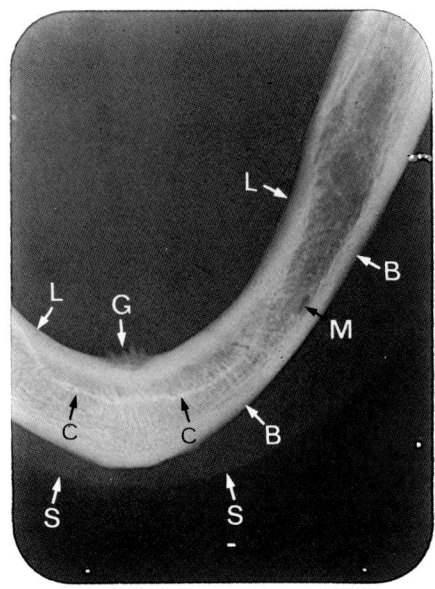

3.38 Lower true occlusal of one side of the mandible (LTO):
 M mental foramen
 G genial tubercle
 S soft tissues of lip and chin
 C crest of alveolar ridge
 B buccal cortical plate
 L lingual cortical plate

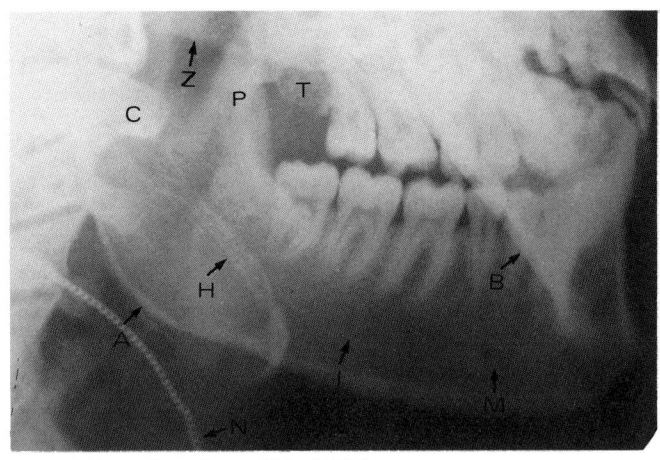

3.39 Oblique lateral mandible (OLM):

- M mental foramen
- I inferior alveolar canal
- H hyoid bone
- A angle of mandible
- C cervical vertebra obscuring condylar process of mandible
- Z zygomatic arch
- P coronoid process
- T maxillary tuberosity
- B inferior border of opposite side of mandible
- N metal necklace

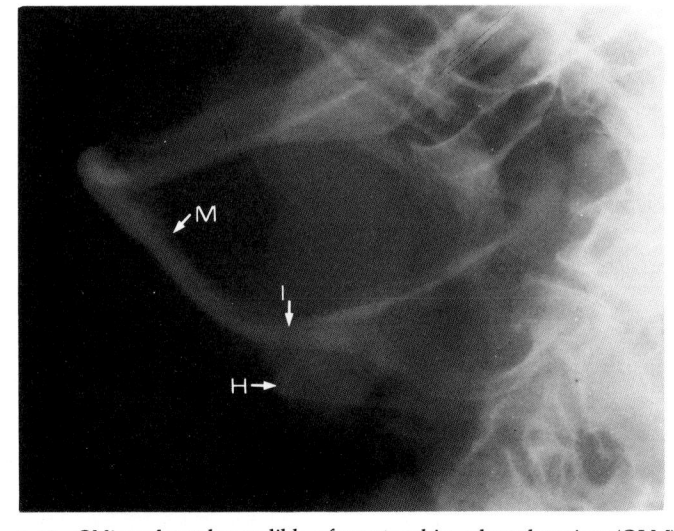

3.40 Oblique lateral mandible of an atrophic, edentulous jaw (OLM):

- I inferior alveolar canal
- M mental foramen
- H hyoid bone

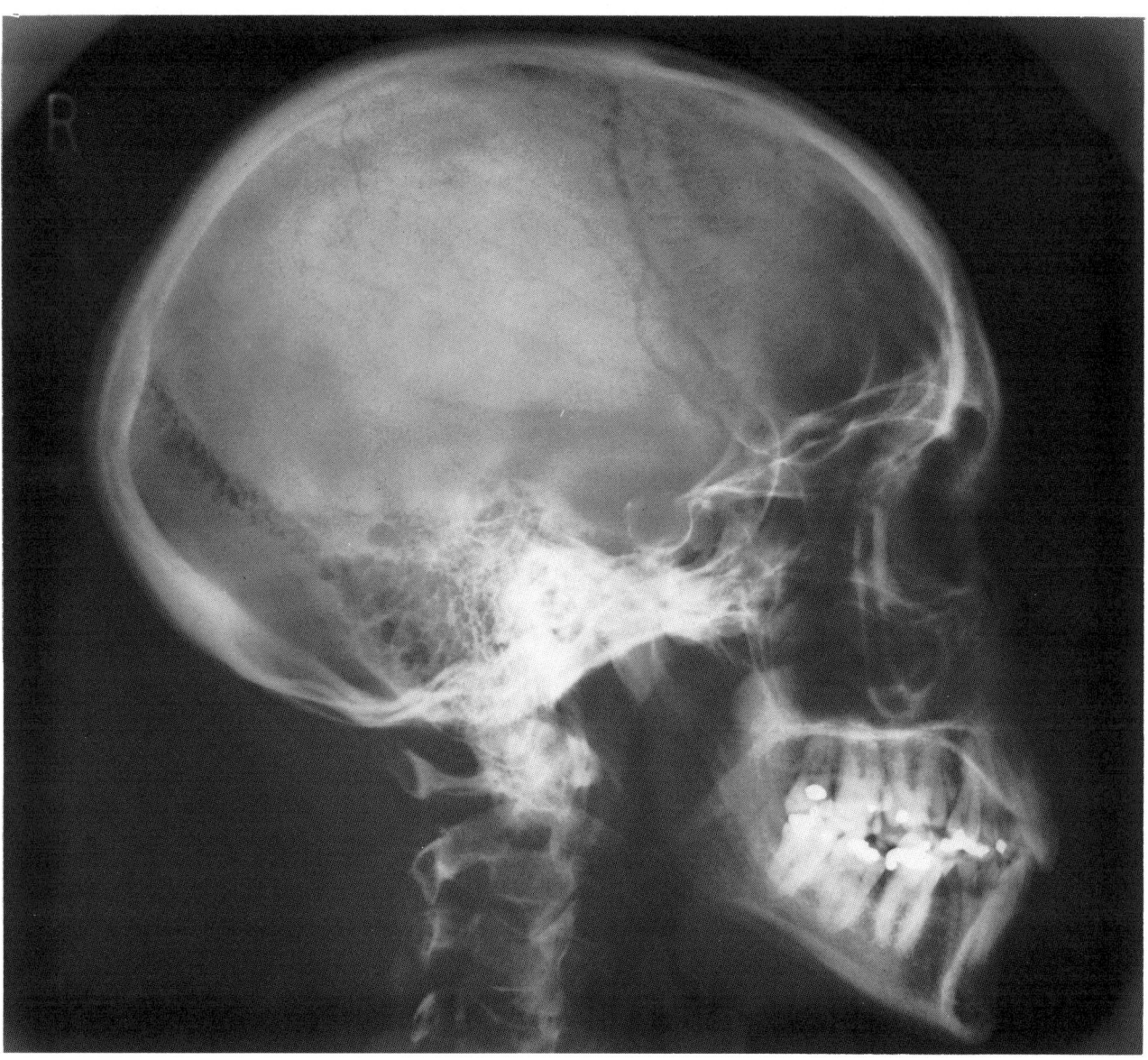

28 *A Radiological Atlas of Diseases of the Teeth and Jaws*

3.41

Normal Radiographic Anatomy 29

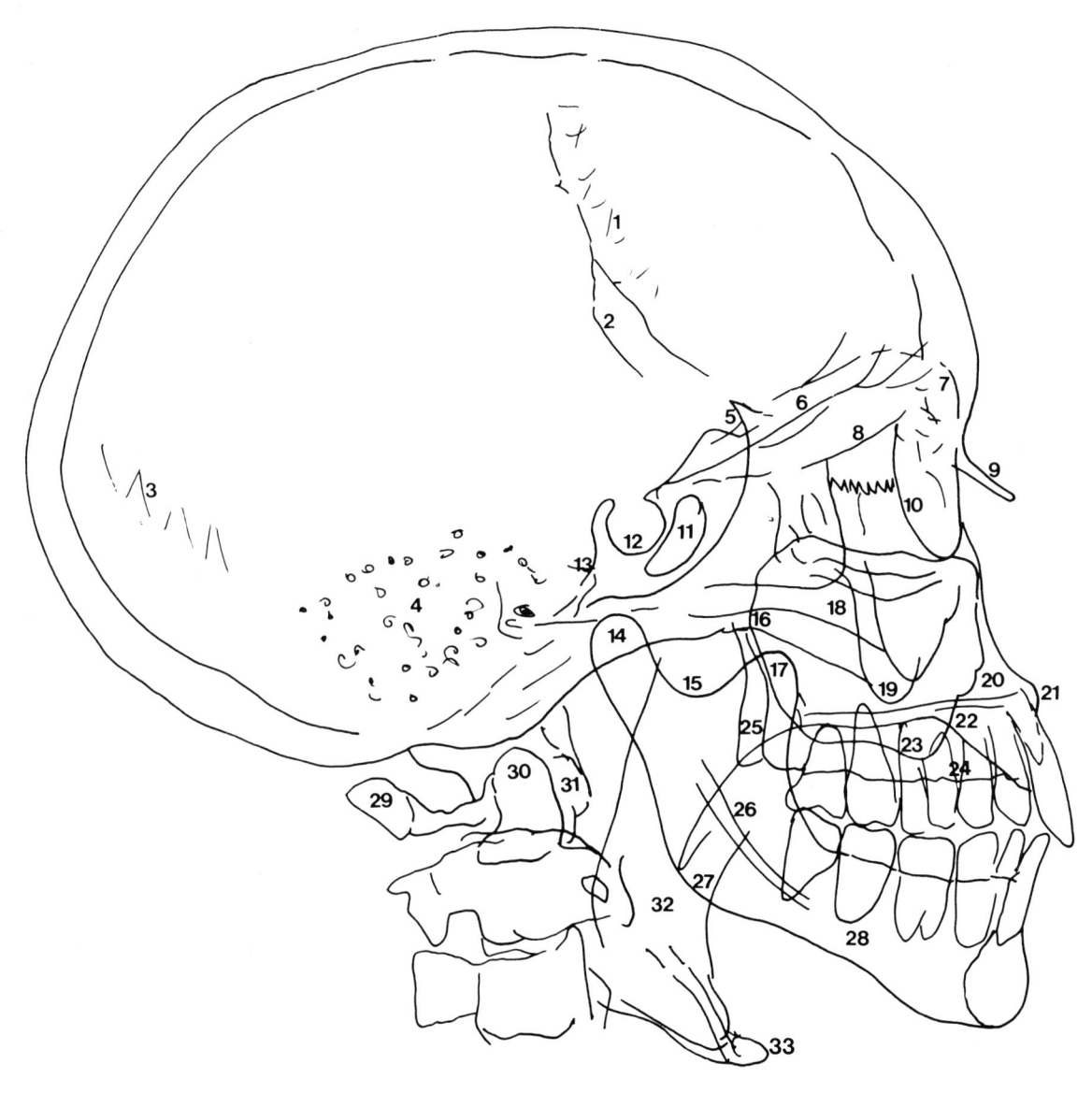

**3.41 (opposite page) and
3.42 (above)** Lateral skull (L):

1. coronal suture
2. meningeal grooves
3. lambdoid suture
4. mastoid air cells
5. anterior wall of middle cranial fossa
6. floor of anterior cranial fossa
7. frontal sinus
8. cribriform plate
9. nasal bones
10. anterior border of lateral wall of orbit
11. sphenoidal sinus
12. pituitary fossa (sella turcica)
13. clivus
14. head of mandibular condyle
15. sigmoid notch
16. posterior wall of maxillary antrum
17. coronoid process of mandible
18. body of zygoma
19. zygomatic process of maxilla
20. anterior wall of maxillary antrum
21. anterior nasal spine
22. hard palate
23. floor of maxillary antrum
24. alveolar ridge of maxilla
25. pterygoid plates
26. inferior alveolar canal
27. angle of mandible
28. body of mandible
29. posterior arch of atlas vertebra
30. odontoid process of axis vertebra
31. anterior arch of atlas vertebra
32. pharyngeal air space
33. hyoid bone

3.43 A cephalometric radiograph (LC) showing the relationship between the maxilla and mandible in a patient with a Class I occlusion, and demonstrating the soft tissue profile of the face. Note the broad, radiopaque band running vertically in the middle of the skull formed by part of the craniostat and the circular ear plugs.

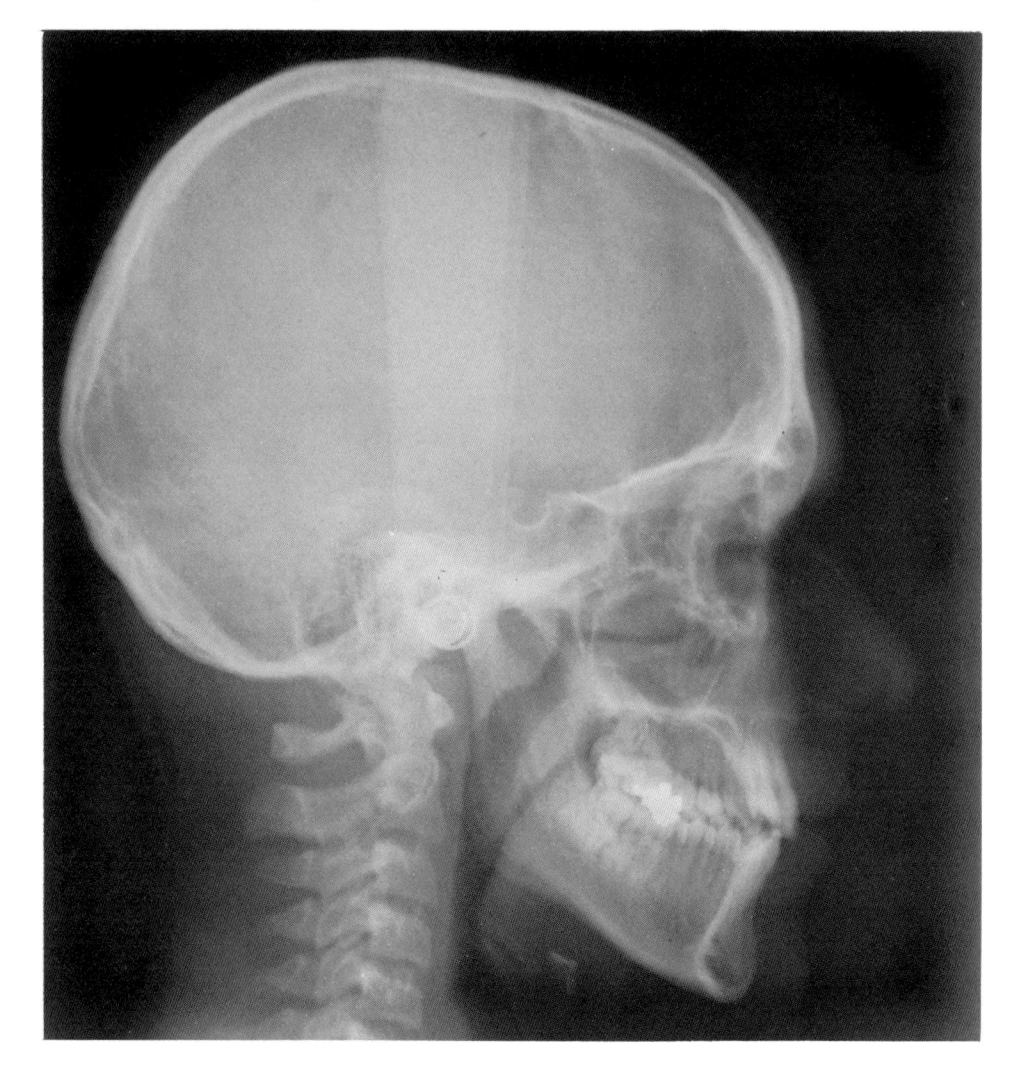

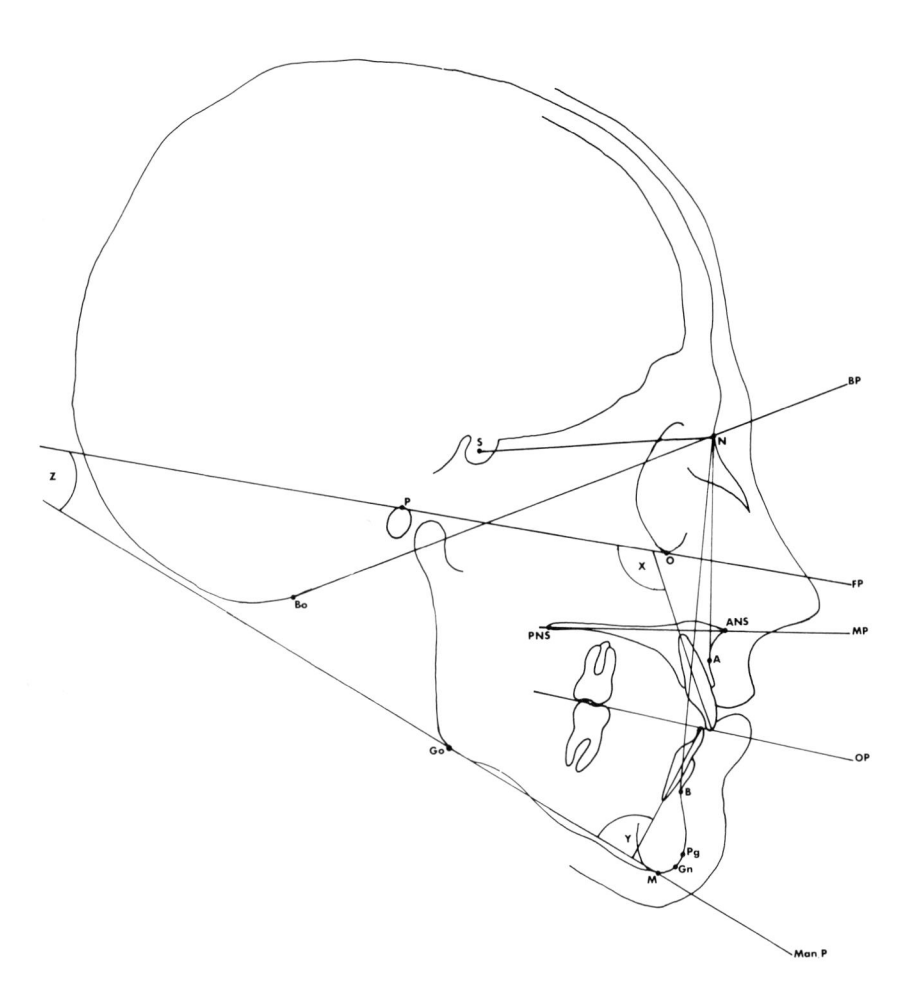

3.44 A line diagram of a cephalometric radiograph (LC) illustrating some of the crucial anatomical landmarks, planes and angles used in cephalometric analysis:

S	sella
P	porion
A	'A' point
B	'B' point
ANS	anterior nasal spine
PNS	posterior nasal spine
Pg	pogonion
Gn	gnathion
M	menton
Go	gonion
N	nasion
O	orbitale
Bo	Bolton point
BP	Bolton plane
FP	Frankfort plane
MP	maxillary plane
OP	occlusal plane
ManP	mandibular plane
X	maxillary incisal angle
Y	mandibular incisal angle
Z	Frankfort–mandibular plane angle
SNA	angle between the anterior part of the maxilla and the base of the skull
SNB	angle between the anterior part of the mandible and the base of the skull

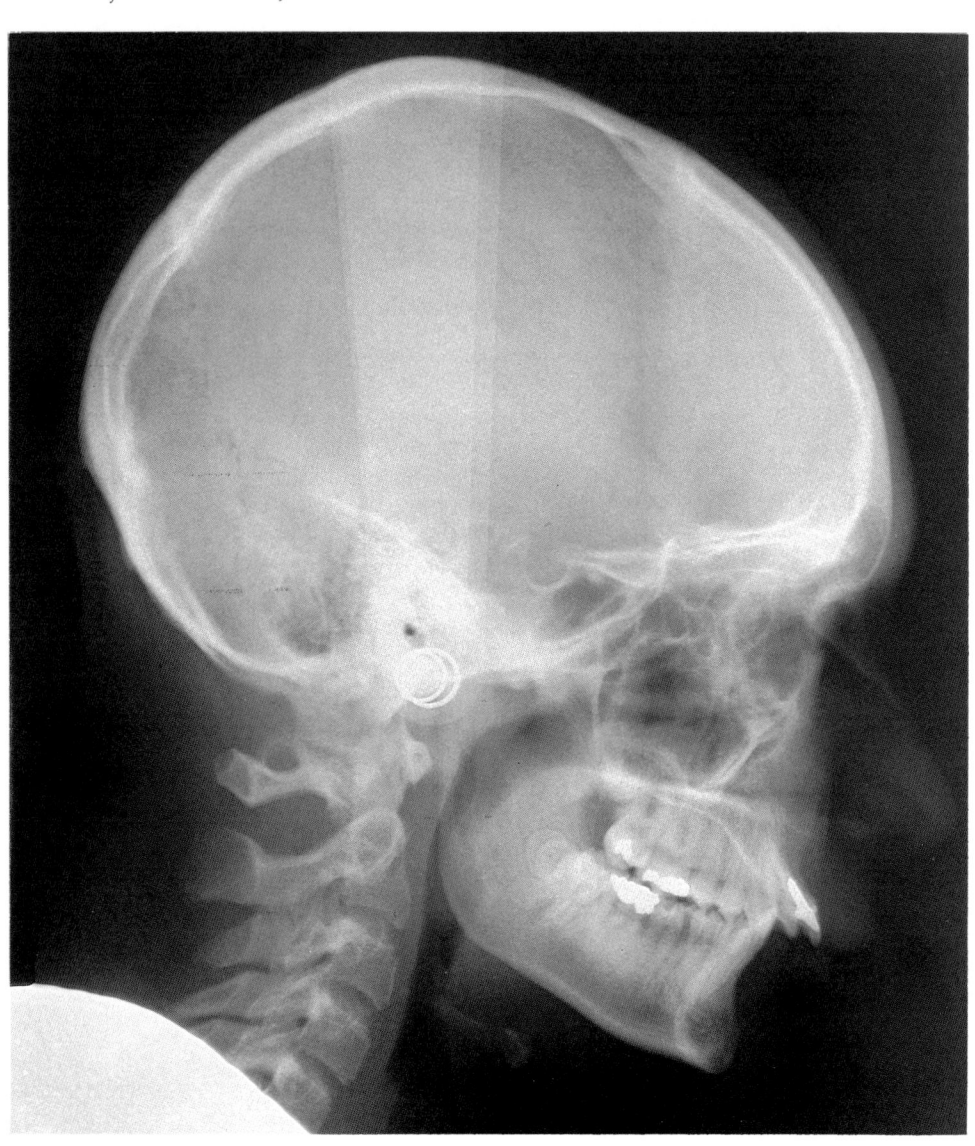

32   *A Radiological Atlas of Diseases of the Teeth and Jaws*

3.45   A similar cephalometric radiograph (LC) in a patient with a Class II occlusion. Note the densely radiopaque lead apron in the lower left corner.

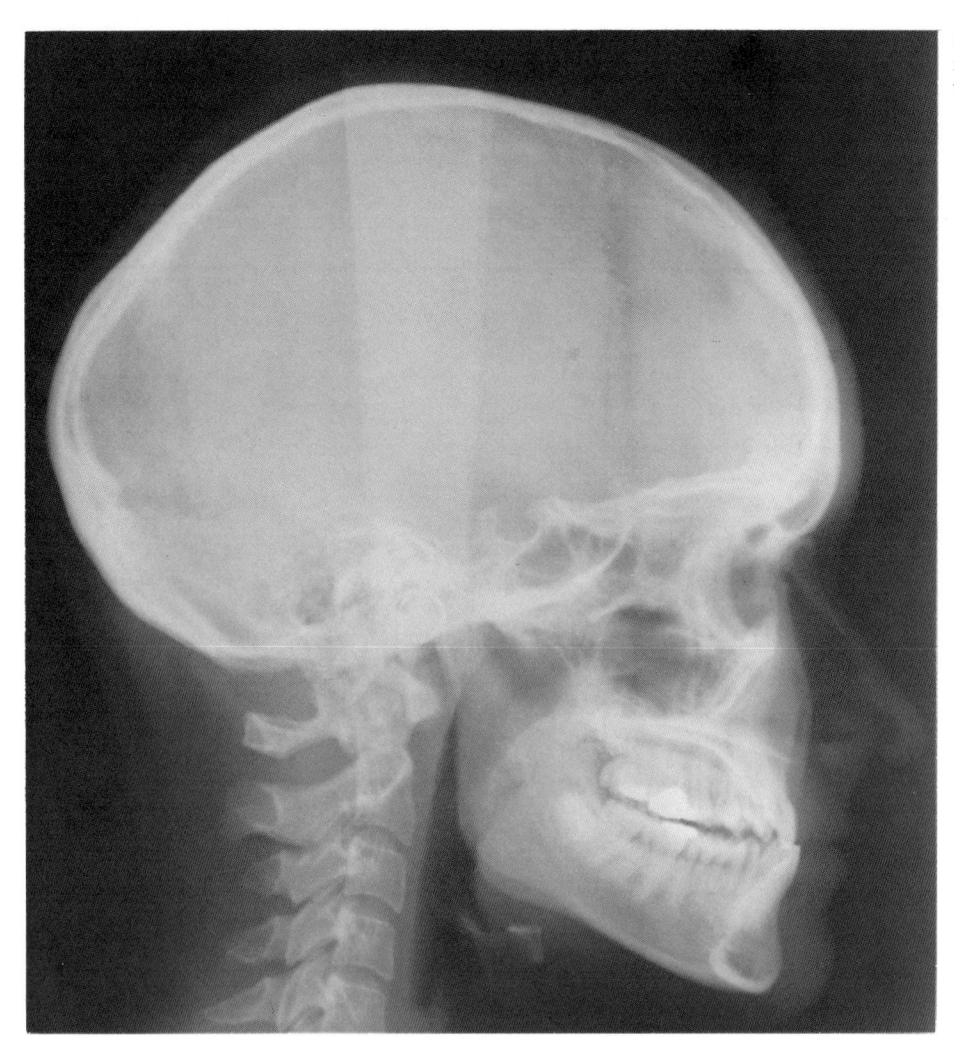

Normal Radiographic Anatomy

3.46 A similar cephalometric radiograph (LC) in a patient with a Class III occlusion.

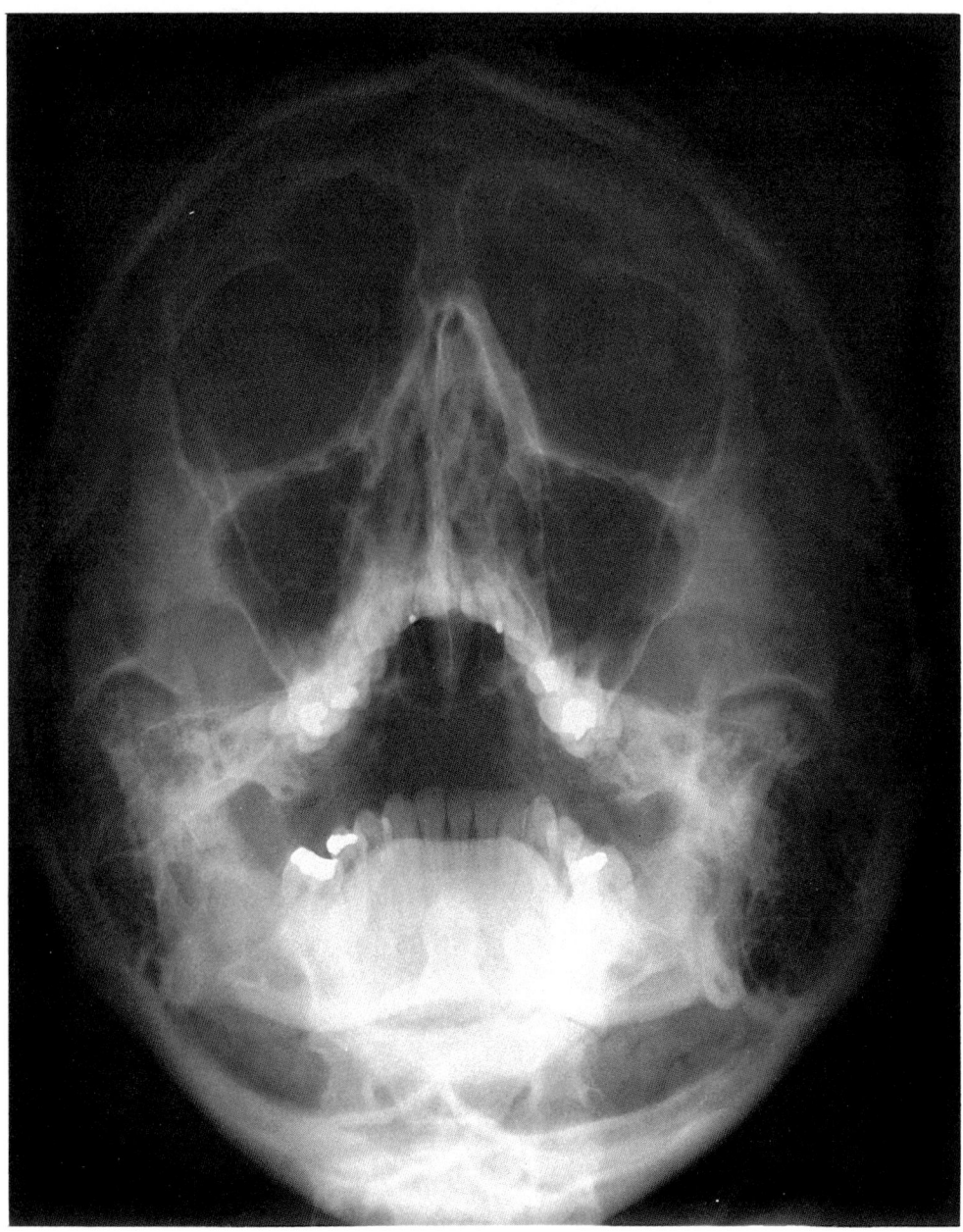

34 *A Radiological Atlas of Diseases of the Teeth and Jaws*

3.47

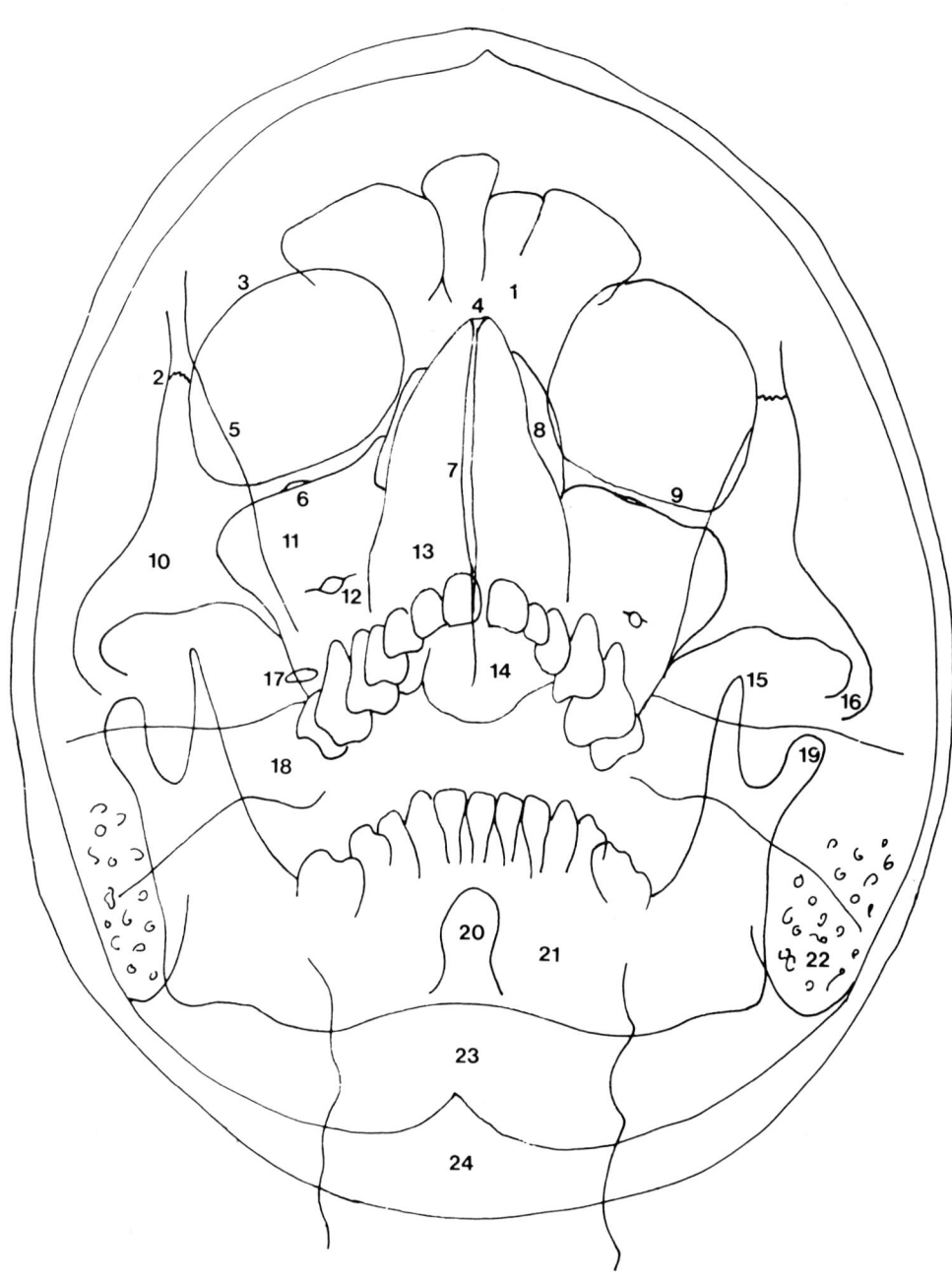

3.47 (opposite page) and 3.48 (left) Occipito-mental (OM):

1. frontal sinuses
2. fronto-zygomatic suture
3. supra-orbital margin
4. nasal bones
5. linea innominata
6. infra-orbital foramen
7. nasal septum
8. anterior ethmoidal sinuses
9. infra-orbital margin
10. zygomatic bone
11. maxillary antrum
12. foramen rotundum
13. nasal cavity and turbinate bones
14. sphenoidal sinus
15. coronoid process of mandible
16. zygomatic arch
17. foramen ovale
18. petrous part of temporal bone
19. condylar head of mandible
20. odontoid process of axis vertebra
21. body of mandible
22. mastoid air cells
23. cervical vertebrae
24. occipital bone

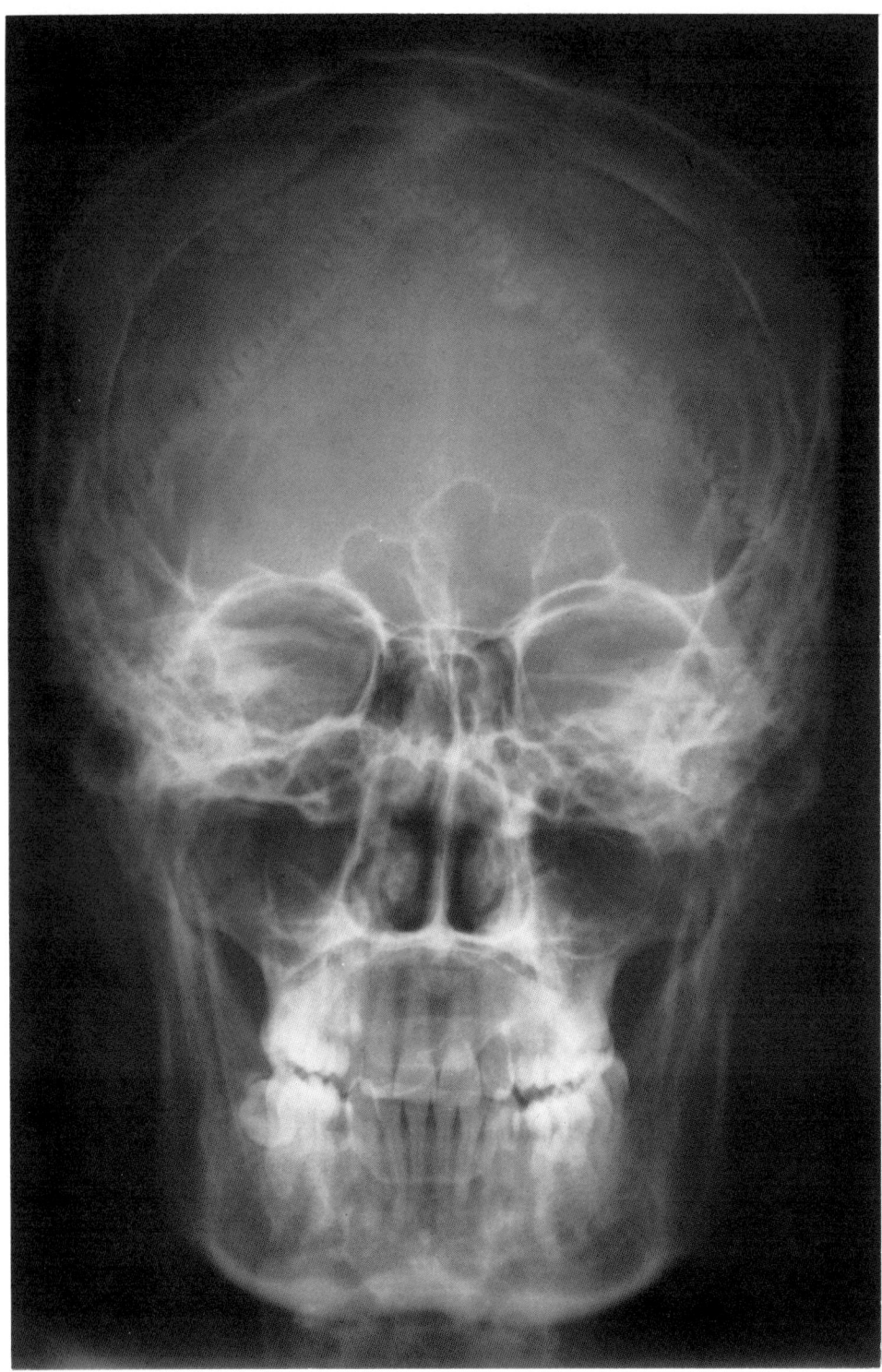

3.49

Normal Radiographic Anatomy 37

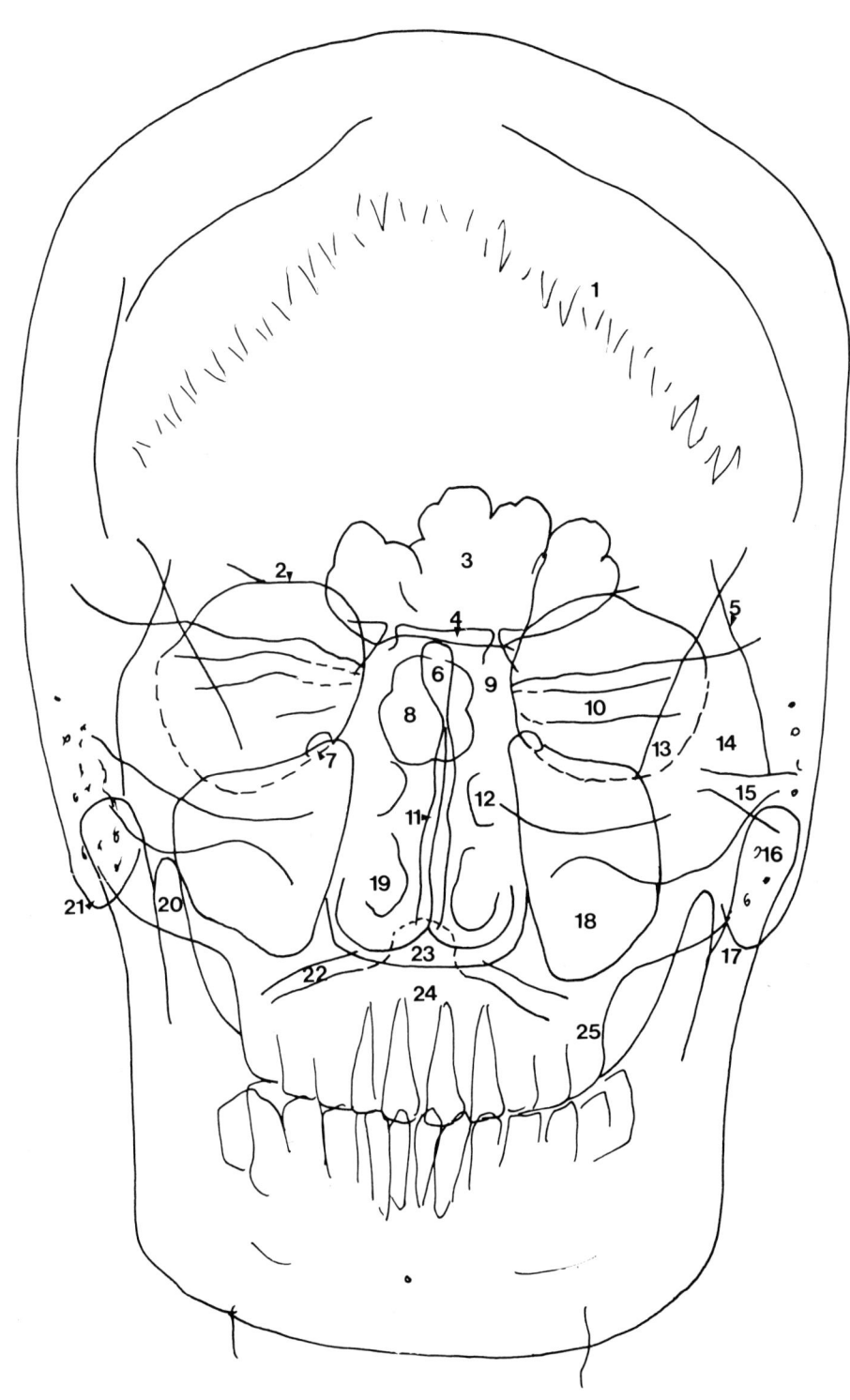

3.49 (opposite page) and 3.50 (left) Postero-anterior (PA):
1. lambdoid suture
2. supra-orbital margin
3. frontal sinuses
4. dorsum sellae
5. zygomatic process of frontal bone
6. crista galli
7. foramen rotundum
8. sphenoidal sinus
9. ethmoidal sinuses
10. internal auditory canal
11. nasal septum
12. middle turbinate bone
13. linea innominata
14. frontal process of zygomatic bone
15. external auditory canal
16. head of mandibular condyle
17. neck of mandibular condyle
18. maxillary antrum
19. inferior turbinate bone
20. coronoid process of mandible
21. mastoid process
22. intervertebral space between atlas and axis vertebrae
23. odontoid process of axis vertebra
24. hard palate
25. alveolar process of maxilla

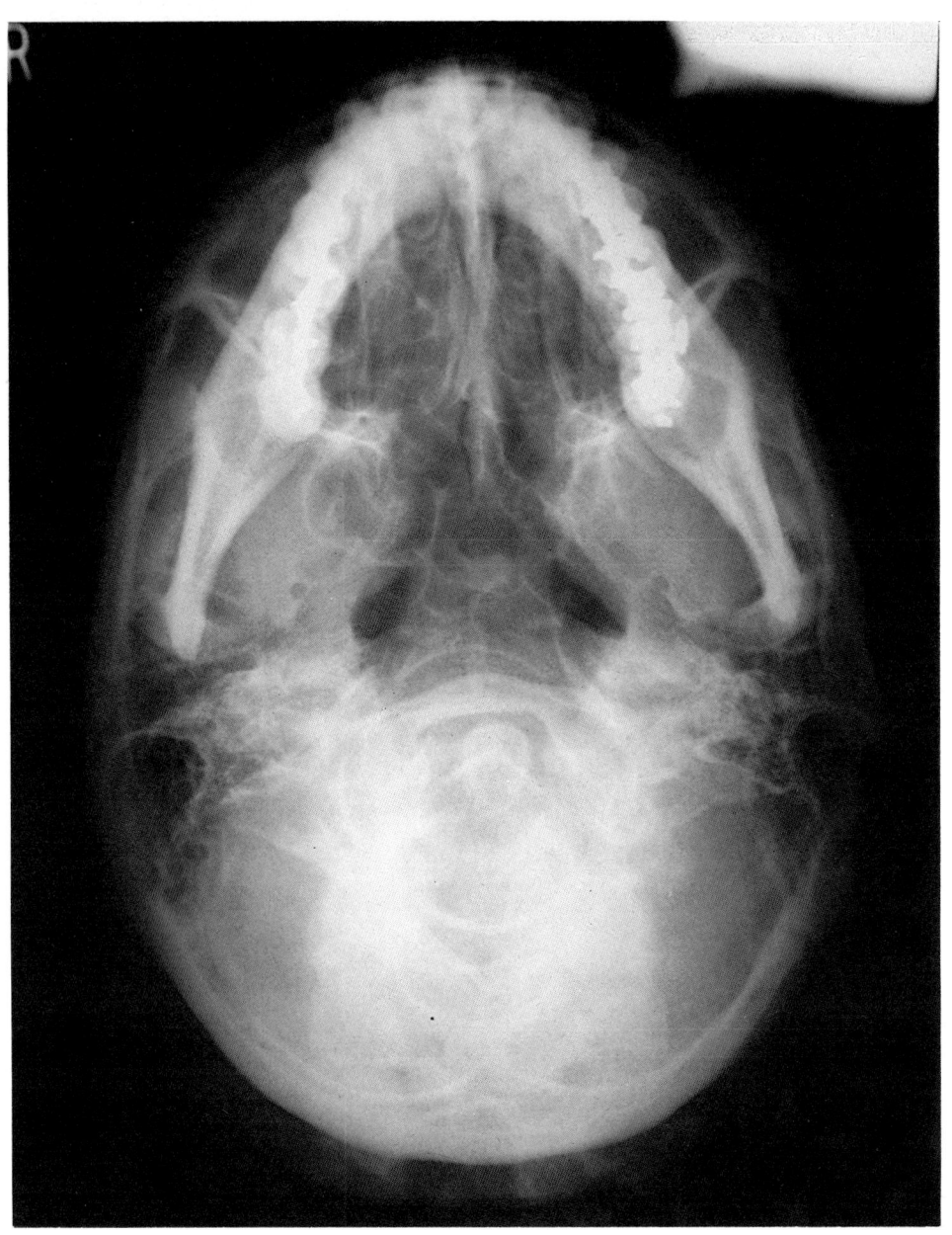

38 *A Radiological Atlas of Diseases of the Teeth and Jaws*

3.51

Normal Radiographic Anatomy 39

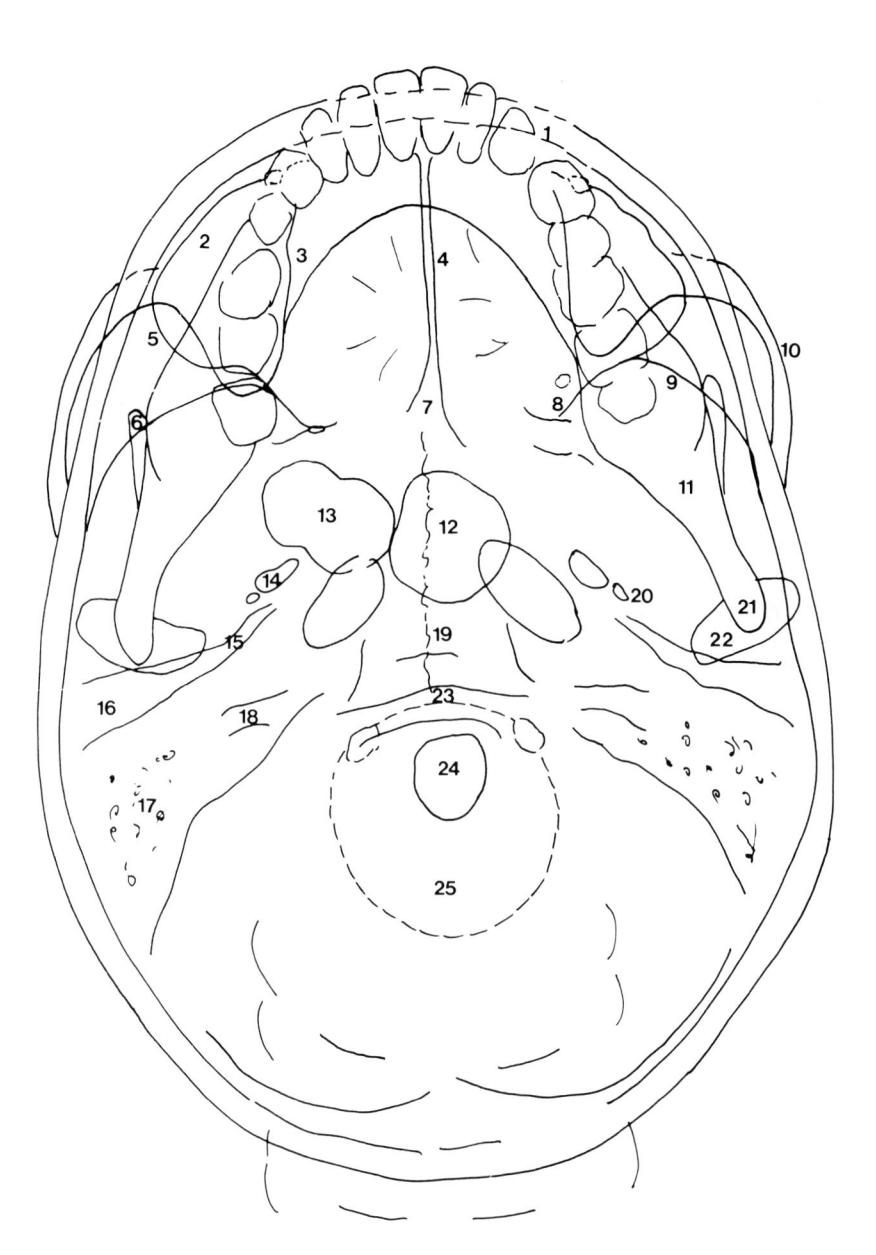

3.51 (opposite page) and 3.52 (left) Submento-vertex (base view) (SMV):

1. frontal bone
2. maxillary antrum
3. medial wall of maxillary antrum
4. nasal septum
5. lateral wall of orbit
6. coronoid process of mandible
7. posterior border of vomer
8. greater palatine foramen
9. anterior wall of middle cranial fossa
10. zygomatic arch
11. ramus of mandible
12. sphenoidal sinus
13. sphenoidal sinus
14. foramen ovale
15. pharyngo-tympanic (Eustachian) tube
16. external auditory canal
17. mastoid air cells
18. internal auditory canal
19. clivus
20. foramen spinosum
21. angle of mandible
22. head of mandibular condyle
23. anterior arch of atlas vertebra
24. odontoid process of axis vertebra
25. foramen magnum

3.53

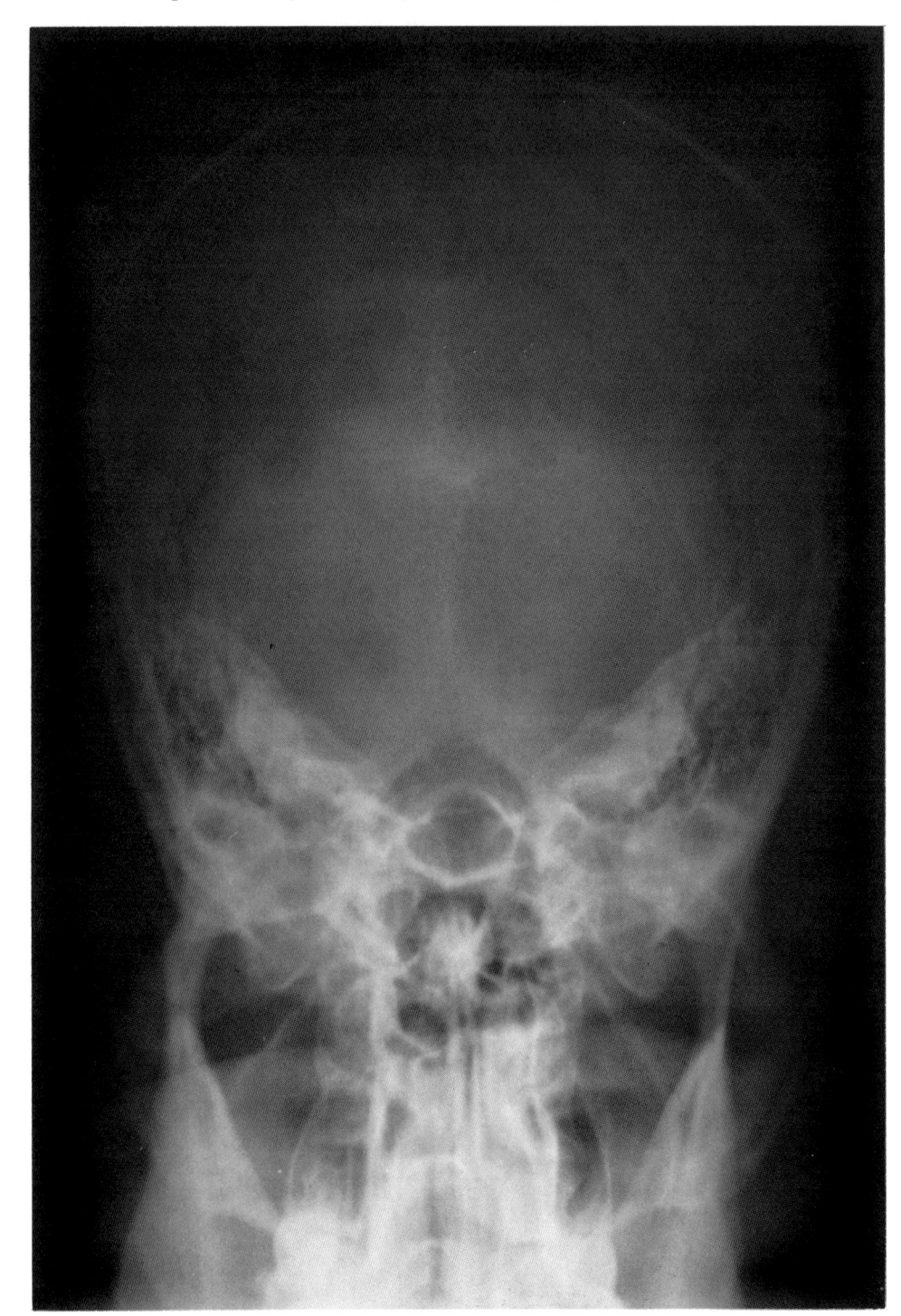

Normal Radiographic Anatomy 41

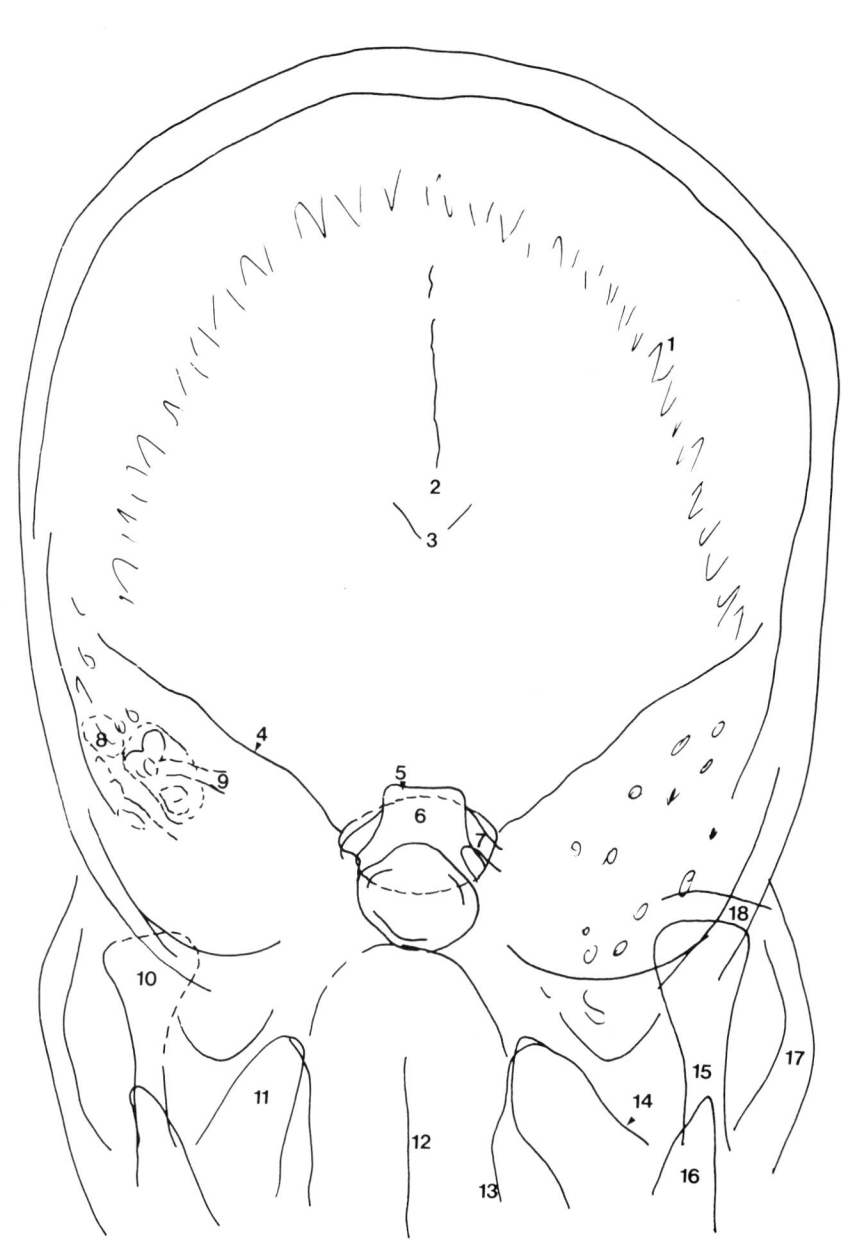

3.53 (opposite page) and 3.54 (left) Fronto-occipital (Towne's view (T)):

1. lambdoid suture
2. internal occipital crest
3. occiput
4. petrous ridge of temporal bone
5. posterior clinoid process
6. dorsum sellae
7. foramen magnum
8. mastoid air cells
9. internal auditory canal
10. head of mandibular condyle
11. maxillary antrum
12. nasal septum
13. medial wall of maxillary antrum
14. roof and wall of maxillary antrum
15. neck of mandibular condyle
16. coronoid process of mandible
17. zygomatic arch
18. temporo-mandibular joint space

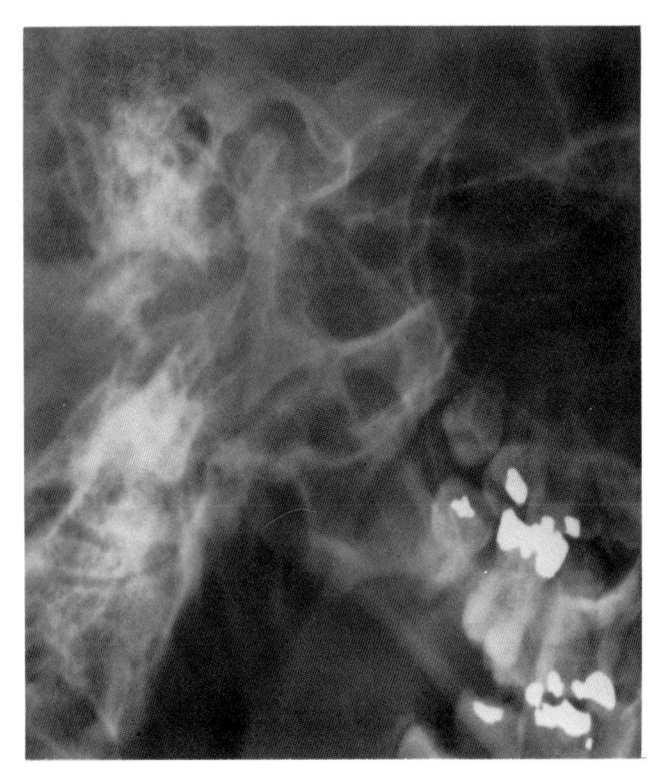

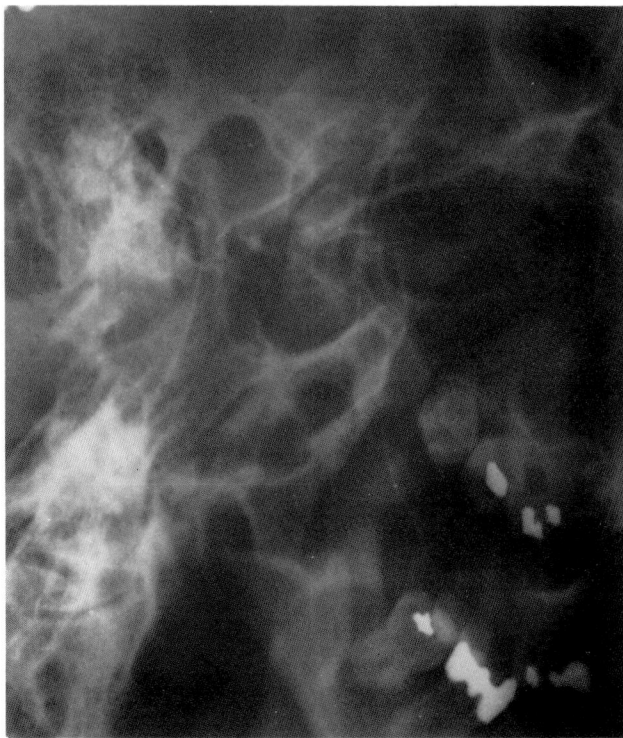

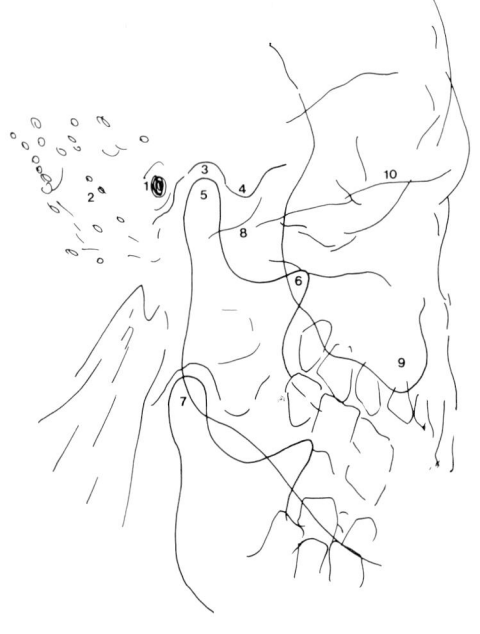

42 *A Radiological Atlas of Diseases of the Teeth and Jaws*

3.55 (top left), 3.56 (bottom left), 3.57 (top right) and 3.58 (bottom right) Transcranial view of temporo-mandibular joint (TMJ), closed (Figs 3.55, 3.56) and open (Figs 3.57, 3.58)

1. external auditory meatus
2. mastoid air cells
3. articular fossa of the temporo-mandibular joint
4. articular eminence
5. head of mandibular condyle
6. coronoid process of mandible
7. mandibular condyle of opposite side
8. medial rim of articular fossa
9. maxillary antrum
10. floor of anterior cranial fossa

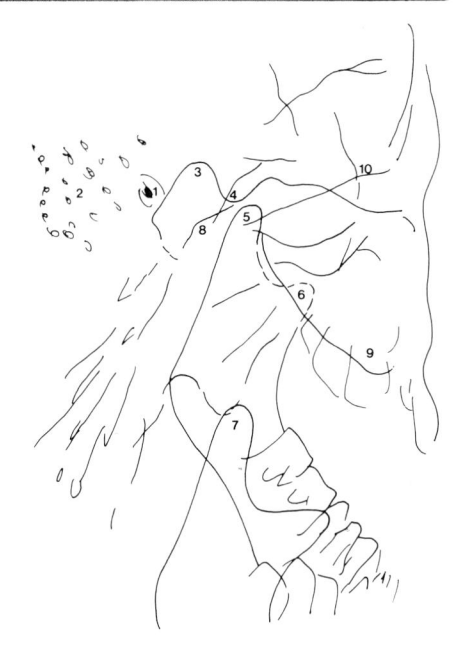

Normal Radiographic Anatomy 43

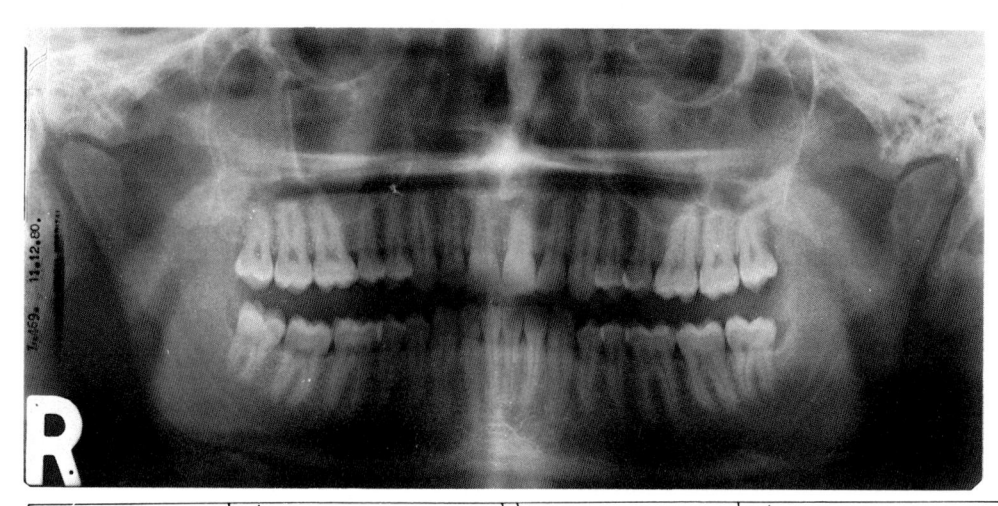

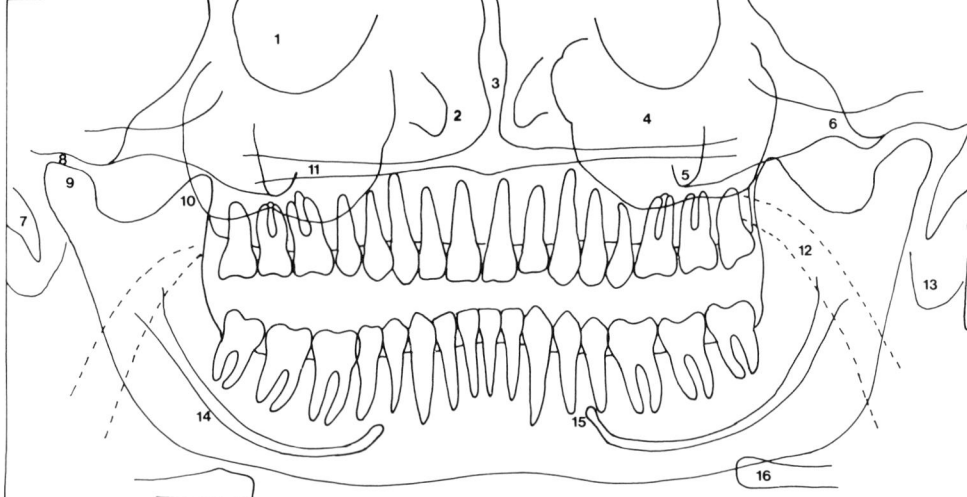

3.59 (left) and 3.60 (below) Panoramic radiograph (PR) of the jaws of an adult:

1. orbital cavity
2. nasal cavity and turbinates
3. nasal septum
4. maxillary antrum
5. root of zygoma
6. zygomatic arch
7. styloid process
8. glenoid fossa
9. head of mandibular condyle
10. coronoid process of mandible
11. hard palate
12. pharyngeal air space
13. pinna of ear
14. inferior alveolar canal
15. mental foramen
16. hyoid bone

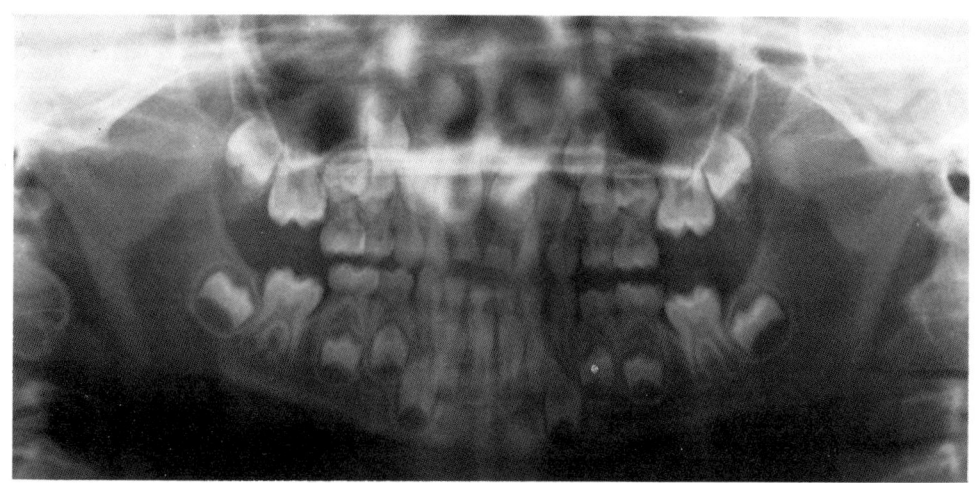

3.61 Panoramic radiograph of jaws (PR). There is substantial variation between individuals in the pattern and chronology of tooth eruption, but Figs 3.61–3.65 illustrate a commonly occurring sequence. In this six-year-old, all the teeth of the primary dentition are erupted and present. All the first permanent molars are erupting into the oral cavity, and the remainder of the permanent teeth, apart from the third molars, are at various stages of development and unerupted. Note the stage of root development of the first permanent molars.

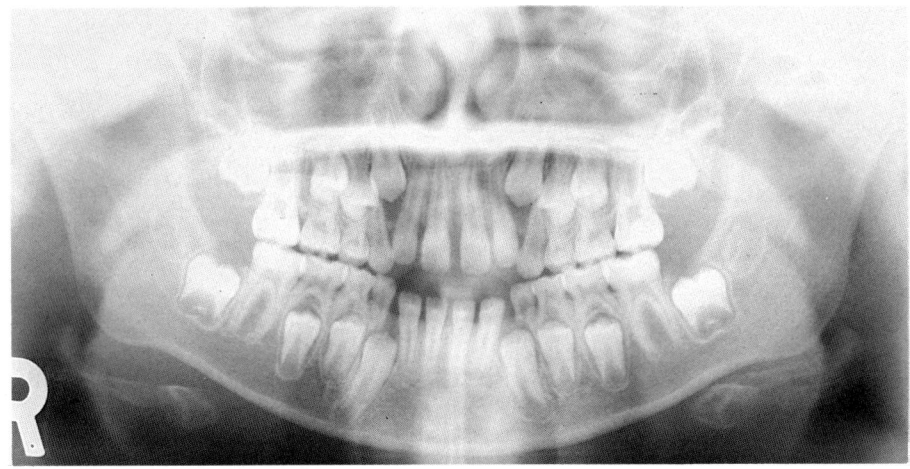

44 *A Radiological Atlas of Diseases of the Teeth and Jaws*

3.62 Panoramic radiograph of jaws (PR) age nine. All the permanent incisors and first molars are erupted, the primary incisors having been shed. The primary canines and molars are still present, their roots being at progressive stages of resorption due to the development of the permanent canines and premolars. Crown formation is complete in the second permanent molars, and just commencing in the third molars. Note the stage of root development of the permanent teeth.

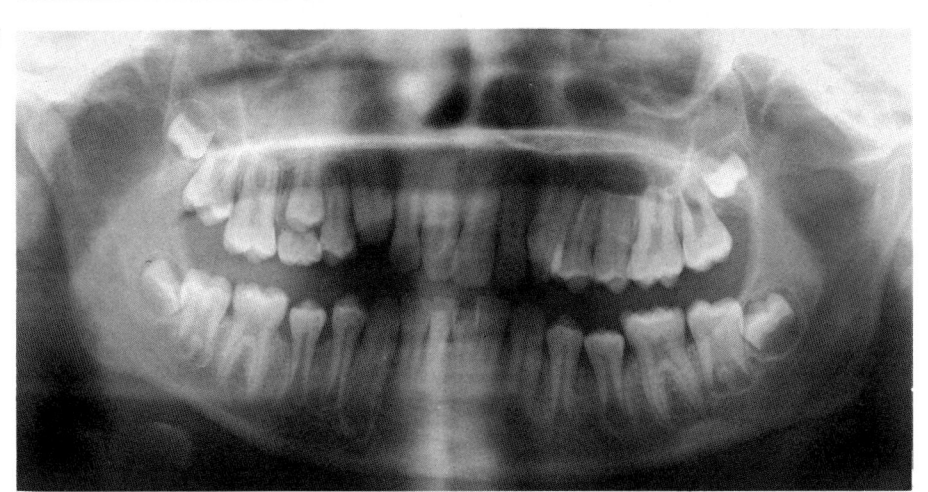

3.63 Panoramic radiograph of jaws (PR) age 12. All the permanent teeth, apart from the four third molars and 5|, are erupted. Only E| remains of the primary dentition. Note the still incomplete root development of the canines, premolars and second molars, and the incomplete crown formation of the third molars.

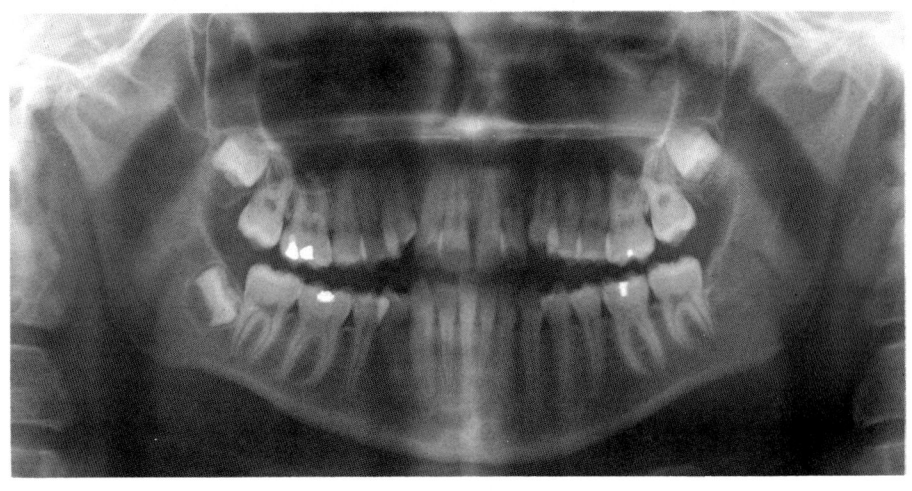

3.64 Panoramic radiograph of jaws (PR) age 15. The root development of most erupted teeth is now complete and is about to commence on the third molars. Note the absence of |8.

Normal Radiographic Anatomy 45

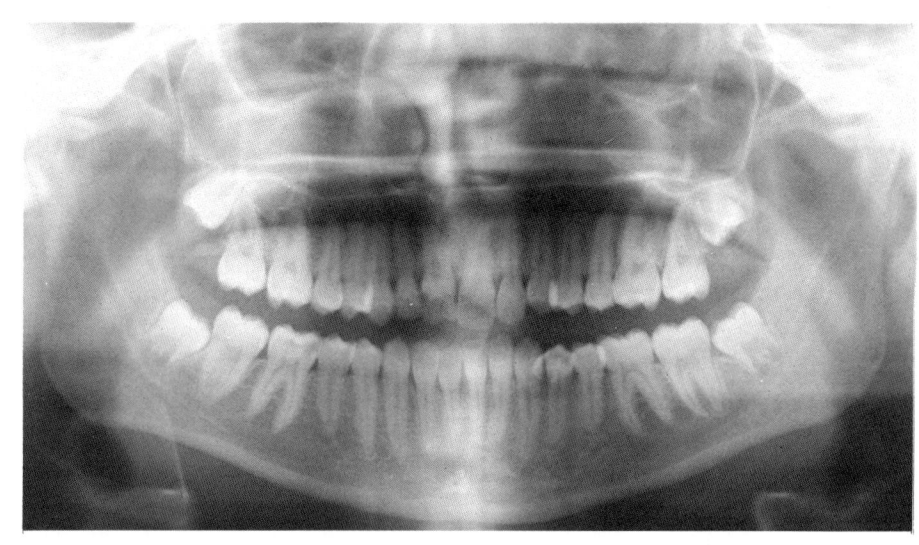

3.65 Panoramic radiograph of jaws (PR) age 18. Root development of all the erupted teeth is complete and the third molars, in which root formation is approximately halfway, are close to eruption into the oral cavity.

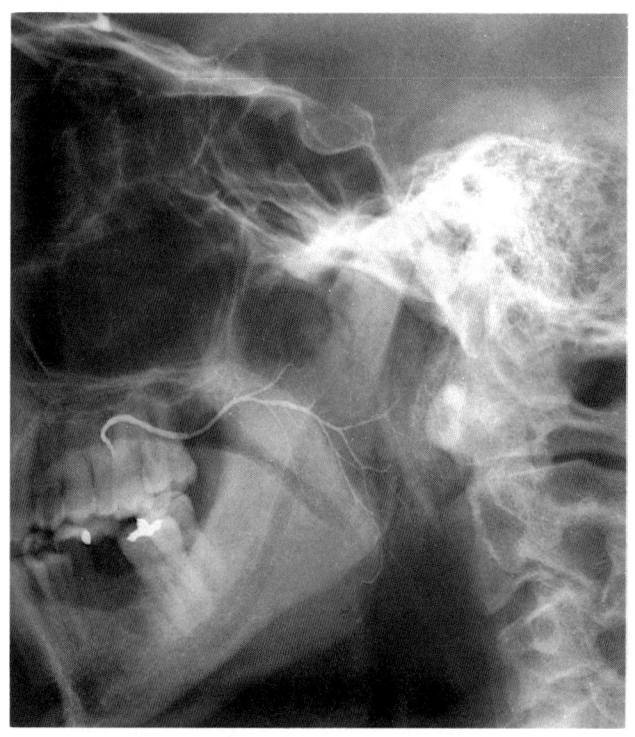

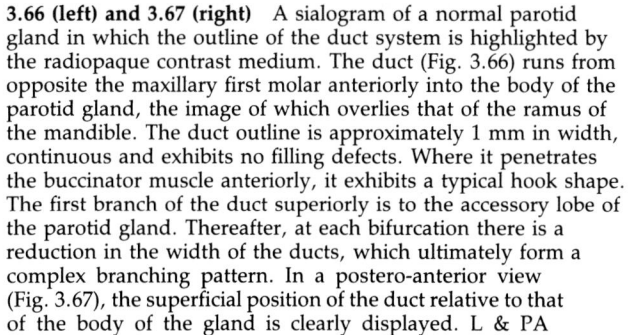

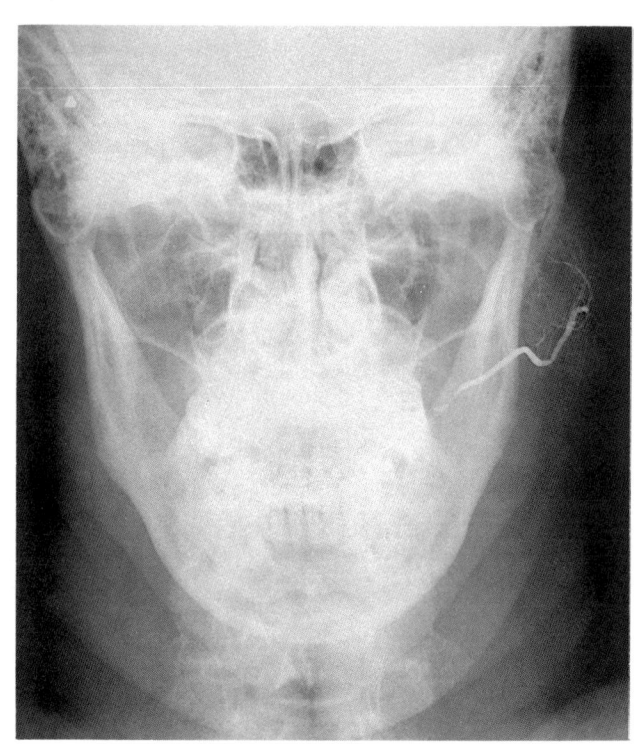

3.66 (left) and 3.67 (right) A sialogram of a normal parotid gland in which the outline of the duct system is highlighted by the radiopaque contrast medium. The duct (Fig. 3.66) runs from opposite the maxillary first molar anteriorly into the body of the parotid gland, the image of which overlies that of the ramus of the mandible. The duct outline is approximately 1 mm in width, continuous and exhibits no filling defects. Where it penetrates the buccinator muscle anteriorly, it exhibits a typical hook shape. The first branch of the duct superiorly is to the accessory lobe of the parotid gland. Thereafter, at each bifurcation there is a reduction in the width of the ducts, which ultimately form a complex branching pattern. In a postero-anterior view (Fig. 3.67), the superficial position of the duct relative to that of the body of the gland is clearly displayed. L & PA

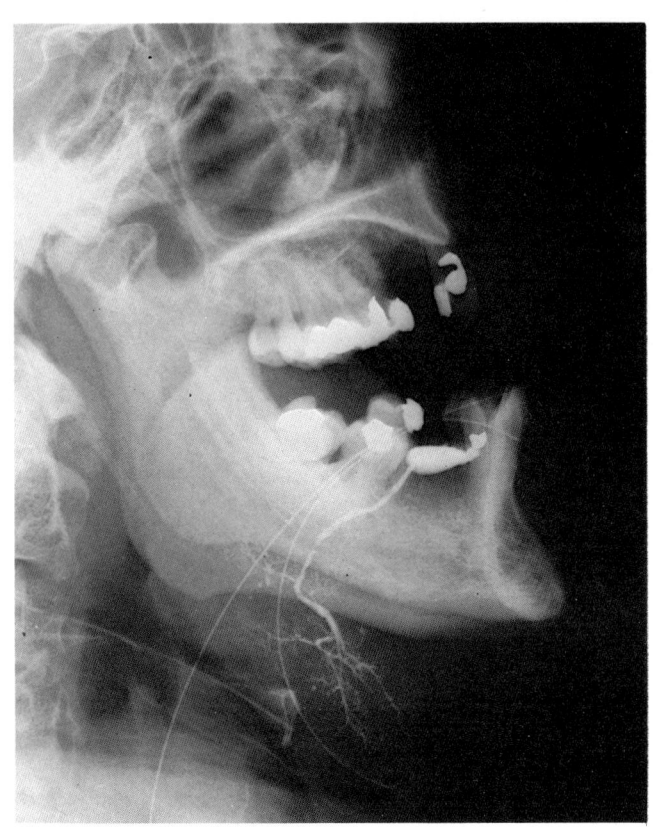

3.68 A sialogram of a normal, right submandibular salivary gland taken immediately after injection of the contrast medium. The main duct, which is of normal and regular width, passes obliquely backwards from its outlet in the anterior part of the floor of the mouth, to a point superimposed upon the inferior border of the mandible where it curves sharply forwards. This point represents the posterior border of the mylohyoid muscle, above which lies the deep part and below which lies the superficial part of the gland. In both parts, there are several smaller branches from which the terminal ramifications of the duct system derive forming a typical branching pattern. Note the smooth, regular, radiopaque arcs formed by the medium in the cannula, which lies on the patient's skin, and the excess of medium which has pooled in the floor of the mouth. L

Chapter 4

Technical Errors

Technical errors may give rise to radiographic appearances which could be misinterpreted unless the viewer is familiar with them. Such errors can arise in the surgery during the time when the radiograph is being taken, or subsequently in the dark room when it is being processed.

Technical Errors 49

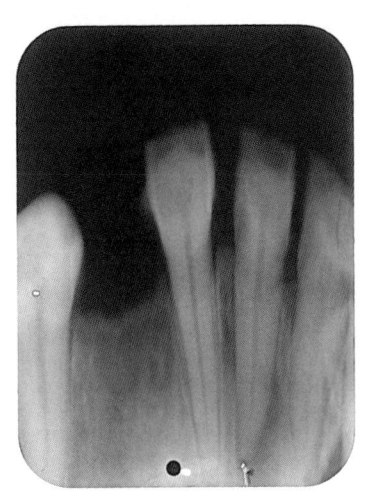

4.1 A common error when using the bisecting angle technique for periapical radiographs arises when the tube is incorrectly angled. If it is placed more occlusally than is necessary to aim the beam at right angles to the bisector, there will be elongation of the images, as in this example, where all the teeth are markedly affected. P

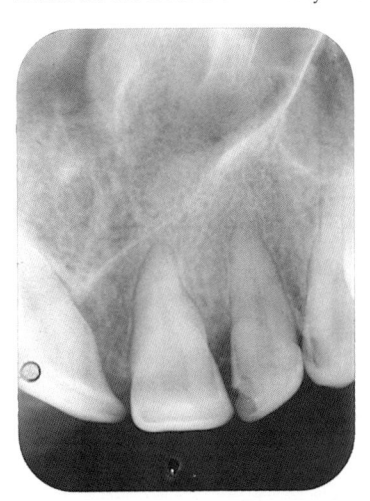

4.2 Conversely, if the tube is placed more apically than is necessary to aim the beam at right angles to the bisector, the images will be foreshortened, as in this example, where all the teeth are affected. Note the embossed dot indicating the front surface of the film overlying the distal incisal edge 1̱|. P

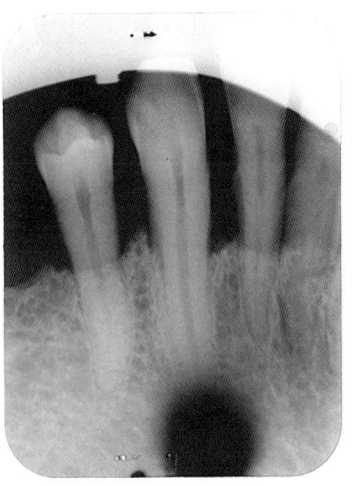

4.3 Coning of the X-ray beam is an important feature in radiation protection, but if the tube is not centred correctly over the tissues to be examined, it may result in a significant part of the field being obscured. In this example, much of the crowns of the mandibular teeth is obscured. In addition, light has reached the film prior to exposure, causing fogging in the apical region 3̄|, thus simulating an apical radiolucency. The distinguishing features of this technical error are its extreme density and its diffuse periphery. It is usually a consequence of damage to the film packet. P

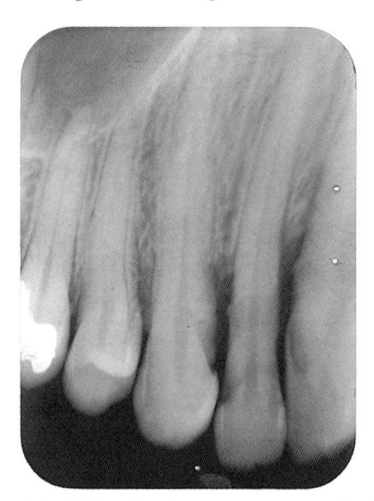

4.4 If the film becomes excessively bent while being held in place by the patient, part of it will be incorrectly aligned in relation to the X-ray beam. Consequently, there may be distortion of the images on only part of the film. In this example, 5̄4̄| are projected normally, but 3̄2̄1̄| are markedly elongated. P

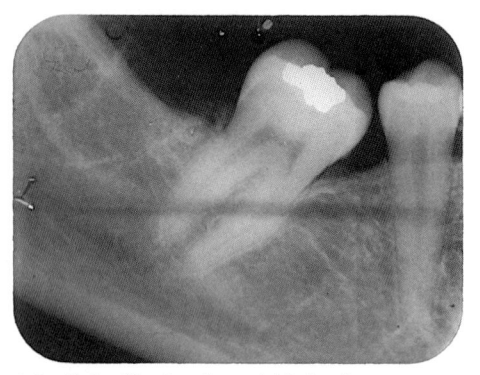

4.5 If the film has been folded prior to exposure, the emulsion may be damaged so that it does not react normally to the X-rays, resulting in a dark line on the film. This fault is more likely to occur on films in the lower jaw, and might be confused with a fracture line. In this example, the line runs horizontally across the film and should not lead to misinterpretation. P

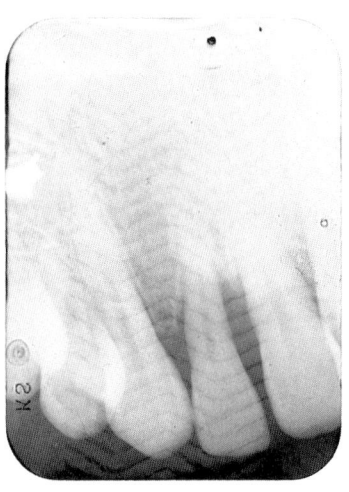

4.6 If the film is placed the wrong way round, it will be underexposed due to the interposition of its lead foil backing between the emulsion and the X-ray source. In addition, the herring bone pattern of the foil will be superimposed upon the film. A similar appearance affecting only part of the film may arise if the lead foil becomes displaced over the front of the film in the packet. P

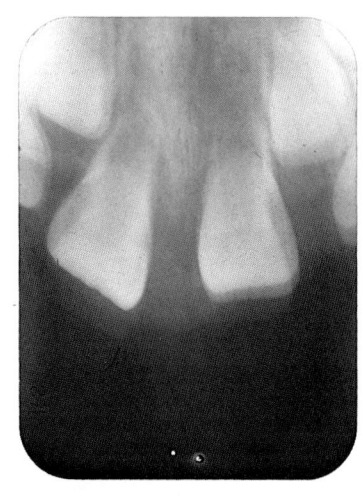

4.7 If the patient moves during exposure of the film, there may be superimposition of several images of the same structure. This is more likely to occur in children, as in this film of the maxillary incisors of a seven-year-old. A similar appearance may also arise if the X-ray tube moves during the exposure. P

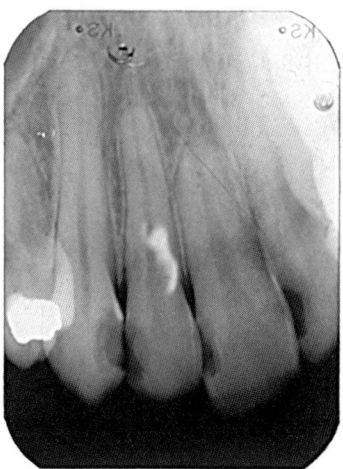

4.8 Rarely, a metallic foreign body may be present in the X-ray tube, producing an unexplained radiopaque image. Exposure of an isolated film will also show such an image, thus confirming the presence of the foreign body in the tube. P

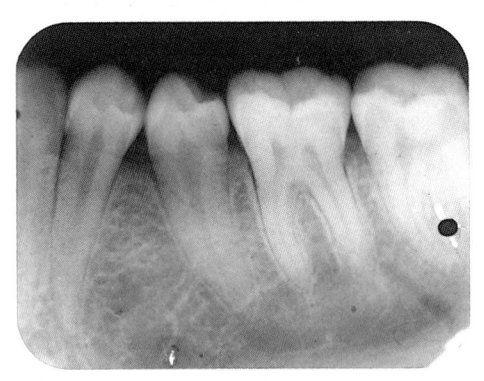

4.9 Another rare form of artefact is a consequence of a hair-line fracture in the cone of the X-ray apparatus. Under these circumstances, a thin, radiolucent line may appear on the film, which could be misinterpreted as a fracture line. In this example, the artefact runs obliquely across the film supero-inferiorly from right to left, and was suspected since it was present in a number of consecutive films. P

Technical Errors 51

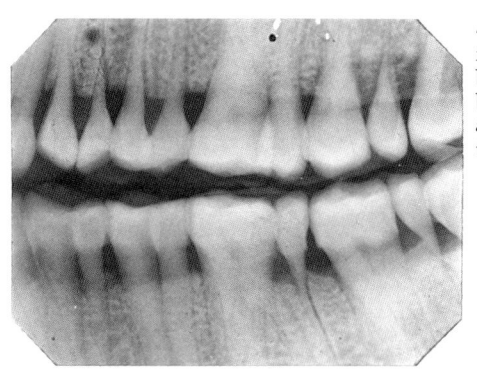

4.10 Double exposure of a film can produce a variety of bizarre appearances, as in this bitewing film in which there is a confusion of images of the teeth. BW

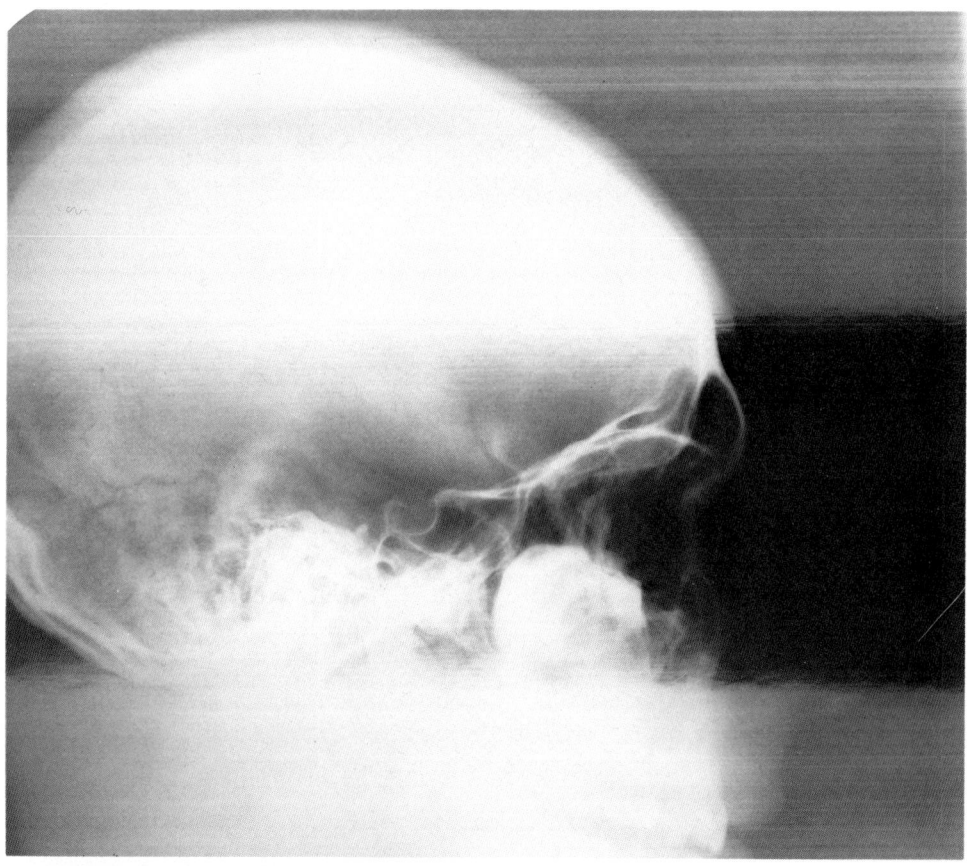

4.11 This appearance results if the grid is positioned the wrong way round when taking extra-oral films. The central part of the film remains reasonably well exposed, but the more peripheral parts are obscured due to incorrect angulation of the oblique lead slats in this part of the grid (see Fig. 2.9), forming a series of linear radiopacities across it. L

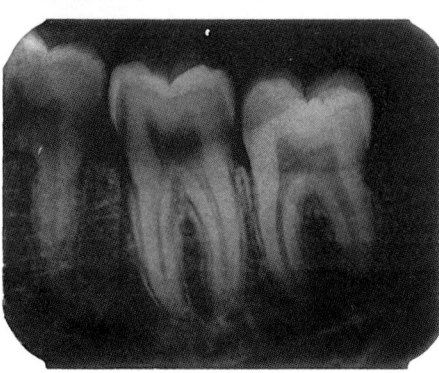

4.12 An overall darkening of the film with lack of contrast can be a consequence of several factors, the most common of which are over-exposure or over-development. The latter may also arise if the temperature is too high during development. P

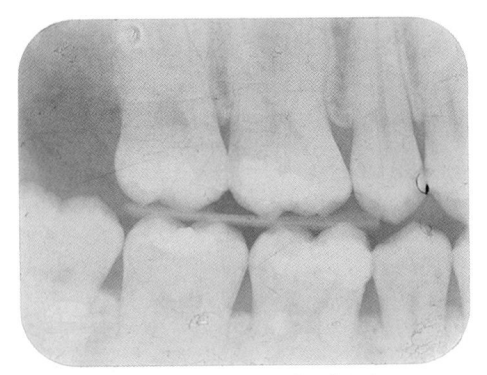

52   *A Radiological Atlas of Diseases of the Teeth and Jaws*

4.13   Under-exposure or under-development can result in a film which has an overall lack of density and contrast. Under-development may arise if the temperature is too low during development. P

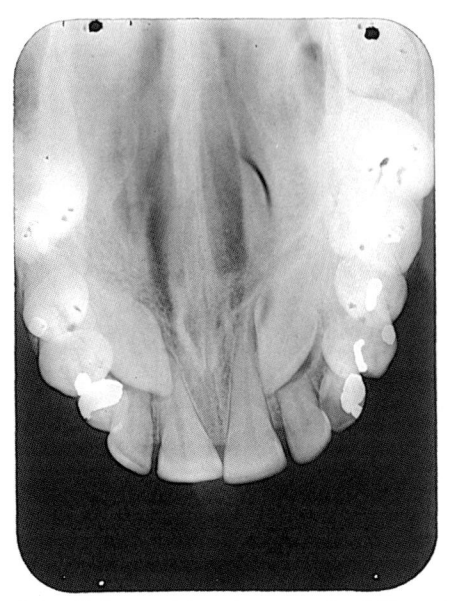

4.14   Defects might arise on occlusal films where the emulsion has been damaged due to the patient biting on the film during the taking of the radiograph. In this example, a number of punctate radiolucent marks due to excessive occlusal force overlie the cusps of the premolar and molar teeth. In addition, there is a densely radiolucent arcuate line overlying the radiolucency of the left nasal cavity due to film damage incurred by finger nail indentation during its removal from the package in the darkroom. USO

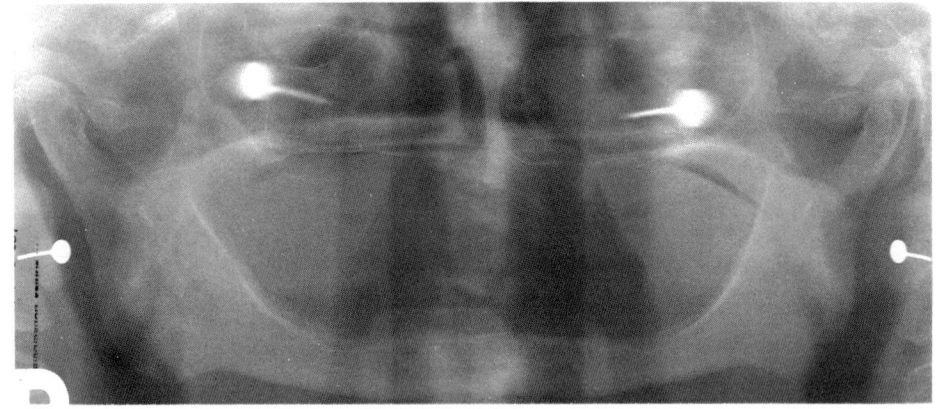

4.15   In panoramic radiographs, the images of extra-oral objects (commonly ear-rings) may be superimposed upon the oral structures. In this patient wearing stud ear-rings, the image of each is clearly displayed on its own side, but in addition a second image is projected onto the opposite side of the jaw at a higher level due to the upward angulation of the X-ray tube. These images are enlarged and blurred and are superimposed upon the maxillary antra bilaterally. Note the densely radiopaque dots scattered over the film, producing a mild snow-storm effect due to the presence of particles of dust on the image-intensifying screen. Also, note the slightly radiopaque rectangular area with rounded superior corners in the inferior midline due to the plastic chin-locating device on the apparatus. PR

Technical Errors 53

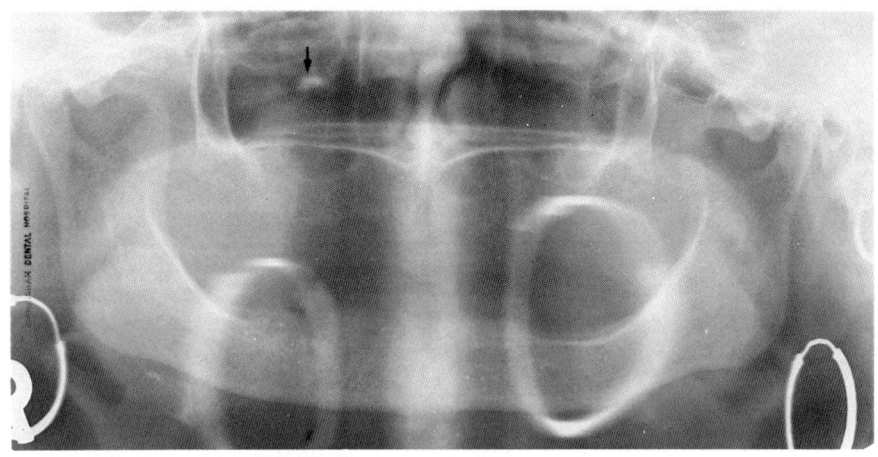

4.16 In this patient wearing annular ear-rings, the projected images are superimposed mostly over the body of the mandible on the opposite side. Again they are enlarged, blurred and at a slightly higher level than the image on the side where they are positioned. In addition, this patient is also wearing a metallic hair clip on the left side, but only a small part of the second image (arrow) projected over the antrum on the right side is apparent. Note that this is also at a higher level. PR

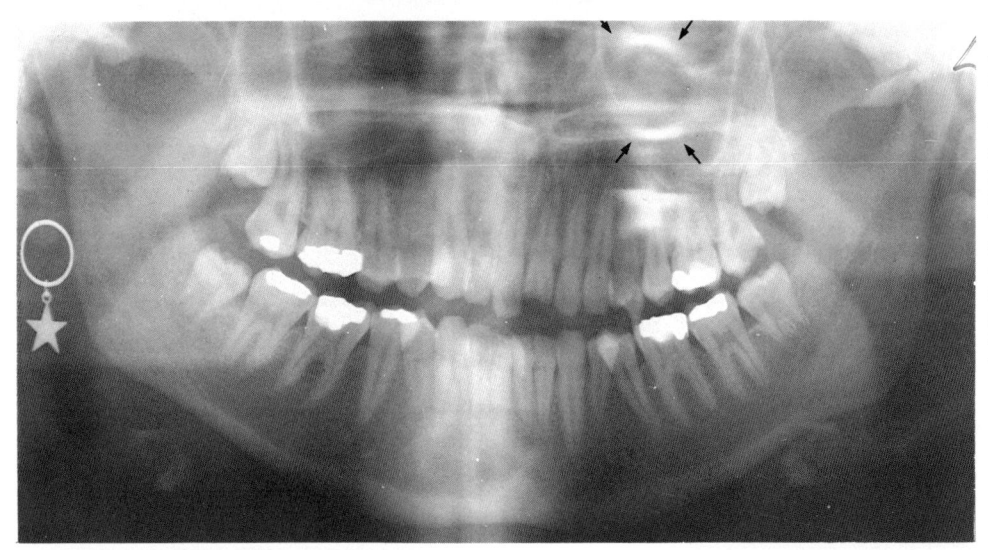

4.17 The projected image of annular ear-rings may be misinterpreted as a cyst ('ear-ring cyst') if it is superimposed over the appropriate part of the maxilla. In this example, there is an 'ear-ring cyst' (arrows) in the left antrum due to the annular ear-ring on the right side. In addition, there is an opacity overlying the apices $\lfloor 456$ due to projection of the image of the star pendant of the ear-ring. PR

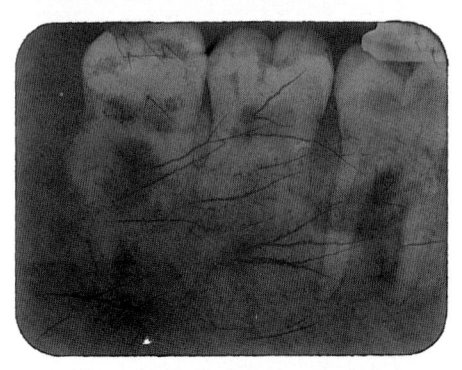

4.18 Electrostatic discharge may rarely occur when the film is removed from its packet in the dark room, so causing a series of irregular, branched, dark tracks. Such discharge results from friction between the film and its packaging, and is more likely to occur in warm, dry environments. P

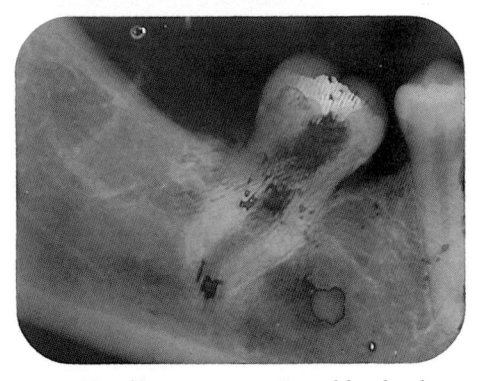

4.19 This film was contaminated by developer prior to processing, both from the operators thumb, producing a dark thumb-print overlying much of the film, and from droplets splashed upon it. P

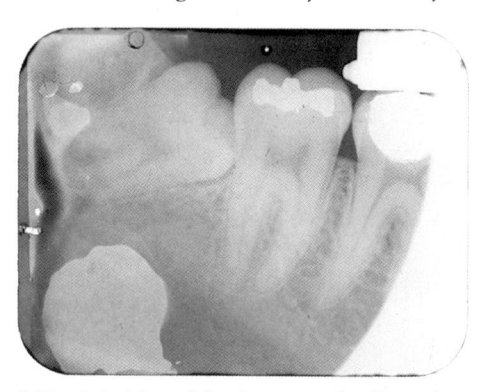

54 *A Radiological Atlas of Diseases of the Teeth and Jaws*

4.20 Splashing of fixative on to the film prior to development causes clear areas lacking in detail. This film is also partly coned-off. P

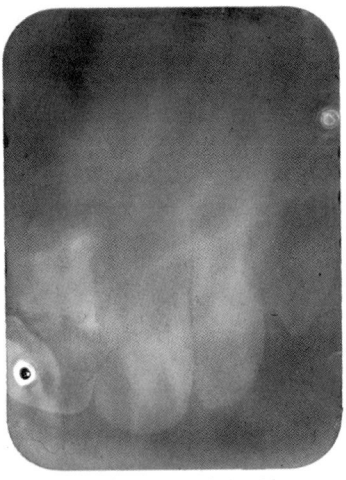

4.21 Development of the film in an insufficiently agitated solution might result in an inadequately developed, poorly defined film. P

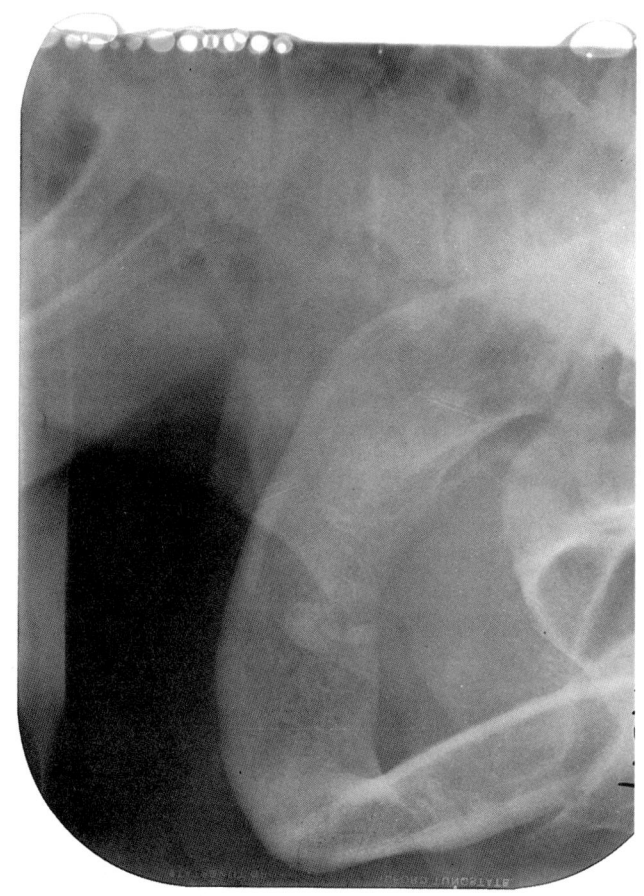

4.22 If the film is incompletely immersed in the developer, that part of the film which remains exposed to the air appears clear. This fault is particularly well demonstrated if there are air bubbles in the surface of the developing fluid, as in this example. OLM

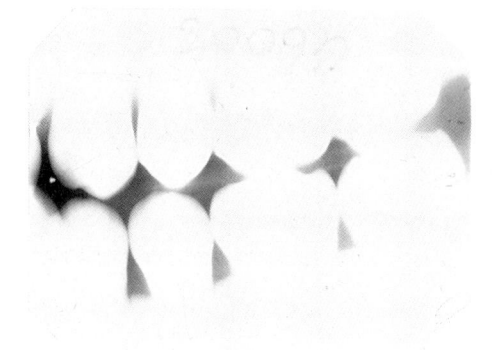

4.23 Over-fixation results in the loss of much of the detail in the affected film. P

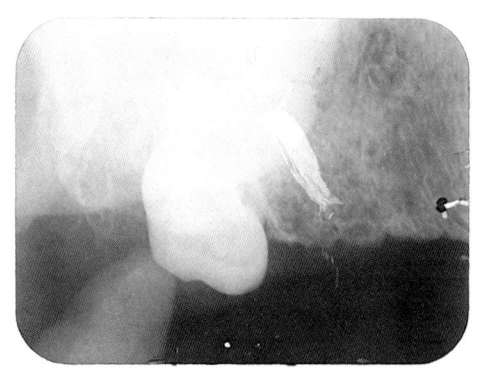

4.24 Scratching of the film—which is most likely to occur after it has been processed, but is still wet—results in clear defects on the film. A common cause is the clip used to suspend the film in the processing fluids, and such small defects can be seen on most hand-processed films, as in the middle of the right-hand margin of this example. P

Chapter 5

The Teeth

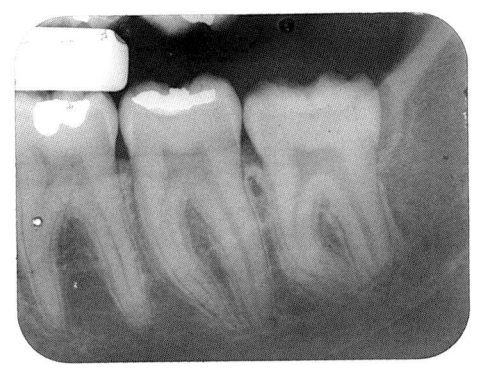

The Teeth 57

Unerupted molar
5.1 Third molar teeth most commonly become impacted and remain unerupted, the mandibular ones more so than the maxillary. Unerupted molars are classified, according to their position, into vertical, mesio-angular, disto-angular, horizontal and transverse impactions. In this vertically impacted ̅8|, the distal aspect of the crown is encased in bone and is surrounded by a normal, radiolucent follicular space and thin, radiopaque cortical lamina. Its occlusal surface is slightly below that of |67̅. The impacted tooth has two mesial roots, the apices of which are curved distally. Note the dense, radiopaque shadow of the film holder above |6̅, which is also present in a number of subsequent films. P

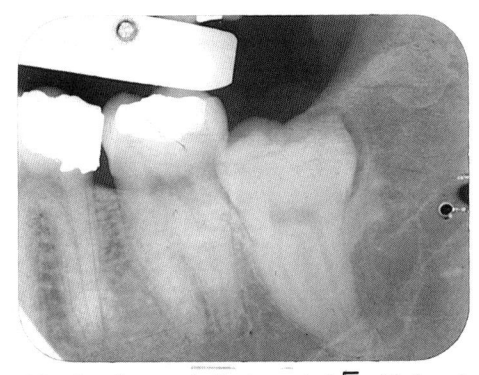

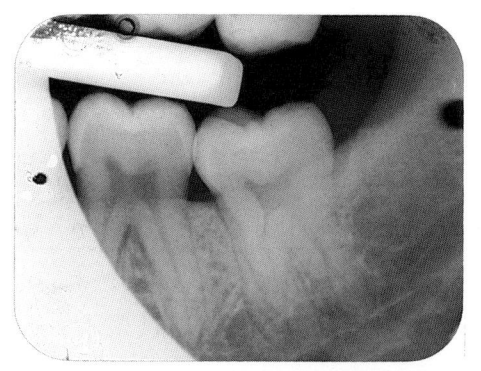

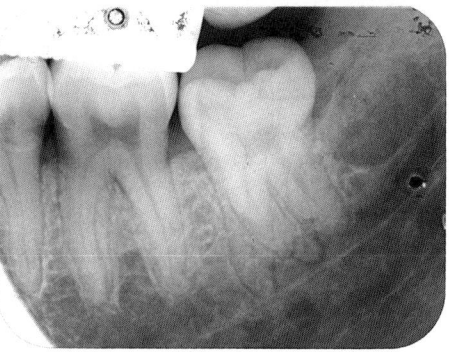

5.3 (top) and 5.4 (bottom) A slightly mesio-angularly impacted |8̅ which is partly erupted and has at least four separate root apices. A faint, soft-tissue shadow of the mucosa overlying the distal aspect of the crown can be seen. The number of roots is better demonstrated (Fig. 5.4) where the tube angulation has been altered upwards in a vertical direction. P

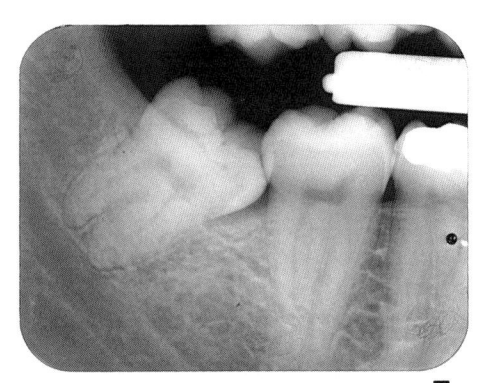

5.2 Another vertically impacted |8̅ with fused roots, the crown of which is covered in bone disto-occlusally. The radiolucent follicular space is of normal width around much of the crown, the mesial part of which slightly overlaps |7̅ cervically. The inferior alveolar canal runs obliquely across the apical part of the root, but shows no evidence of narrowing. P

5.5 A markedly mesio-angularly impacted 8|, in which the distal part of the crown is partially erupted. It has two stout roots, whereas 7| has a single, conical root. P

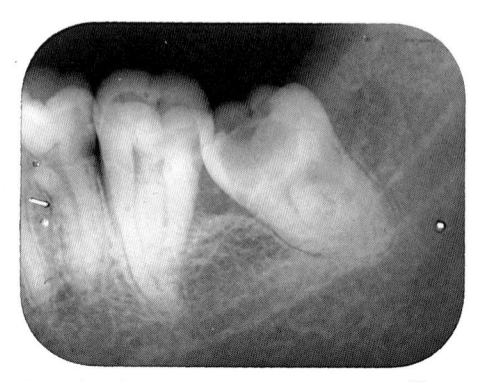

5.6 Another mesio-angularly impacted 8| with a large, carious lesion occlusally in its crown. There is also bone loss interdentally |78 where the alveolar crest is radiolucent, being further evidence of stagnation around the impacted tooth. The roots of |78 are both conical and the inferior alveolar canal runs obliquely across the apex 8|, although there is no evidence of narrowing. P

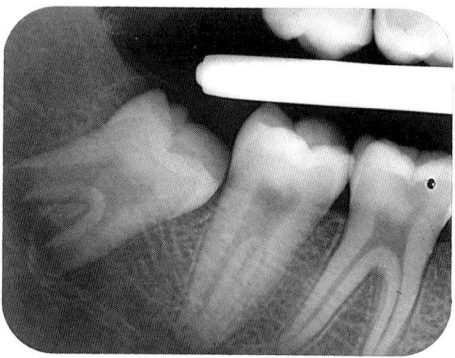

5.7 A mesio-angularly positioned, still erupting 8| with incomplete root formation, which is impacting into the distal aspect 7|. The crown of 8| is surrounded by a normal, radiolucent, follicular space and a thin, radiopaque, cortical lamina. P

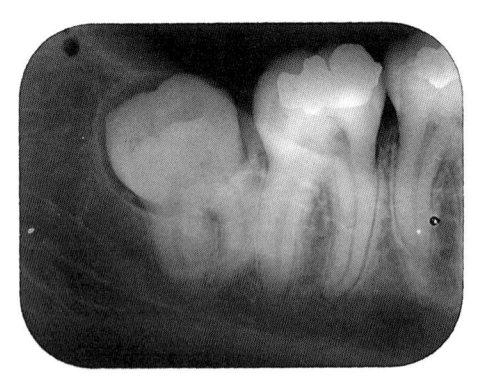

5.8 A disto-angularly impacted 8| with a well defined, radiolucent, follicular space and a thin, radiopaque, cortical lamina around the crown. The tooth is two-rooted, the apical part of the mesial root being curved distally. P

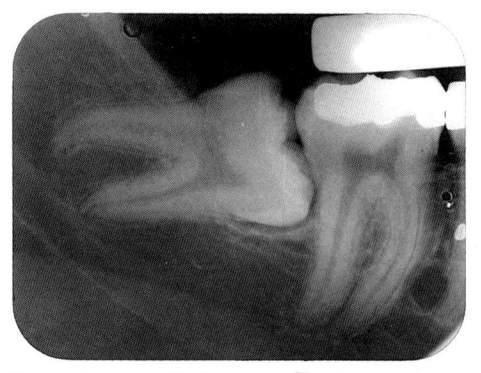

5.9 A horizontally impacted 8|, the distal portion of its crown being erupted to the same occlusal level as 7|. It is two-rooted, the apex of the distal root being slightly hooked. P

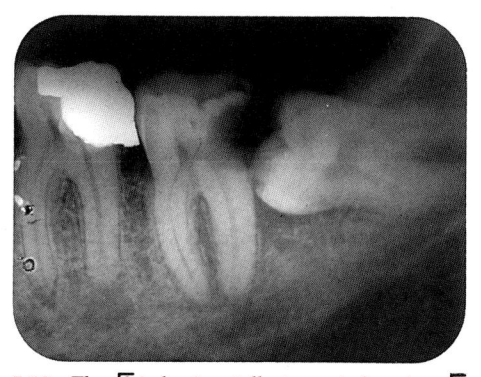

5.10 The |8 is horizontally impacted against |7, which has a large, carious cavity distally. |8 is two-rooted, but the apices are not demonstrated on this radiograph. Note the large, cervical overhang in the disto-occlusal amalgam restoration |6, which has a periapical radiolucency with loss of lamina dura on the distal root. The interdental crest |67 is irregularly radiolucent, indicating early bone loss of chronic periodontitis. P

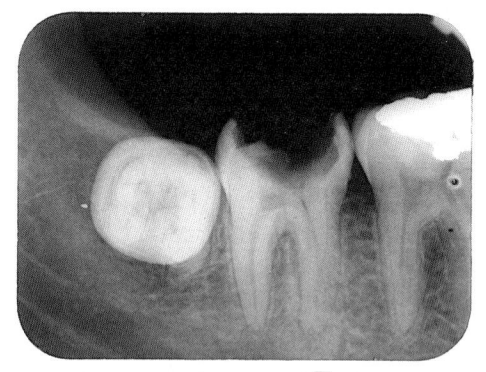

5.11 A transversely impacted 8|, distal to a grossly carious 7|. It is not possible to be certain from this radiograph whether the crown of 8| lies on the buccal or lingual side of the alveolus, but since the crown is more clearly defined than the roots, it is probable that it lies closer to the film, i.e. lingually. To confirm this, a lower occlusal view is required. P

The Teeth 59

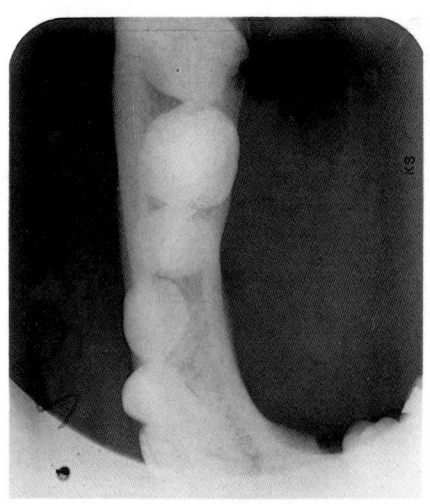

5.12 An occlusal film from another patient in which the position of the crown of the transversely impacted 8| is shown to be lying lingually. LTO

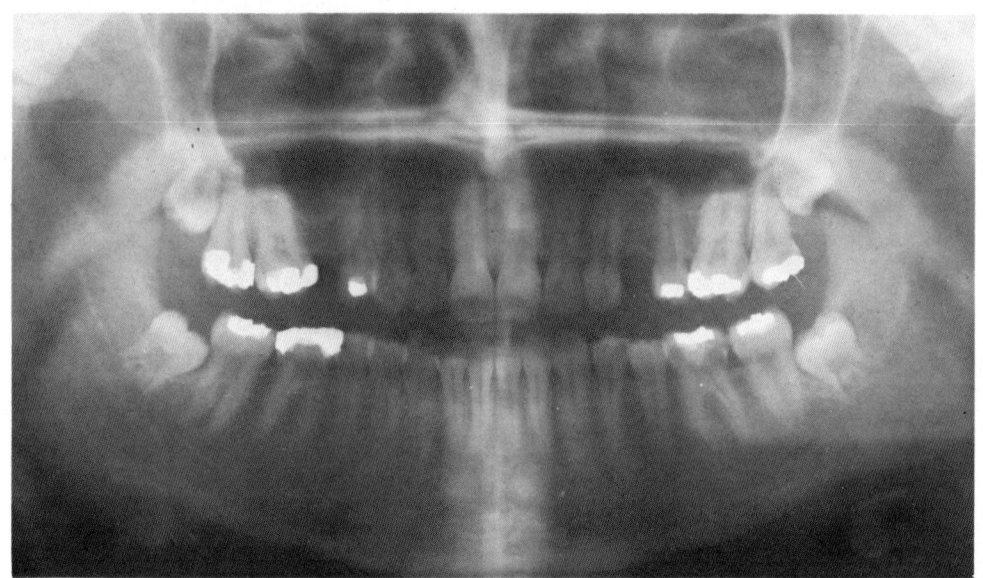

5.13 In this patient, there are four unerupted third molars, all with in-completely formed roots. 8|8 are mesially inclined and 8|8 distally inclined, |8 being higher than 8|. Intra-oral films would be necessary to obtain better definition. Note the presence of numerous carious lesions in the other teeth, the periapical radiolucencies |6, and that 5|4 are missing. PR

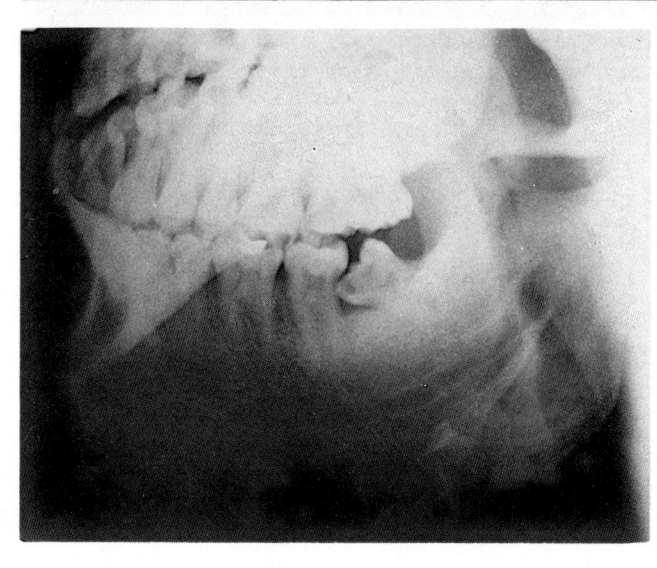

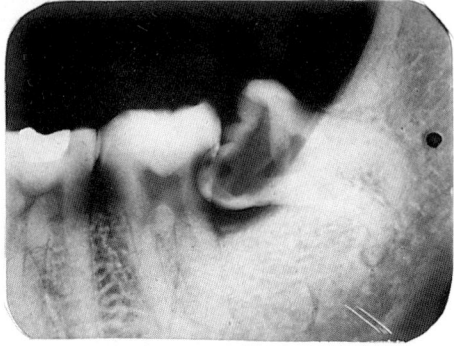

5.14 (left) and 5.15 (above) A mesio-angular |8 with grossly carious crown impacted into a cavity on the distal aspect |7. |8 has two roots, both of which exhibit marked mesial curvature apically (Fig. 5.15). The surrounding bone is densely radiopaque with increased trabeculations. Note the greater detail available on the intra-oral film. OLM & P

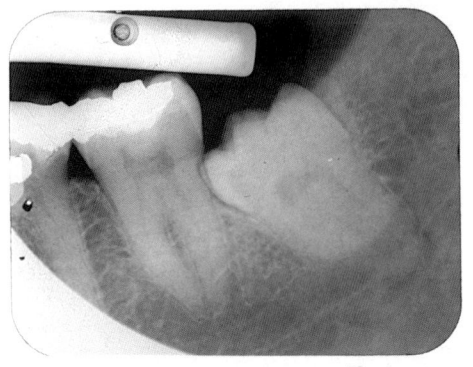

60 *A Radiological Atlas of Diseases of the Teeth and Jaws*

5.16 A mesio-angularly impacted 8̵ with a conical root over the apical part of which the inferior alveolar canal runs transversely. The radiopaque laminae demarcating the bony walls of the canal are continuous across the root and exhibit slight narrowing. In addition, the root is less radiopaque in this region, suggesting that its surface is indented by the canal. P

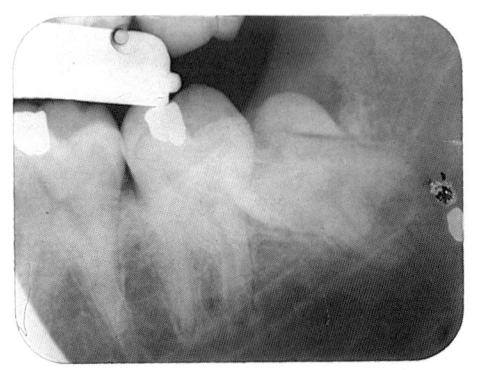

5.17 Another mesio-angularly impacted 8̵ with more marked narrowing of the laminae of the walls of the inferior alveolar canal as it crosses both roots. Again, there is a marked reduction in the radiodensity of the roots in these regions, suggesting that they are deeply grooved. There is a large, radiolucent follicle space and radiopaque lamina on the distal aspect of the crown. The dark line running obliquely across the distal part of the crown 8̵ is a finger nail indentation (see Fig. 4.14). P

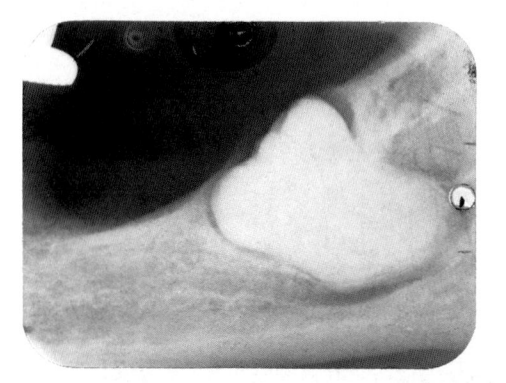

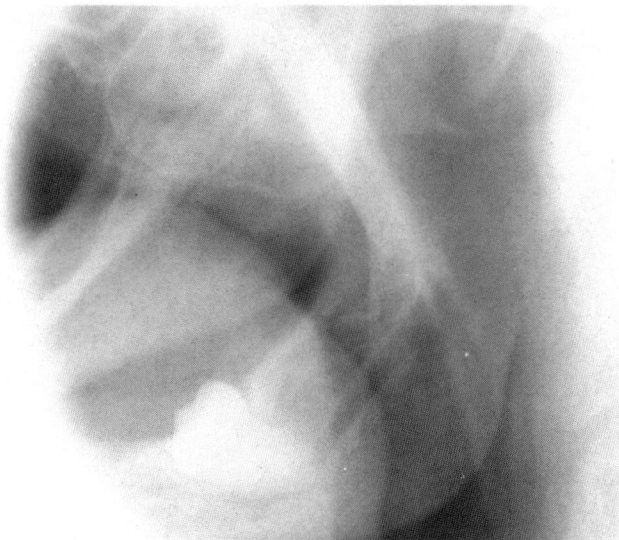

5.18 (top) and 5.19 (bottom) A deeply placed, mesio-angularly impacted 8̵ in an otherwise edentulous mandible. Its fused root has caused narrowing and deviation of the inferior alveolar canal inferiorly. P & OLM

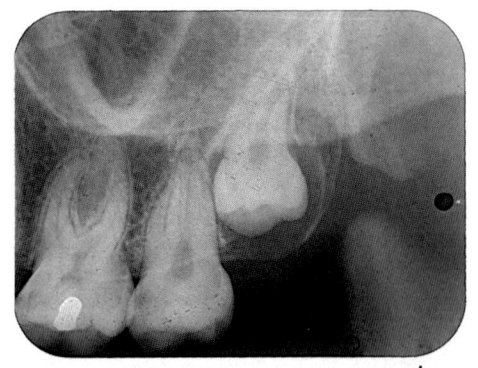

5.20 An almost fully formed, unerupted 8̲ in the maxillary tuberosity. Its crown is surrounded by a normal, radiolucent, follicular space and a thin, radiopaque layer of cortical bone. The root of the zygoma lies above 6̲ and running posteriorly from it is the zygomatic arch, its inferior border crossing 8̲ cervically. Note the pterygoid plate distal to the tuberosity and the coronoid process of the mandible. P

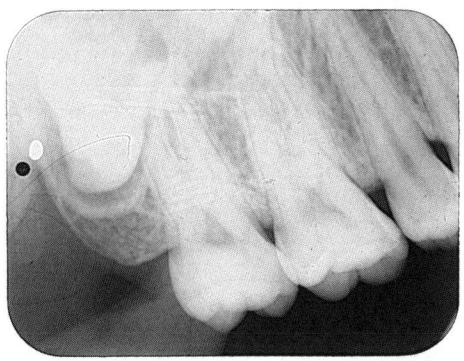

The Teeth 61

5.21 An unerupted, incompletely formed 8⌋ deeply buried in bone and with marked distal inclination. There is a normal, radiolucent, follicular space and thin, radiopaque lamina around its crown. P

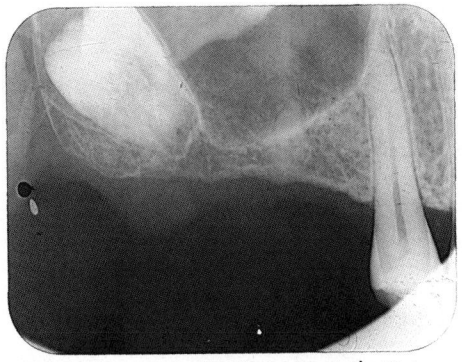

5.22 An inverted, distally inclined 8⌋with incomplete root formation and totally enclosed in bone. Note its close proximity to the floor of the maxillary antrum and the presence of a retained root 6⌋. The soft-tissue shadow of the mucosa overlying the tuberosity is clearly shown. P

Unerupted canine
5.23 (far right) and 5.24 (right) Two differently angled views of the same mesially inclined, unerupted ⌊3 demonstrate that its crown lies palatally (parallax, see Fig. 2.8). The X-ray tube was positioned more distally in the second film (Fig. 5.24), and the crown of the unerupted tooth has moved in the same relative direction. Note the crown and inadequate root filling 1⌋, with part of the gutta percha point projecting beyond the apex. P

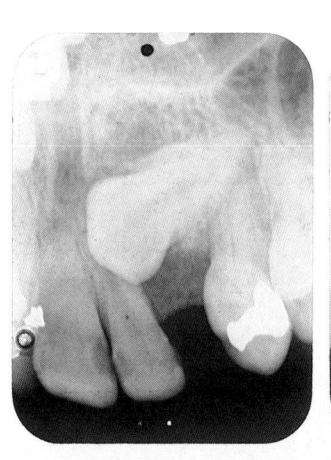

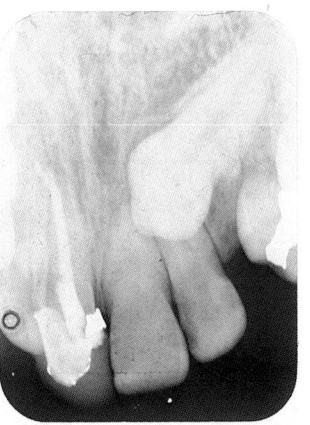

5.25 (right) and 5.26 (far right) Another mesially inclined, unerupted ⌊3, lying palatally as demonstrated by these two differently angled views (parallax). In one (Fig. 5.25), the tube was centred over the midline, as demonstrated by the clear contact 1⌋1 mesially, and in the other (Fig. 5.26) between ⌊2 4. Again, the crown of the unerupted tooth has moved in the same direction as the tube. Note that both naso-lacrimal canals are clearly demonstrated. USO & UOO

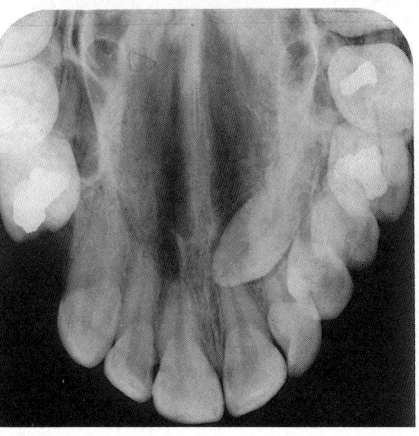

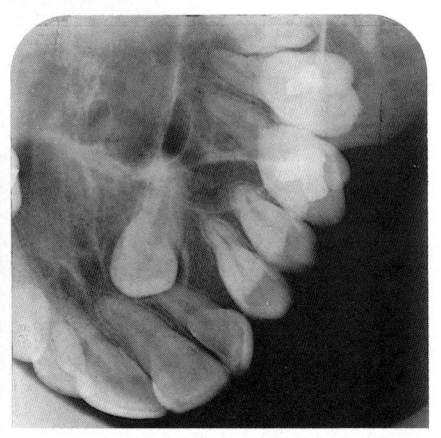

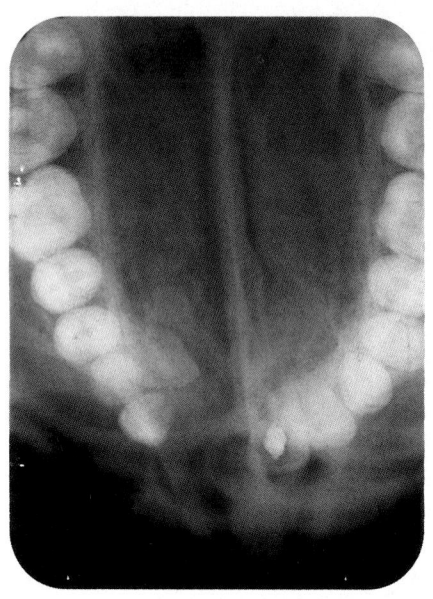

5.27 The position of an unerupted, maxillary canine can also be demonstrated on a vertex-occlusal view. In this example, the crown 3| is displayed palatally to 4C2|, but little other information can be obtained. Note that 1| is missing. VO

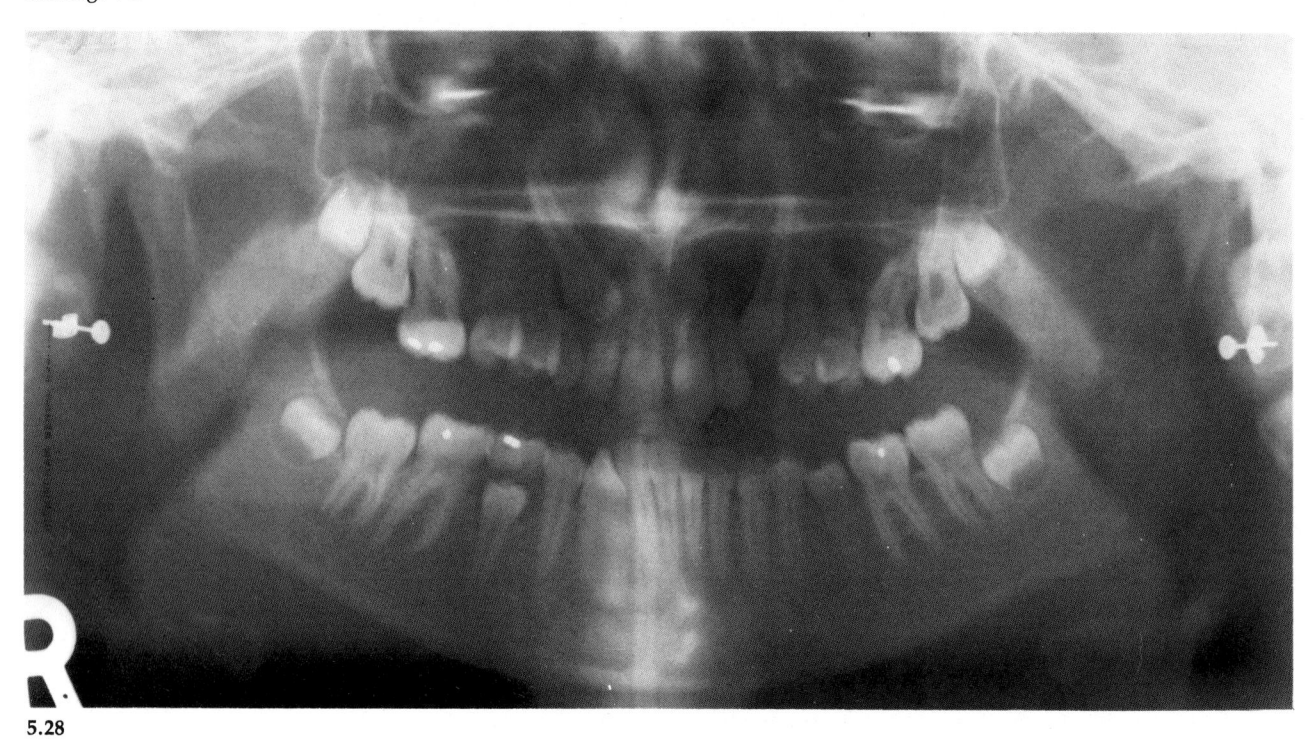

5.28

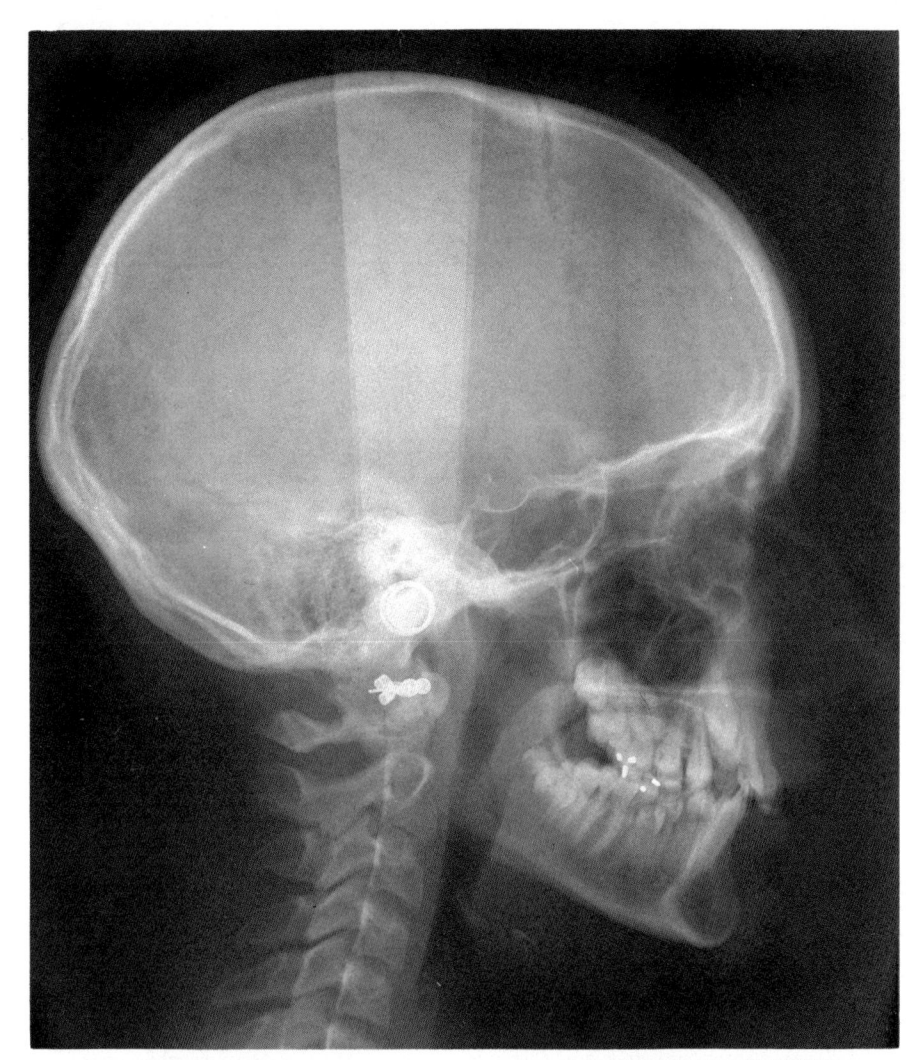

5.28 (opposite page), 5.29 (left), 5.30 (bottom left) and 5.31 (bottom right) The first two of these four radiographs of a 12-year-old patient were taken for orthodontic assessment and show $\frac{87\ \ 3|3\ \ 78}{87\ 5\ \ \ \ \ \ \ \ 8}$ to be unerupted, and $\underline{C|}$ and $\overline{E|}$ retained. $|3$ is in a favourable position to erupt, but there is insufficient space in the arch. On the other hand, $\underline{3|}$ is unfavourably positioned, being mesially inclined, with a large, radiolucent, follicular space around its crown. Its apex lies above $\underline{5|}$, close to the floor of the nose, as demonstrated in the lateral film (Fig. 5.29) in which the two unerupted canines are superimposed. In the latter two films taken with the X-ray tube at different angles (Figs 5.30 and 5.31), treatment has started with the patient wearing a fixed, orthodontic appliance $|3$ has erupted and $\underline{3|}$ is still unerupted in a palatal position (parallax). Note the stud ear-rings (Fig. 5.28) which have also caused linear opacities bilaterally at the lower border of the orbits (see Fig. 4.15). PR, LC, UOO & USO

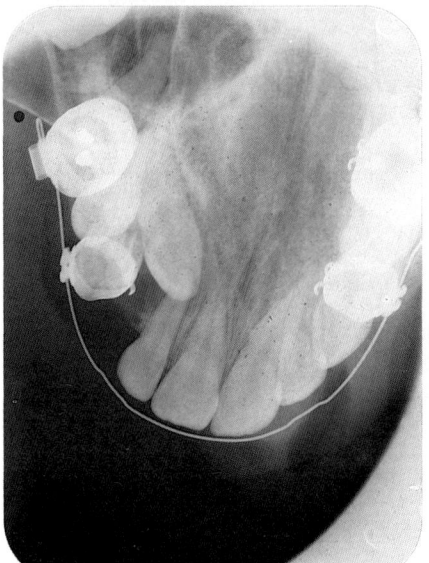

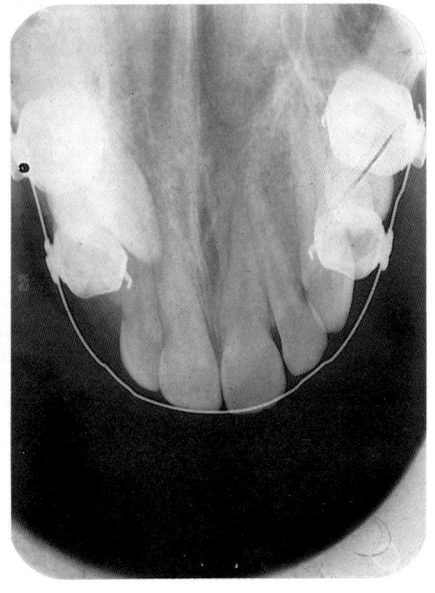

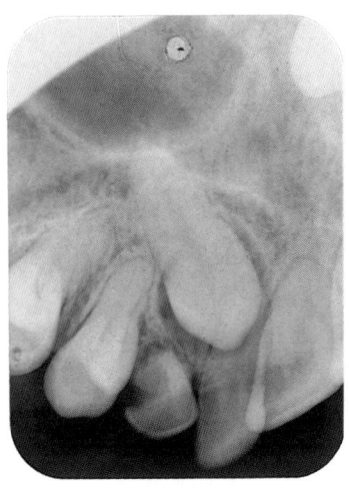

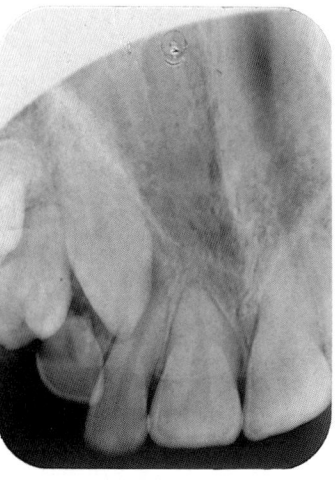

64   *A Radiological Atlas of Diseases of the Teeth and Jaws*

5.32 (left) and 5.33 (right)   Two views of an unerupted 3|, taken with the X-ray tube more mesially placed in the second film, demonstrating that its crown lies buccally to the adjacent teeth (parallax) and is surrounded by a normal, radiolucent, follicular space. C| is retained with a large, carious cavity distally and there is advanced resorption of the root. P

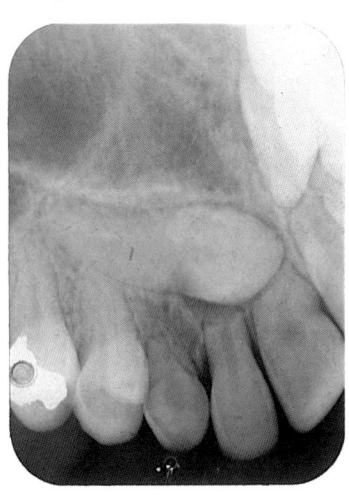

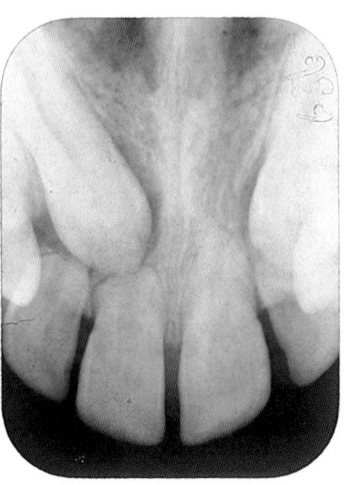

5.35   Root resorption caused by unerupted teeth usually slows down and eventually ceases when the normal age of completed eruption of the impacted tooth has been reached. In this example in an adult, the unerupted 3| has cause apical resorption of the roots 21| which are shortened and flattened. Both roots are surrounded by a distinct radiolucent periodontal ligament space and radiopaque lamina dura, and the crown 3| by a normal, follicular radiolucency, suggesting that the resorptive process is no longer active. P

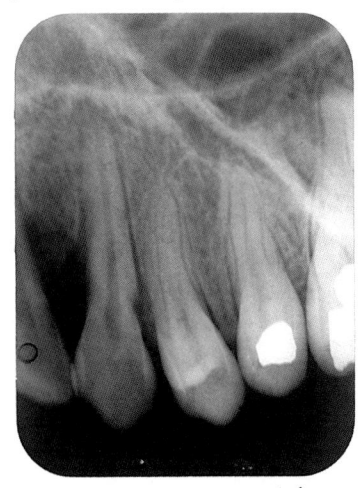

5.34   An unerupted, impacted 3| which has caused apical resorption 2| in a 14-year-old. The apex of the resorbed tooth is irregularly blunted and lacks a distinct periodontal ligament space and lamina dura, so that the follicular radiolucency around the crown 3| abuts directly onto the root, suggesting that the resorptive process is active. On the other hand, the root of the retained C|, although irregularly shortened, is surrounded by a periodontal ligament space and lamina dura indicating that any resorption is proceeding slowly. Note the dilaceration 1| apically, indicated by the curvature of its root canal, and that |3 is also unerupted. P

5.36   A previously impacted |3 transplanted into |C socket six months before in a 15-year-old. A lamina dura and periodontal ligament space has formed around much of its root surface, although there are several areas of external resorption, one of which is superimposed over the middle third of the root canal. In addition, there is incomplete infilling of bone mesially into the crestal part of the prepared socket. P

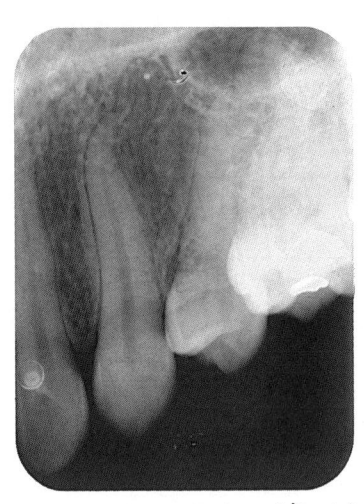

5.37 Another transplanted |3, eight years after operation, showing complete restoration of the alveolar bone with a normal periodontal ligament space and lamina dura around the entire root. P

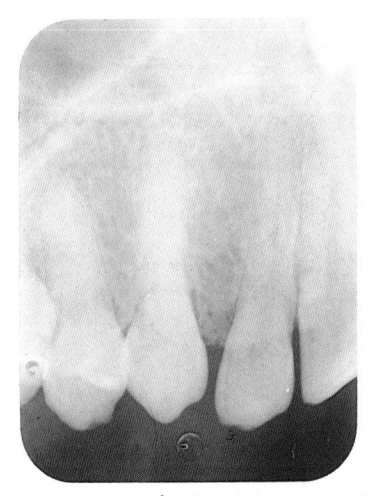

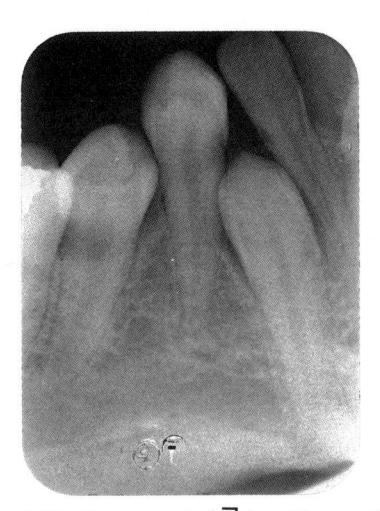

5.39 An unerupted 3| in a 12-year-old, vertically impacted between 4| and 2|, which have drifted mesially and distally, respectively. There is a normal follicular radiolucency around the crown 3| and its slightly hooked apex lies close to the inferior border of the mandible. P

5.38 In this 3| which was transplanted nine years previously, there is now complete sclerosis and obliteration of its root canal, although the surrounding alveolar bone is quite normal and there is no evidence of periapical inflammation. P

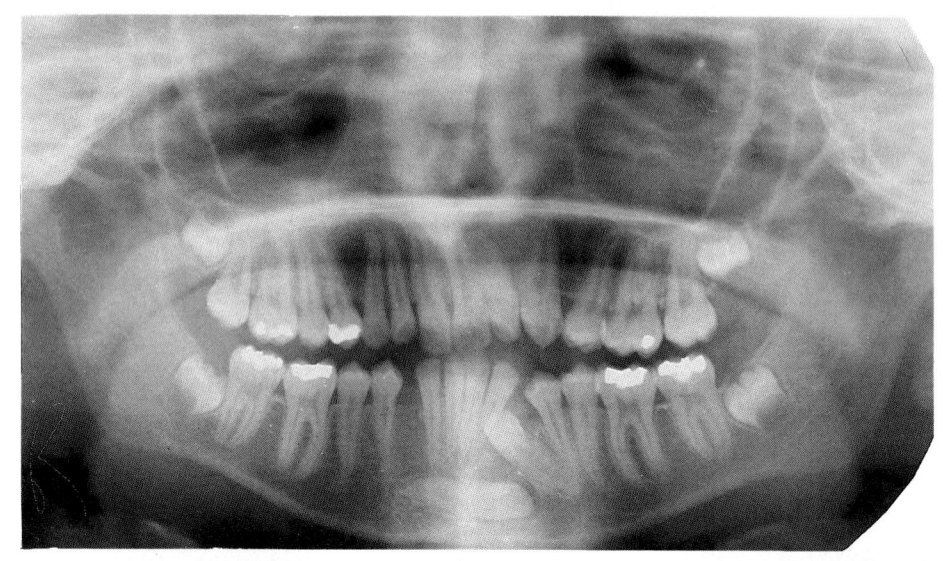

66 *A Radiological Atlas of Diseases of the Teeth and Jaws*

5.40 Bilateral, unerupted, impacted, mandibular canines with resultant diastemas in a 15-year-old. 3| lies horizontally beneath the incisors and |3 is mesio-angularly impacted against |2, the crown of which is tilted distally. The follicular space around the crown 3| is enlarged and is contiguous superiorly with that surrounding |3. Note the four unerupted third molars, and that |4 is missing. PR

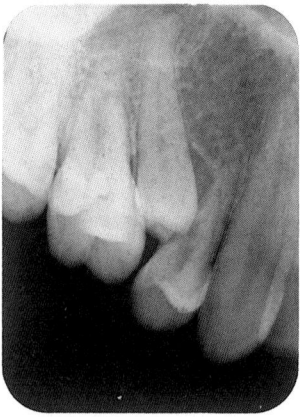

Unerupted premolar
5.41 An unerupted, mesio-angularly impacted 5|, lying between 6| and 4| which are tilted mesially and distally, respectively. A normal follicular space surrounds the crown 5| and there is a slight curvature of its root apex. P

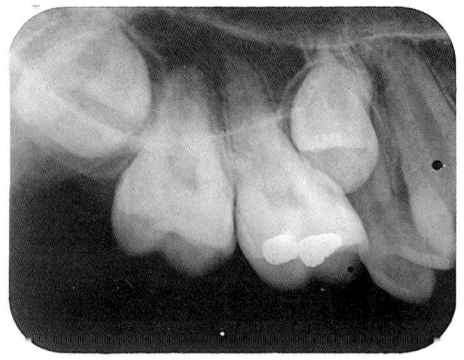

5.42 In this 13-year-old patient, the image of the unerupted 5| is markedly foreshortened due to the palatal inclination of its crown which lies in roughly the same plane as that of the X-rays. Its root is dilacerated and has an open apex. 6| is mesially tilted, the root formation 7| is incomplete, and 8| only partially formed and unerupted. P

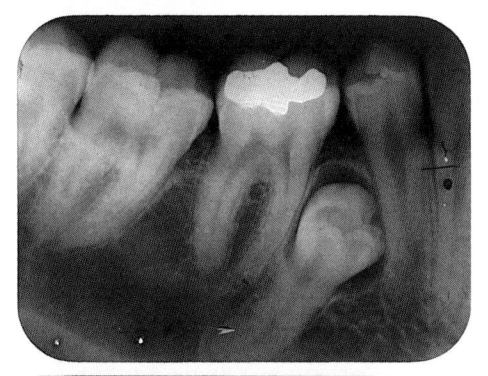

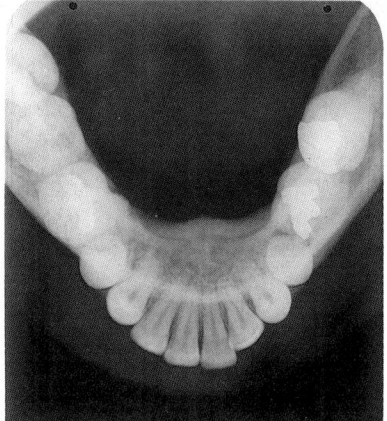

5.43 (top) and 5.44 (bottom) An unerupted, mesio-angularly inclined 5| lying between 6| and 4|, which are tilted mesially and distally, respectively. There is a normal follicular radiolucency around its crown and a slight distal curvature to the root. It is difficult to be certain on periapical films whether the crown of such an unerupted tooth lies lingually or buccally to the adjacent teeth. However, the greater definition of the crown compared with that of the root, suggests that the crown is closer to the film, i.e. lingually. Its position is confirmed on the occlusal film (Fig. 5.44). P & LTO

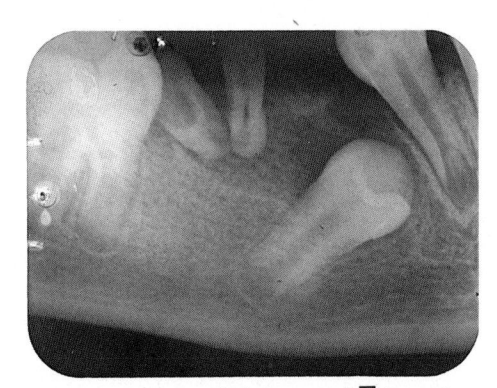

The Teeth 67

5.45 A mesio-angularly impacted 5̄| in a 13-year-old. The 4̄| is tilted distally and has an incompletely formed root which exhibits apical bifurcation of the root canal, suggestive of taurodontism. Both roots of 6̄| are retained and carious. There is a normal follicular space around the crown 5̄| inferiorly, but superiorly there is an enlarged, poorly defined, radiolucent area which is confluent with a periapical radiolucency around 6̄| roots. A cortical lamina is continuous from the distal aspect of the distal root 6̄| to the distal cervical region of the 5̄|. 7̄| roots are not completely formed. P

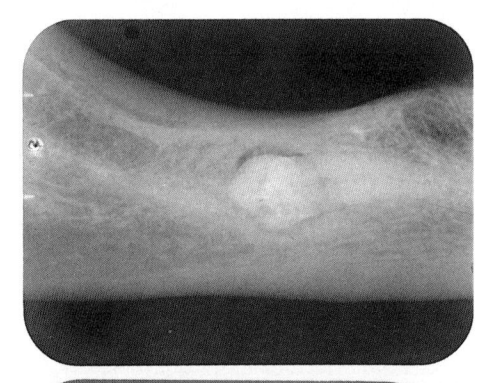

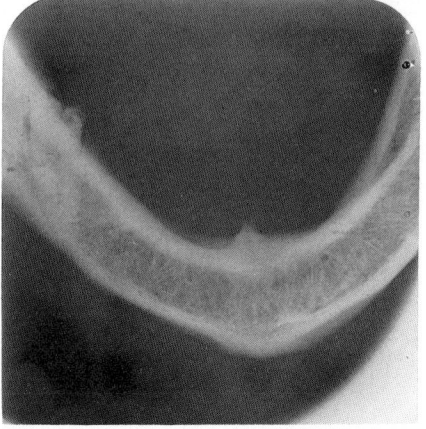

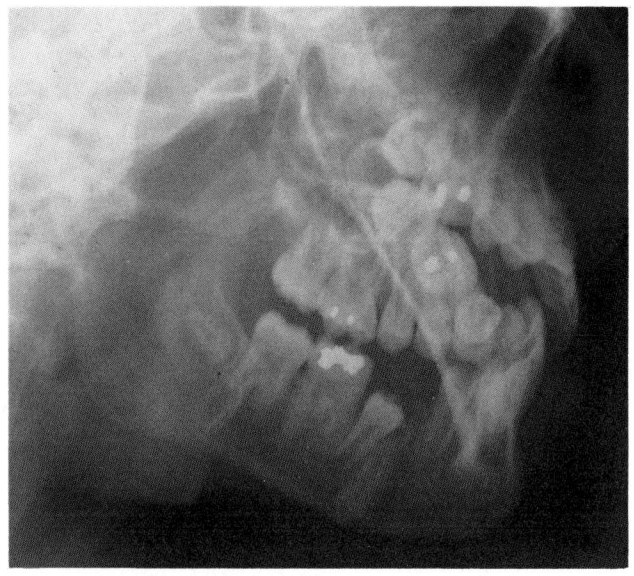

5.48 An inverted, unerupted 4̄| in a 13-year-old. The crown has perforated the inferior border of the mandible and its root is incompletely formed. 5̄| is also unerupted and has an incompletely formed root. Note that the roots of 3̄| and 7̄| are also incompletely formed and the crown 8̄| is at an early stage of mineralisation. OLM

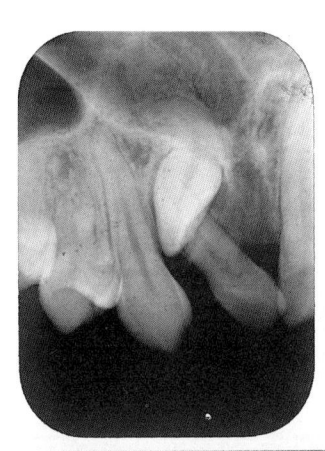

Unerupted incisor
5.49 (left) and 5.50 (below) An unerupted 1| with a dilacerated root, which appears foreshortened on the periapical film (Fig. 5.49). The tooth is rotated and lies with its crown buccally and its root palatally (parallax). 3|2| are tilted mesially and 2| has migrated towards |1, although a diastema is still present. A true lateral view of the region may help in determining the vertical inclination of such unerupted teeth. Note the outlines of the antrum and nasolacrimal canal (arrow) on the right side of the maxilla (Fig. 5.50). P & USO

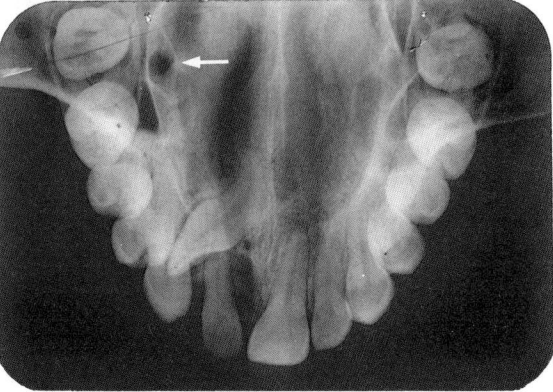

5.46 (top) and 5.47 (bottom) · An unerupted 5̄| lying horizontally in an edentulous mandible. The definition of the crown (Fig. 5.46) is better than that of the root, suggesting that the former is lingually positioned. The tooth appears to be lying anterio-posteriorly in the jaw, but its oblique position is indicated in the occlusal view (Fig. 5.47). The lingual position of the crown is also confirmed, it having perforated the cortical plate and become carious. P & LTO

Tooth transposition

5.51 Tooth transposition most commonly involves the canine teeth. In this example, |34 are transposed, and |3 is rotated and impacted between |45. In addition, this patient has partial anodontia, 3|, |2 and 5| being missing and 2|, 8| and |8 being smaller than usual. 4| is unerupted, lying above the retained C|, and |5 is impacted. All four third molars are at an early stage of development. PR

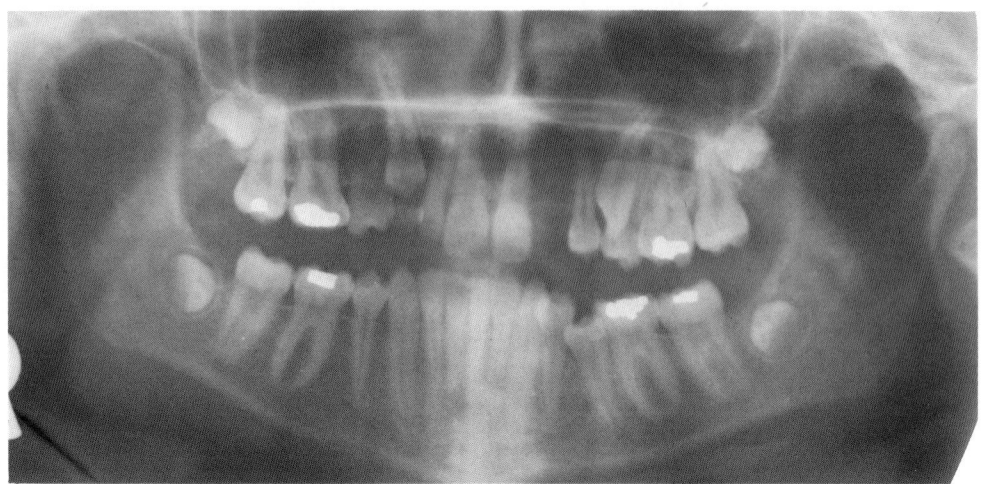

Supernumerary teeth

5.52 Supernumerary teeth most commonly occur in the anterior maxilla, as in this example (mesiodens), in the midline of the maxilla in a five-year-old. It has a conical crown and its root formation is complete, whereas that of the unerupted 21|12, the images of which are superimposed, has only just started. |A is missing and root resorption A| is advanced. P

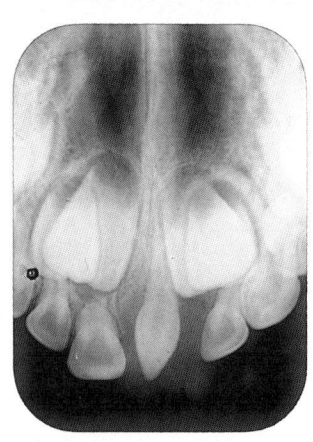

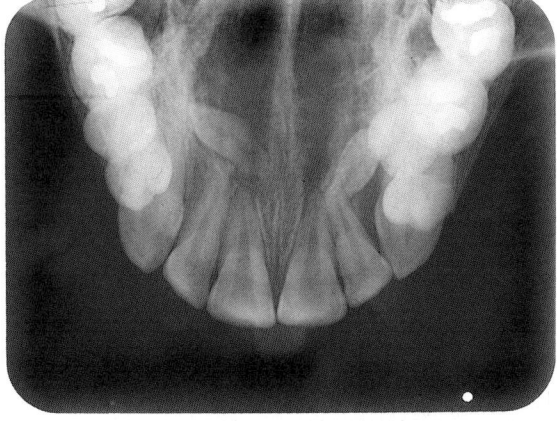

5.53 An erupted supernumerary tooth (mesiodens) with a conical crown, lying between 1|1. Note the radiolucent interstitial restorations 2| mesially, 1| mesially, |1 mesially and distally, and |2 distally, and the carious cavity |2 mesially. P

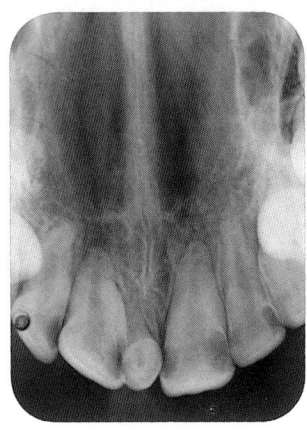

5.54 Two unerupted, distally inclined, inverted, supernumerary teeth with conical crowns lying above the apices of the maxillary incisors. The apex of the right tooth is hooked. It is not uncommon for supernumerary teeth in the anterior maxilla to be inverted and/or bilateral. Note the instanding |5. USO

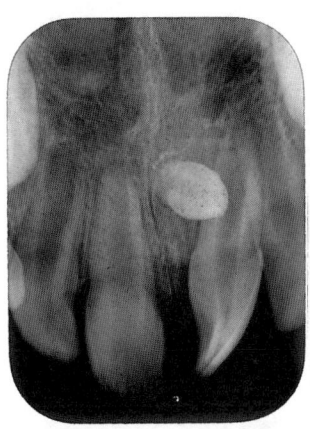

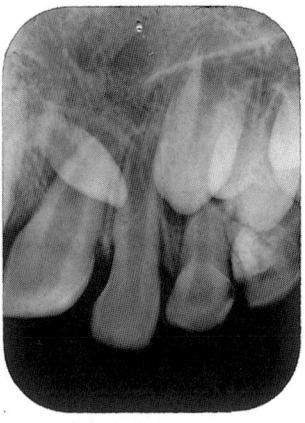

The Teeth 69

5.55 (far left) and 5.56 (left) An unerupted, supernumerary tooth (mesiodens), the crown of which is inclined disto-occlusally, in the midline of the maxilla of a nine-year-old. Its root is dilacerated (Fig. 5.56) with its apex pointing occlusally. The crown lies palatally and the root buccally to |1 (parallax), which is rotated (Fig. 5.55). Note the incomplete root development of the permanent teeth. P

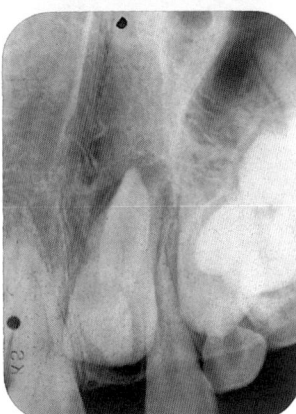

5.57 (left) Two unerupted, supernumerary teeth inhibiting the eruption |1 in a ten-year-old. The more apically placed is inverted, conically shaped and has a complete root. The more occlusally placed is tuberculate, incompletely formed and probably the cause of the delayed eruption |1. Root formation |1 is nearly complete and the space between 1| and |2 is partly closed. Note the unerupted |345. P

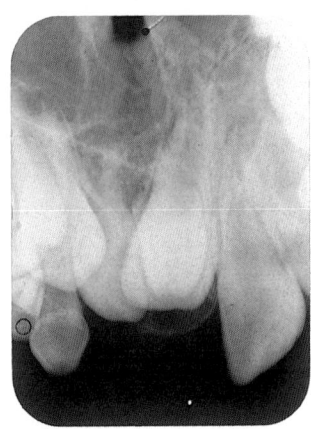

5.58 An unerupted, tuberculate, supernumerary tooth in the anterior maxilla, which has caused delayed eruption 1| in a nine-year-old. The outline of the supernumerary tooth overlies 1|, the root of which is more fully formed than that of the supernumerary tooth. Note the unerupted 32| and erupted C|. P

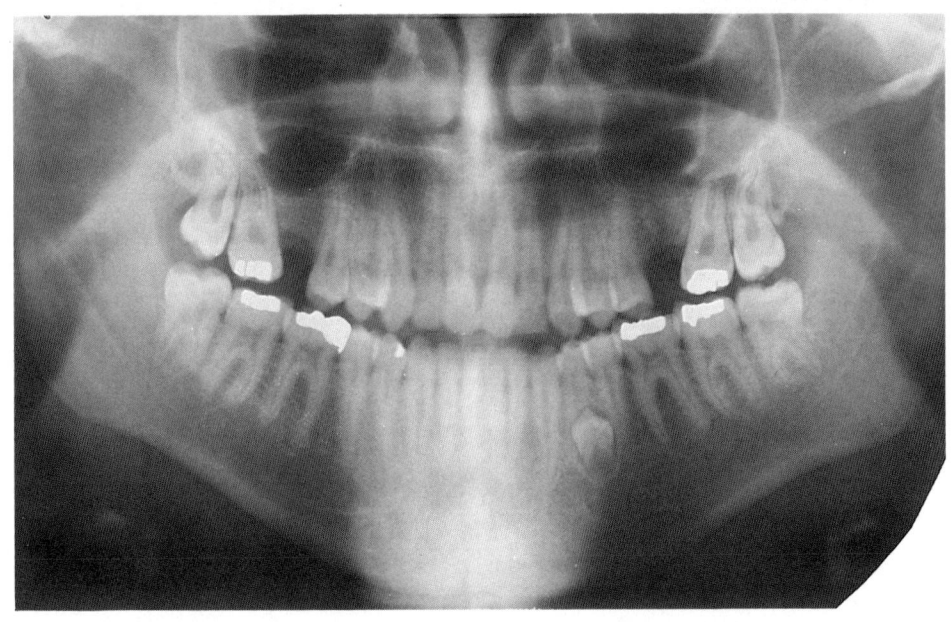

Supplemental teeth
5.59 In contrast to supernumerary teeth, supplemental teeth are morphologically similar to the normal dentition. In this 21-year-old patient, there is an incompletely formed, unerupted, supplemental, left mandibular premolar. The developing tooth is surrounded by a radiolucent follicular space and a thin, radiopaque lamina. Note the healing sockets 6|6. PR

5.60 Two unerupted, vertically impacted, supplemental, right mandibular premolars. Note that $\overline{5|5}$ are rotated, $\overline{8|}$ is unerupted and $|\underline{8}$ is partially erupted, and the proximity of the antral floor to the crest of the edentulous ridge bilaterally and to the $|\underline{8}$. PR

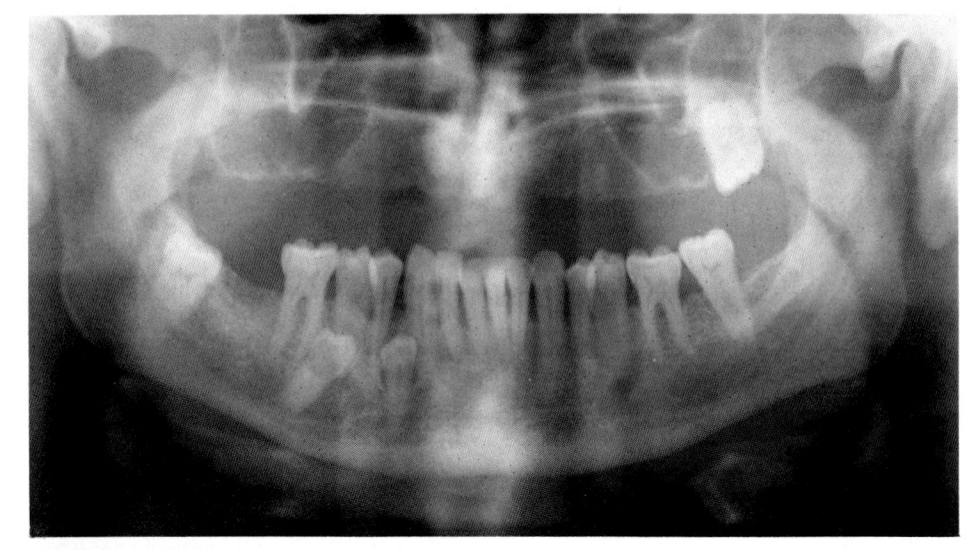

5.61 A horizontally impacted, supplemental molar lying occlusally to an unerupted third molar which is also horizontally impacted. Note the recurrent carious lesion mesially $|\overline{7}$ beneath the amalgam restoration. OLM

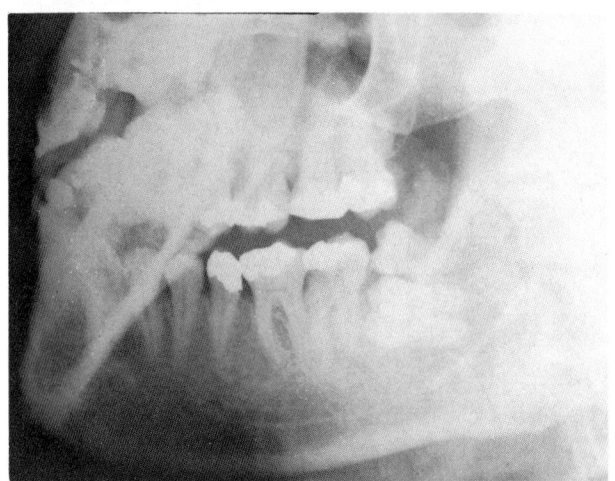

5.62 Supplemental upper molar teeth in a 14-year-old. In addition to the developing upper third molars, two extra molars are forming in each quadrant. The lower arch has a normal complement of molar teeth. PR

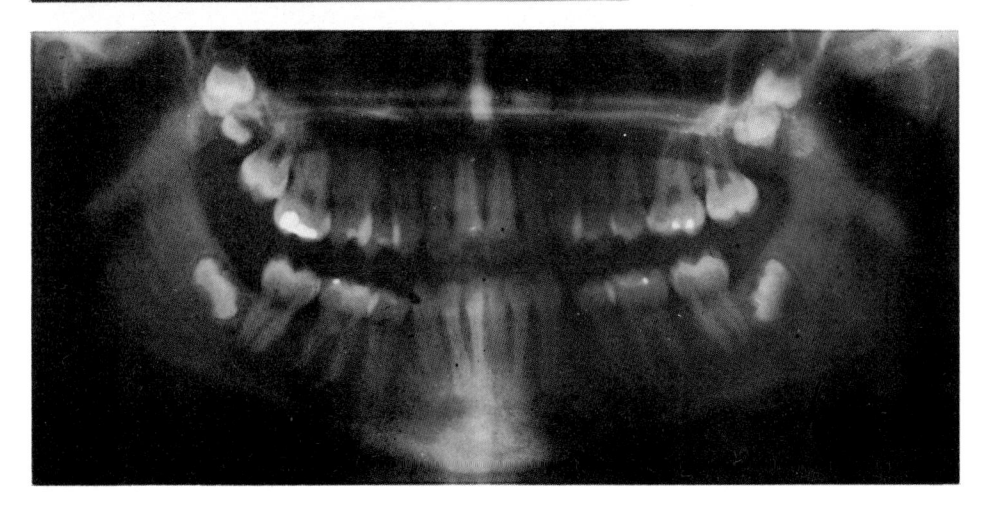

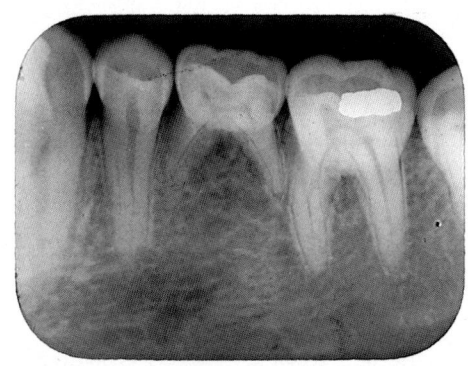

Retained primary molar
5.63 A mandibular, second primary molar in an adult, retained due to the absence of the second premolar. There is some sclerosis of the inter-radicular bone close to the tooth roots, possibly a consequence of occlusal trauma due to the inadequate root size of the primary tooth. P

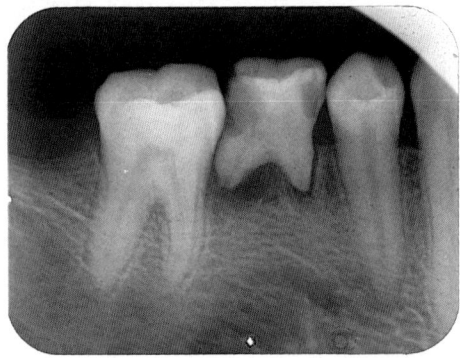

5.64 Another mandibular, second primary molar in an adult, retained due to the absence of the second premolar. The roots are markedly shortened, indicating past resorption. There are large mesial and distal carious cavities together with periapical radiolucencies on both roots. The outline of the radiolucent areas is indistinct. P

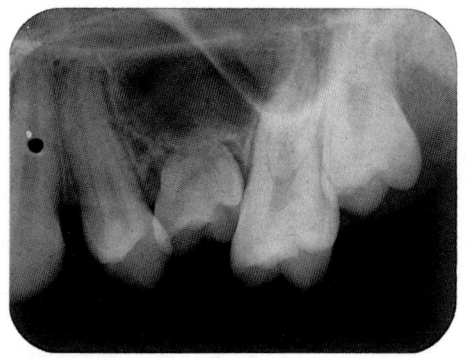

Submerged primary molar
5.65 A submerged maxillary, second primary molar with absence of the second premolar. There is complete resorption of the roots of the primary molar and only the crown remains. The boundary between the tooth and the surrounding bone is indistinct and no lamina dura is present, indicative of bony ankylosis. The occlusal level of the crown |E is apically positioned relative to that of |4 and |6, which are distally and mesially inclined, respectively. Note the outline of the root of the zygomatic arch and the proximity of the antral floor to the submerged tooth. P

72 *A Radiological Atlas of Diseases of the Teeth and Jaws*

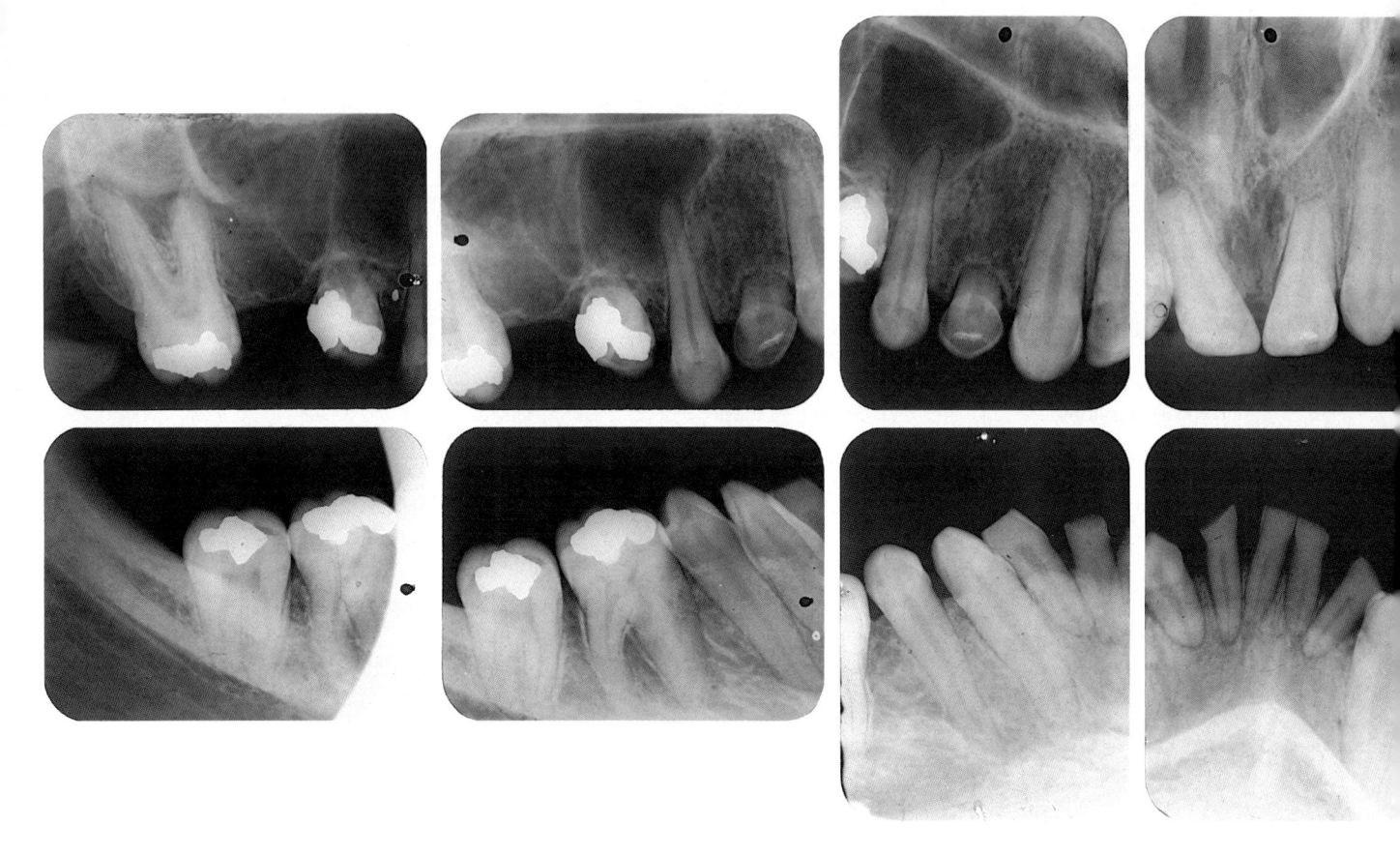

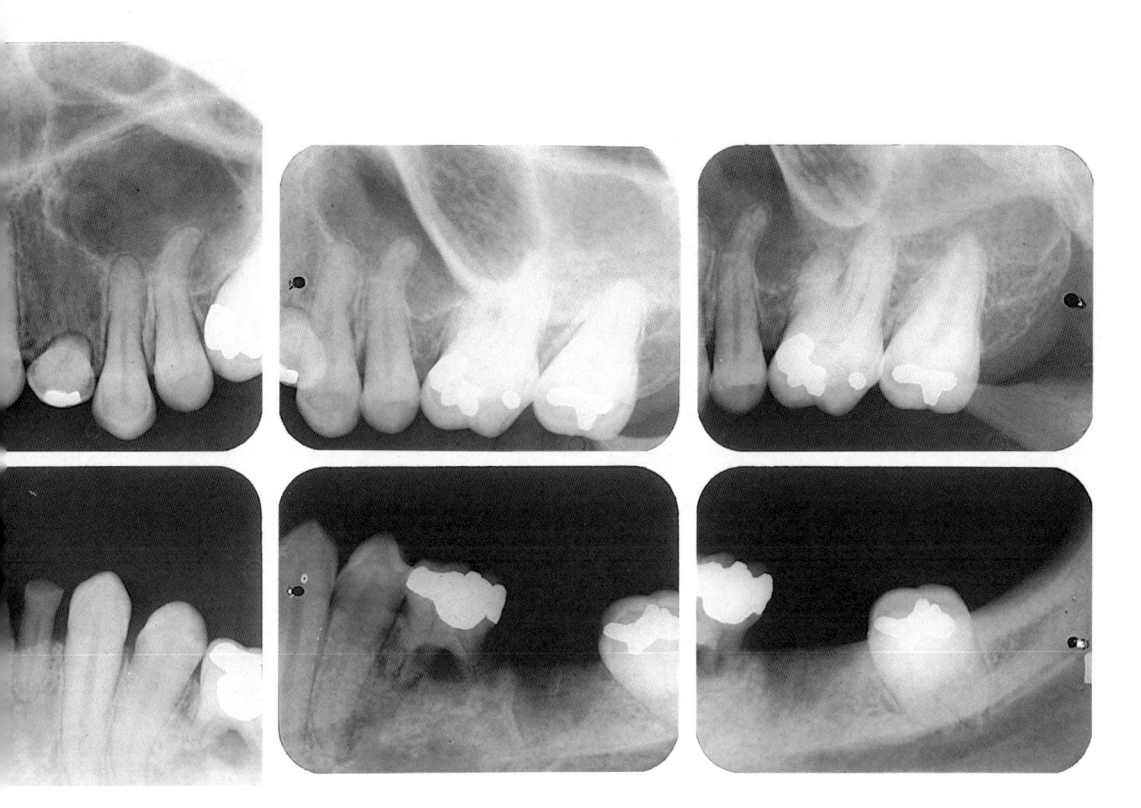

Partial anodontia

5.66 In partial anodontia (hypodontia), there may be a varying number of missing teeth, and several examples of the absence of one or two teeth are illustrated elsewhere. In this quite severe example, all the permanent lateral incisors and third molars, together with three second premolars and both mandibular first incisors, are absent. There is retention of $\frac{E\ C\ \ |\ \ C\ \ }{CBA\,|\,AB\ \ E}$, and the maxillary canines have erupted into the position of the lateral incisors. The absence of so many teeth has resulted in spacing of those present, with multiple diastemas. There is blunting of the apical part of the roots of the maxillary central incisors, probably indicative of past resorption. Note the distally hooked root $\underline{5}$ and the closeness of the antral floor to the posterior maxillary teeth. P

74 A Radiological Atlas of Diseases of the Teeth and Jaws

Ectodermal dysplasia
5.67 In this genetically determined condition, adnexal structures of ectodermal origin may be abnormal or absent, and the teeth are affected to a varying extent. In this five-and-a-half-year-old with severe involvement of the dentition, many teeth are absent, and those that have developed exhibit pronounced conical form and bulbosity of their crowns. The only teeth present are $\frac{6E\ CB\ |1BC\ E6}{6\ \ \ \ \ |\ \ \ \ 6}$, none of the permanent teeth having yet erupted. Note how the absence of teeth has resulted in failure of the aveolar bone to develop, so that the jaws have less height than normal. PR

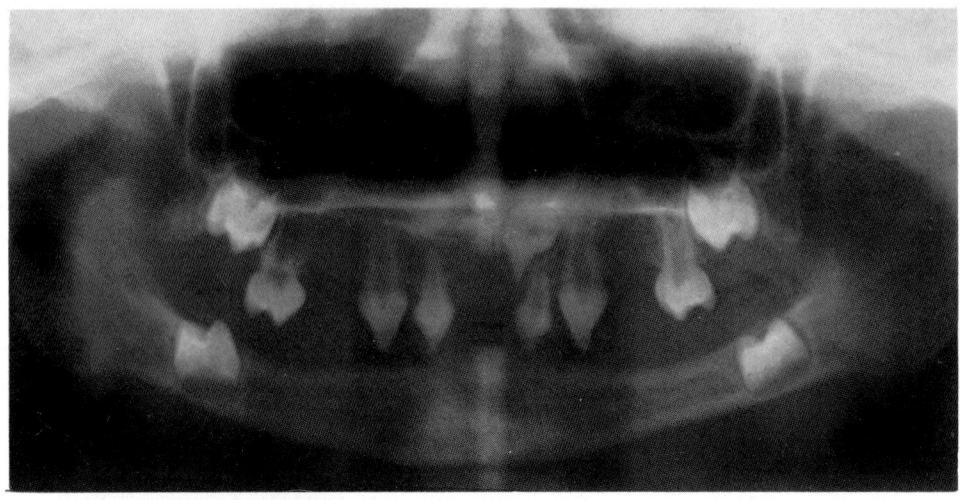

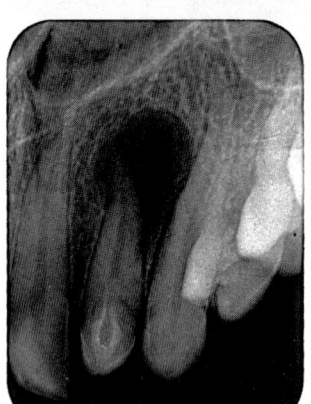

Invaginated odontome
5.68 A lesion of the dens in dente type which most commonly affects the maxillary lateral incisors. In this |2, the crown is conical in outline and contains an invaginated mass which is lined by a densely radiopaque layer of enamel. The root is of normal structure. Pulpal necrosis occurs commonly in this condition as a result of direct bacterial penetration of the invagination, and consequently periapical lesions form. In this example, there is a large, clearly defined, periapical radiolucency, with absence of the lamina dura apically. P

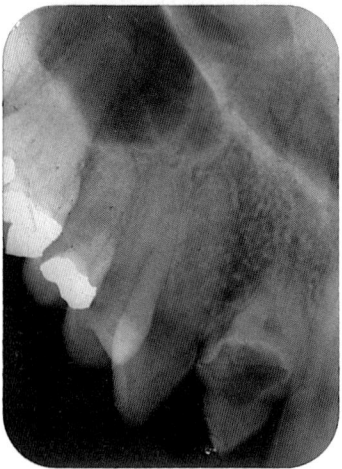

5.69 A dilated type of odontome 2|, in which the crown is conical and the cervical part of the root is widened by a radiolucent dilatation lined by a thin, radiopaque layer of enamel. The invagination has displaced the pulp chamber into the apical half of the root. Such invaginations may weaken the tooth considerably and, in this example, a thin, radiolucent fracture line is present, running obliquely across the widest part of the invagination. P

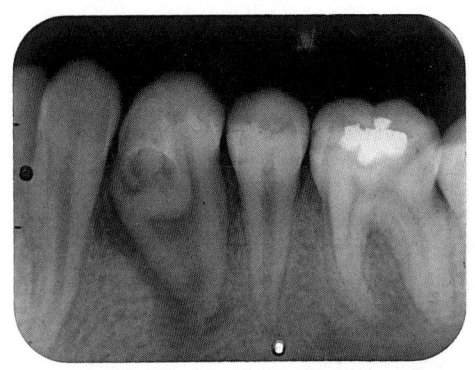

The Teeth 75

5.70 This invaginated odontome $\overline{4|}$ has arisen on the mesial aspect of the tooth. The crown is enlarged and mesially contains a convoluted mass of dental tissues which projects into the coronal part of the pulp chamber. The root is also enlarged and contains a widened root canal. As a consequence of pulpal necrosis, there is a periapical radiolucency which extends along the entire mesial aspect of the root up to the alveolar crest with loss of the lamina dura. P

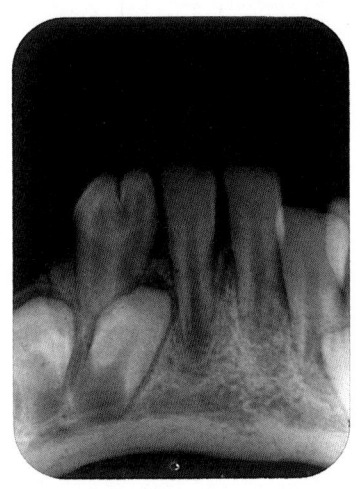

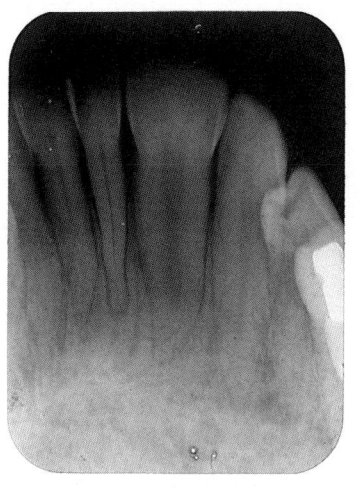

5.72 This odontome in the lower incisor region has probably arisen from the fusion of the tooth germs of $|\overline{1}$ and $|\overline{2}$. In their place is a single tooth structure with a large incisiform crown (megadontia), and a single, large root canal and pulp chamber with two elongated pulp horns. Note the bone loss crestally and widened periodontal ligament space, indicative of occlusal trauma. P

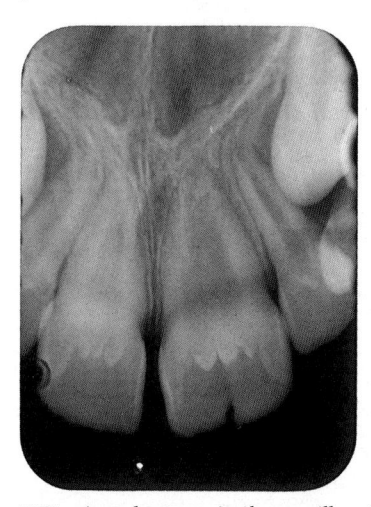

Geminated odontome
5.71 An odontome replacing $\overline{B|}$ in an eight-year-old, which has two distinct crowns, each with its own pulp chamber, and a common root containing two separate root canals. There is only slight resorption of the root of the odontome, part of the surface of which is irregular. $\overline{2|}$ is missing and the unerupted $\overline{43|}$ have drifted mesially, $\overline{3|}$ lying beneath the odontome. P

5.73 An odontome in the maxillary left incisor region, which has a large crown partially separated by a centrally placed, vertical cleft. There is a large pulp chamber with two prominent pulp horns and a single wide root canal in the greatly enlarged root. The cingulum is composed of several small tubercles. $\underline{1|}$ is also larger than normal and may be a mild expression of a geminated odontome. Note the pronounced horizontal cervical radiolucency overlying the odontome, caused by the contrast of the relatively radiodense crown incisally and the crest of the alveolar bone apically. P

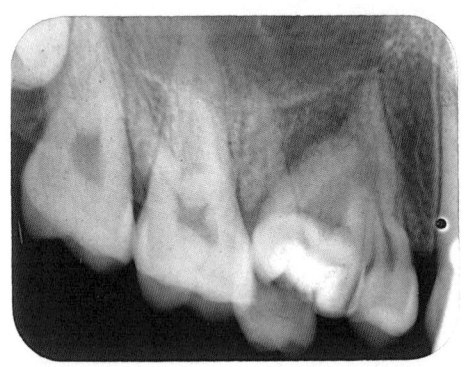

5.74 An odontome in the maxillary first premolar region, which has two separate crowns, each with its own pulp chamber, which are joined approximately half way along their roots. At this level, the two separate root canals become joined, forming a single, common root canal in the apical half. The occlusal part of the distal crown is densely radiopaque due to the convoluted pattern of the surface enamel. 5| has been displaced buccally by the odontome and thus its crown appears at a lower occlusal level than that of the adjacent teeth. P

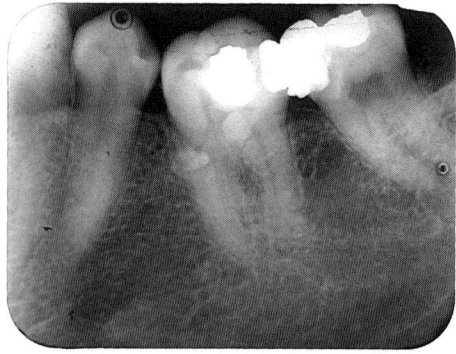

Enameloma (Enamel pearl)
5.75 This lesion occurs most commonly on molars, usually at the level of the furcation of the roots. In this example, on the mesio-cervical aspect of the root |6 there is a small, irregularly ovoid, densely radiopaque mass. Note the overhanging restoration and recurrent caries mesially |7. P

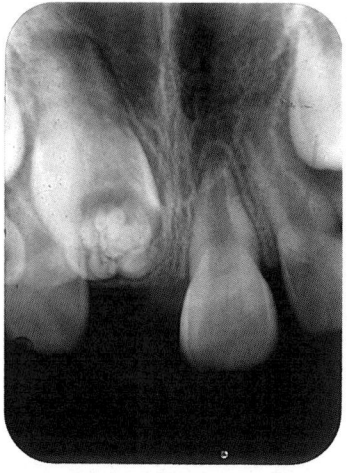

Compound composite odontome
5.76 An odontome preventing the eruption 1| in a ten-year-old. The odontome is circumscribed by a clearly defined, capsular radiolucency and thin, radiopaque lamina, and is composed of numerous small discrete, radiopaque, tooth-like structures (denticles). The mass overlies the crown 1|, which appears wider and less clearly defined than that of |1, suggesting that it is more buccally placed. Note the stage of root development |12. P

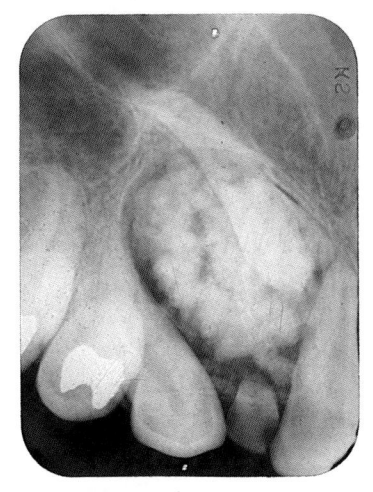

5.77 A large odontome which has prevented the eruption of and displaced 2| . It is surrounded by a capsular radiolucency and thin, radiopaque lamina, and is composed of numerous denticles superimposed upon each other forming a mass of variable radiopacity. The root 3| is displaced distally, and B| is retained and exhibits advanced root resorption. P

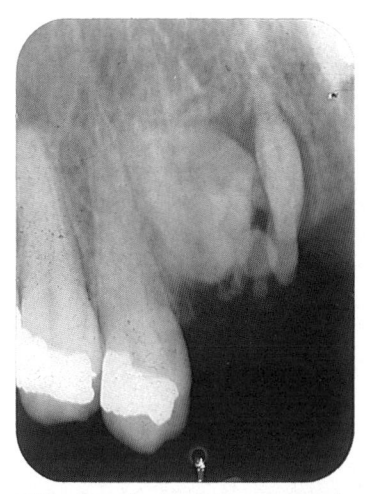

The Teeth 77

5.78 An odontome in an edentulous part of the anterior maxilla. The mass consists of a number of denticles of varying size, several of them showing a root canal, enamel and dentine. It is clearly defined anteriorly where there is a radiolucent capsular space and radiopaque lamina, but less so superiorly and posteriorly, probably as a consequence of infection. The occlusal surface of the mass lies in soft tissue. P

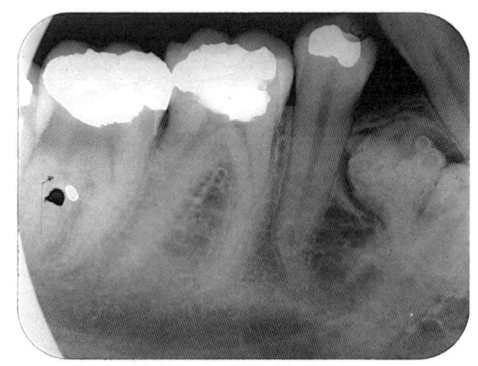

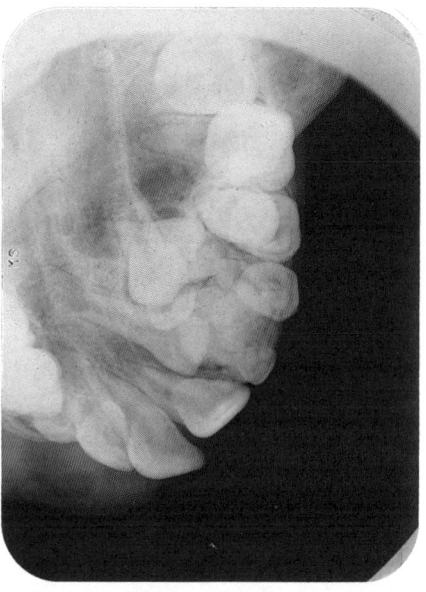

5.80 A larger lesion in an 11-year-old, which has displaced and prevented the eruption of |23C4. The mass is variably radiopaque and approximately circular in outline. [B and [D are retained. The root |1 has been displaced mesially and [E is still present, [5 developing normally beneath it. UOO

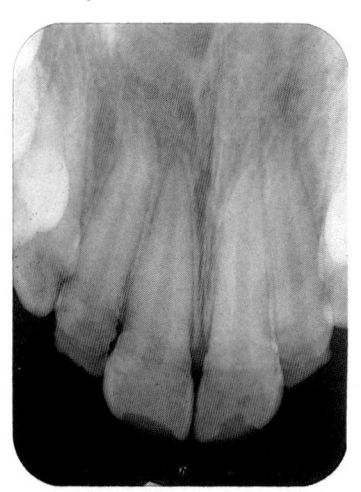

Complex composite odontome
5.79 In complex odontomes, the disordered mass of mineralised dental tissues bears no morphological resemblance to a tooth. This lesion, which has displaced and prevented the eruption of 4|, is variably radiopaque and clearly defined, being surrounded by a radiolucent capsular space and thin radiopaque lamina. The root 3| is displaced mesially and 5| distally. P

Enamel hypoplasia
5.81 Hypoplasia resulting from environmental disturbances of either local or systemic origin during amelogenesis results in horizontally placed, ring-like defects of the enamel which may be single or multiple according to the aetiology. Depending upon the age of the patient and the duration of the disturbance, a varying number of teeth may be affected. In this example, the enamel is generally thinner and less radiopaque than normal, and is virtually absent from the incisal edges of the lateral incisors which are malformed. Superadded attrition to the central incisors has resulted in the formation of concave incisal edges. Several bands of radiolucency run horizontally across the crowns of all the teeth, particularly in their cervical halves, due to the presence of multiple rings of hypoplastic enamel. P

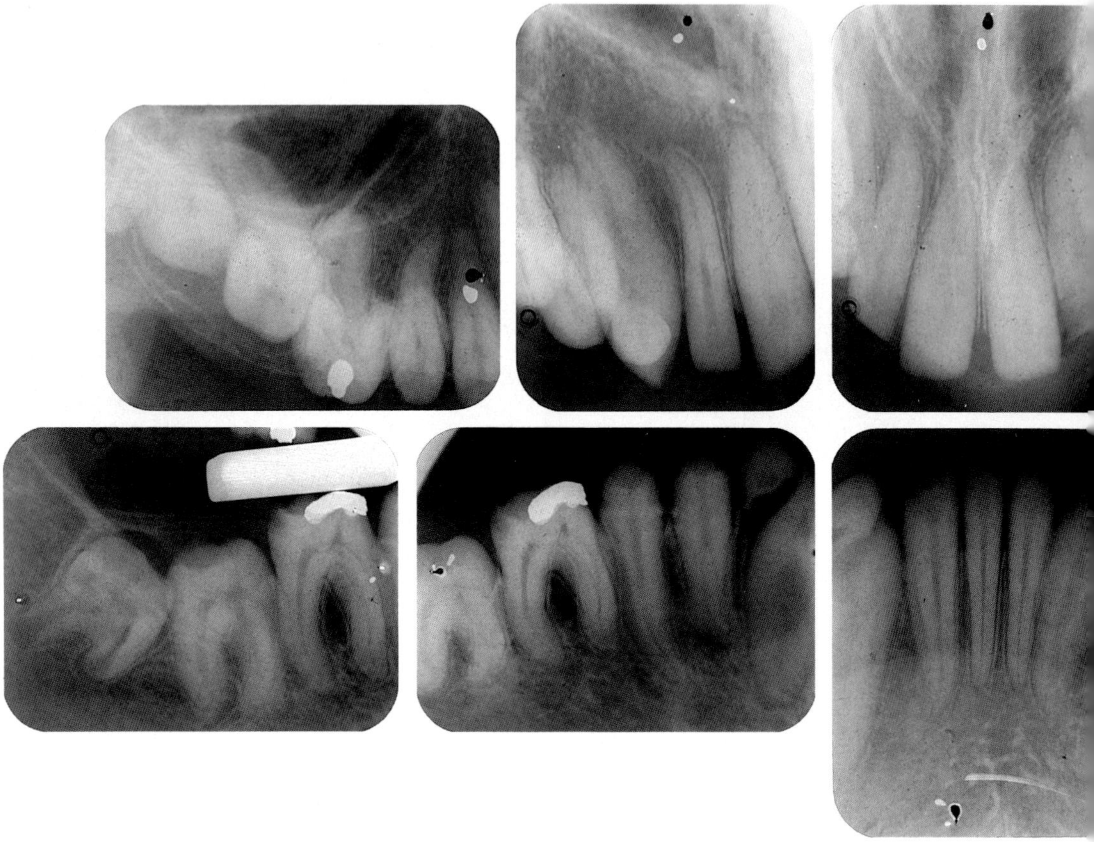

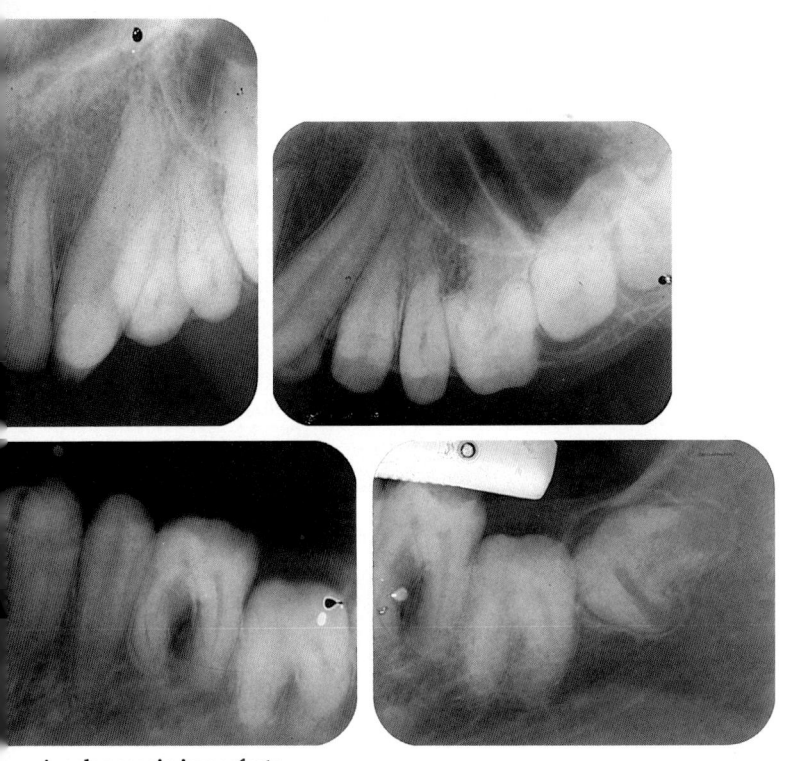

Amelogenesis imperfecta
5.82 In this genetically determined condition, the enamel of the entire permanent dentition is usually defective or absent. In this severe case, there is no radiographic evidence of enamel on the crowns of any of the teeth, thus giving the appearance of spacing. The absence of enamel is also apparent on the unerupted second and third molars. All four primary canines are retained and exhibit advanced root resorption, and they too show an absence of enamel, although involvement of the primary dentition is not always a feature. The mandibular permanent canines are only partially erupted and the third molars, which are of abnormal shape, incompletely formed. The buccal roots of the maxillary molars are markedly foreshortened due to incorrect radiographic technique. P

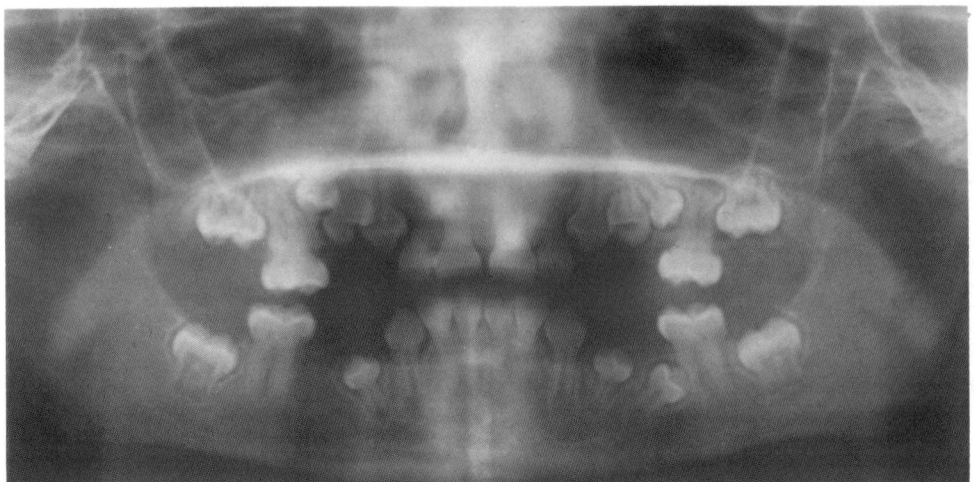

80 A Radiological Atlas of Diseases of the Teeth and Jaws

Dentinogenesis imperfecta
5.83 This genetically determined condition primarily affects dentine formation in both the primary and permanent dentition. In this nine-year-old, many of the teeth are still incompletely formed with large papillary spaces apically, but the characteristic features of the disorder are clearly displayed. The crowns of all the teeth are markedly bulbous, and the pulp chambers and root canals of those teeth approaching the completion of development are becoming narrowed and obliterated. The third molars and 5| are missing. PR

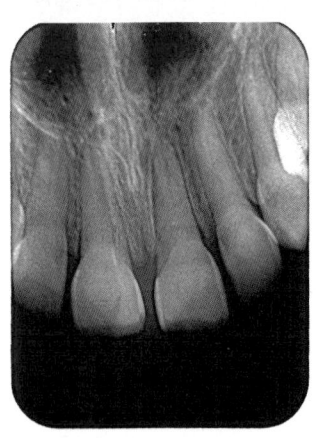

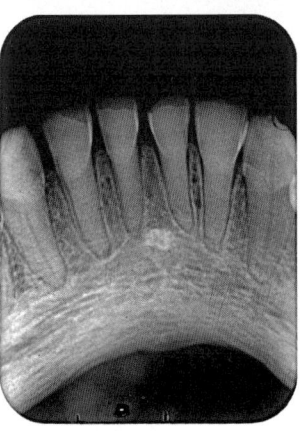

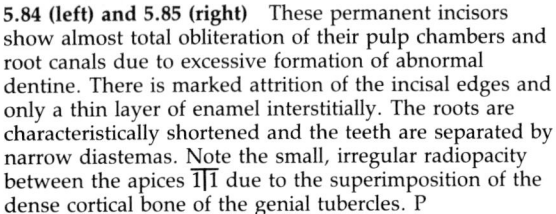

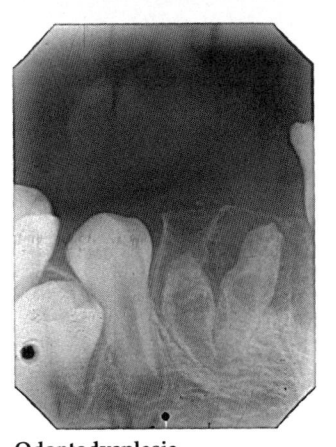

5.84 (left) and 5.85 (right) These permanent incisors show almost total obliteration of their pulp chambers and root canals due to excessive formation of abnormal dentine. There is marked attrition of the incisal edges and only a thin layer of enamel interstitially. The roots are characteristically shortened and the teeth are separated by narrow diastemas. Note the small, irregular radiopacity between the apices 1|1 due to the superimposition of the dense cortical bone of the genial tubercles. P

Odontodysplasia
5.86 This condition can affect any number of contiguous teeth and might involve teeth to each side of the midline. The enamel and dentine of the affected teeth are markedly hypoplastic and thus they are only a shadow of their normal selves, an appearance often referred to as 'ghost teeth'. In this example in a ten-year-old, 32| are unerupted and affected. There is no evidence of enamel on their crowns, and the roots have only a thin outline of dentine and are shortened with wide pulp chambers. The radiolucent follicular space around the crowns is wide due to the proliferation of odontogenic tissue which is a feature of the condition. P

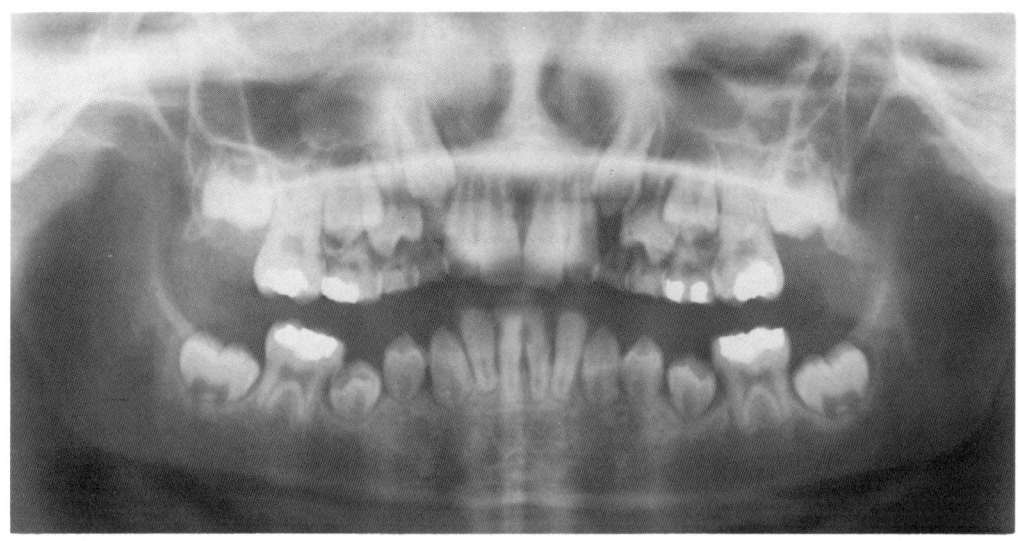

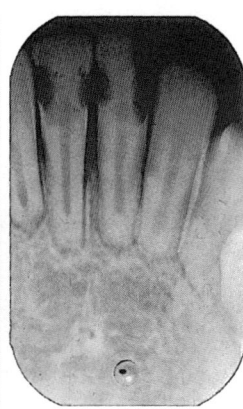

Irradiation

5.87 (left) and 5.88 (right) Arrested development of the mandibular teeth in a nine-year-old who received radiotherapy to the cervical lymph nodes some eighteen months previously for the treatment of Hodgkin's disease. There has been arrest of the development of the roots at the approximate stage they had reached at the time of irradiation. The roots are stunted and blunted, and the apical foramina narrowed. The periodontal ligament space is widened and the lamina dura indistinct around some of the teeth. The nature of the apical changes is more clearly demonstrated on the intra-oral film (Fig. 5.88). The apical foramina of the incisors are almost completely obliterated. There are also numerous interstitial and labial cavities in the mandibular incisors (irradiation caries) as a result of reduced salivary secretion from the affected glands. Contrast the appearance of the mandibular teeth with that of the maxillary ones which were not affected by the irradiation. PR & P

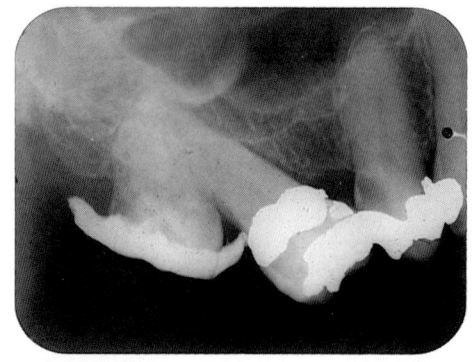

Concrescence

5.89 Concrescence may occur between the roots of adjacent teeth, usually as a consequence of chronic irritation. In this example, there is concrescence of the roots of $\underline{87|}$, $\underline{7|}$ being tilted mesially with its root contiguous with that of $\underline{8|}$. There is no periodontal ligament space between the roots of the two teeth, although this is apparent around the fused roots mesially and distally. $\underline{8|}$ contains an excess of temporary dressing material which is overhanging the crown. Note the recurrent carious lesion $\underline{5|}$ distally. P

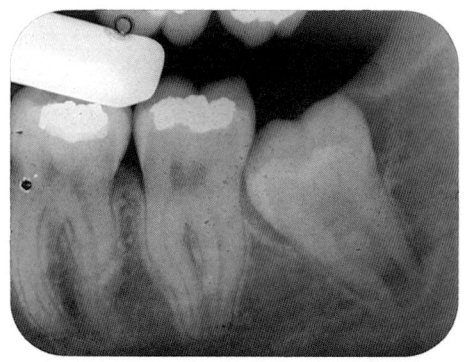

Pulp stone

5.90 Pulp stones occur with increasing frequency with age and in the presence of chronic inflammation, but are visible radiographically only when they have reached substantial size, as in $\overline{|78}$. Discrete radiopaque masses are present in the pulp chamber $\overline{|7}$ coronally and in the incompletely formed root canal $\overline{|8}$. Note that $\overline{|8}$ is mesio-angularly impacted and has a normal follicular radiolucency around the crown. P

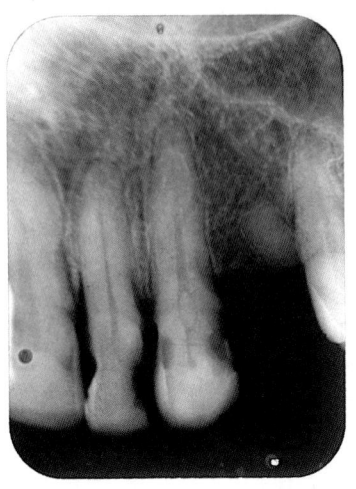

82   A Radiological Atlas of Diseases of the Teeth and Jaws

5.91   A large pulp stone |3 lying in a dilatation of the root canal cervically. There are radiolucent fillings mesially and distally |3, and a large carious lesion distally |2. Note the root fragment near the surface of the alveolus, just mesial to |5. P

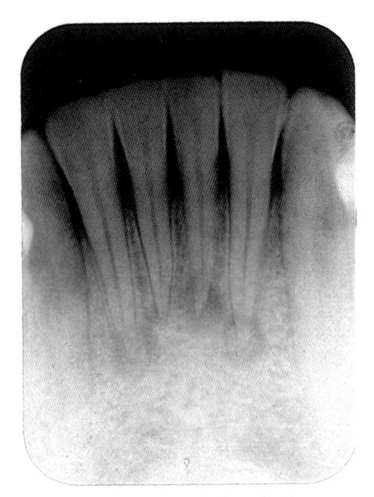

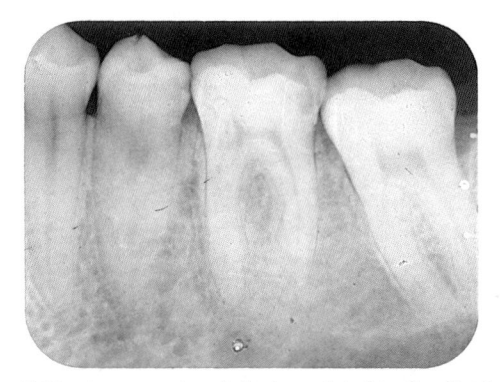

5.93   A more sclerotic lesion related to the distal root |6. The outline of the apical part of the root is indistinct and is surrounded by a radiodense area which has a finely granular appearance and a poorly defined periphery. There has been some resorption of the apical part of the root. More commonly, such lesions are more clearly defined from the surrounding bone. P

Periapical cemental dysplasia
5.92   This condition may affect one or, as in this example, multiple teeth. At the apices of 2|12, there are approximately circular, clearly defined, periapical radiolucencies. The central surface of each area is relatively radiopaque due to the deposition of cementum. In this condition, the early lesion is radiolucent and is similar in appearance to a periapical inflammatory lesion. However, the teeth retain their vitality in periapical cemental dysplasia. In this case, there is also slight loss of bone at the crests of the interdental septa, indicative of early chronic periodontitis. P

The Teeth   83

Gigantiform cementoma
5.94 Multiple cementum masses in the edentulous jaws of a patient with gigantiform cementomas. This condition commonly affects negresses, and lesions may be found in all four quadrants. The radiodense masses are present in the alveolar part of the jaws and are each surrounded by a radiolucent capsule and thin, radiodense lamina of cortical bone. Such lesions may become infected, as in the mass in the right mandibular premolar region in this patient. PR

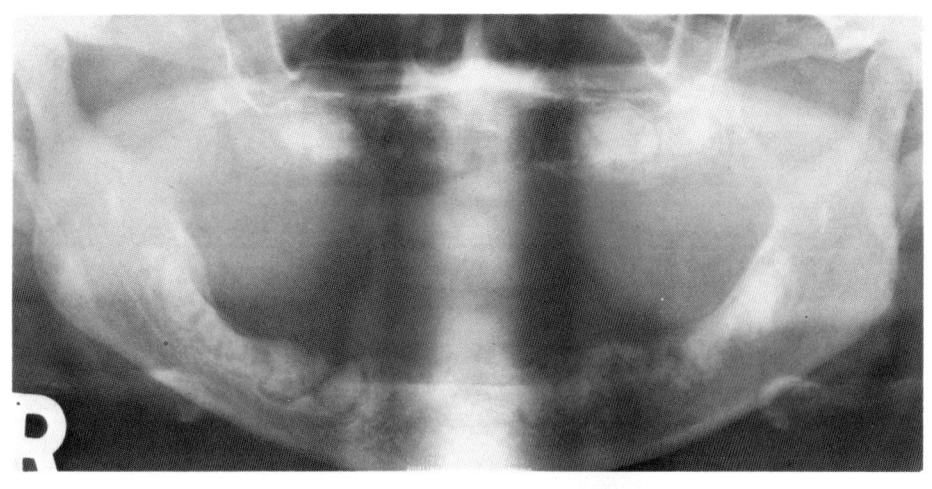

Cementifying fibroma
5.95 This neoplasm consists of fibrous tissue containing a variable amount of mineralised cementum and thus may present a range of radiographic appearances. In this large lesion in the left maxilla, the mass is oval in outline and clearly defined, being of uniform radiopacity. Around its superior and lateral margins there is a distinct radiolucent capsular space and thin, radiopaque cortical lamina. PA

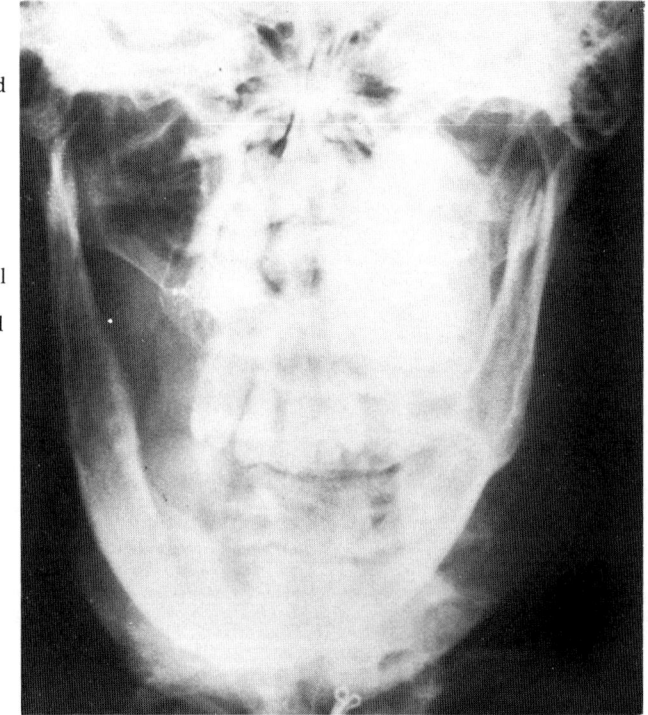

Benign cementoblastoma
5.96 This lesion typically develops on the mesial root of mandibular molars in adolescents. There is an approximately circular mass of uniform radiopacity overlying and obscuring the mesial root 6| and circumscribed by a radiolucent capsular space. There is blunting of the apex of the distal root, indicating early resorption. Unusually, in this example there is some radiopacity of the surrounding bone due to reactive osteosclerosis. P

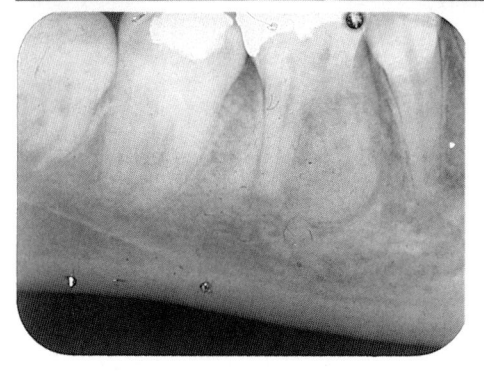

Dentinoma

5.97 This lesion arises from the abnormal proliferation of odontogenic mesenchyme, within which increasing amounts of mineralised dentine matrix are laid down. In this 16-year-old patient with an immature lesion, which arose in a most unusual site on the buccal aspect of the molar region of the left mandible, an approximately circular radiolucent mass which contains randomly arranged radiopacities is present. At the base of the lesion superiorly, there is a triangular area of reactive, subperiosteal bone formation. Note the hair grips in the upper left corner. PAC

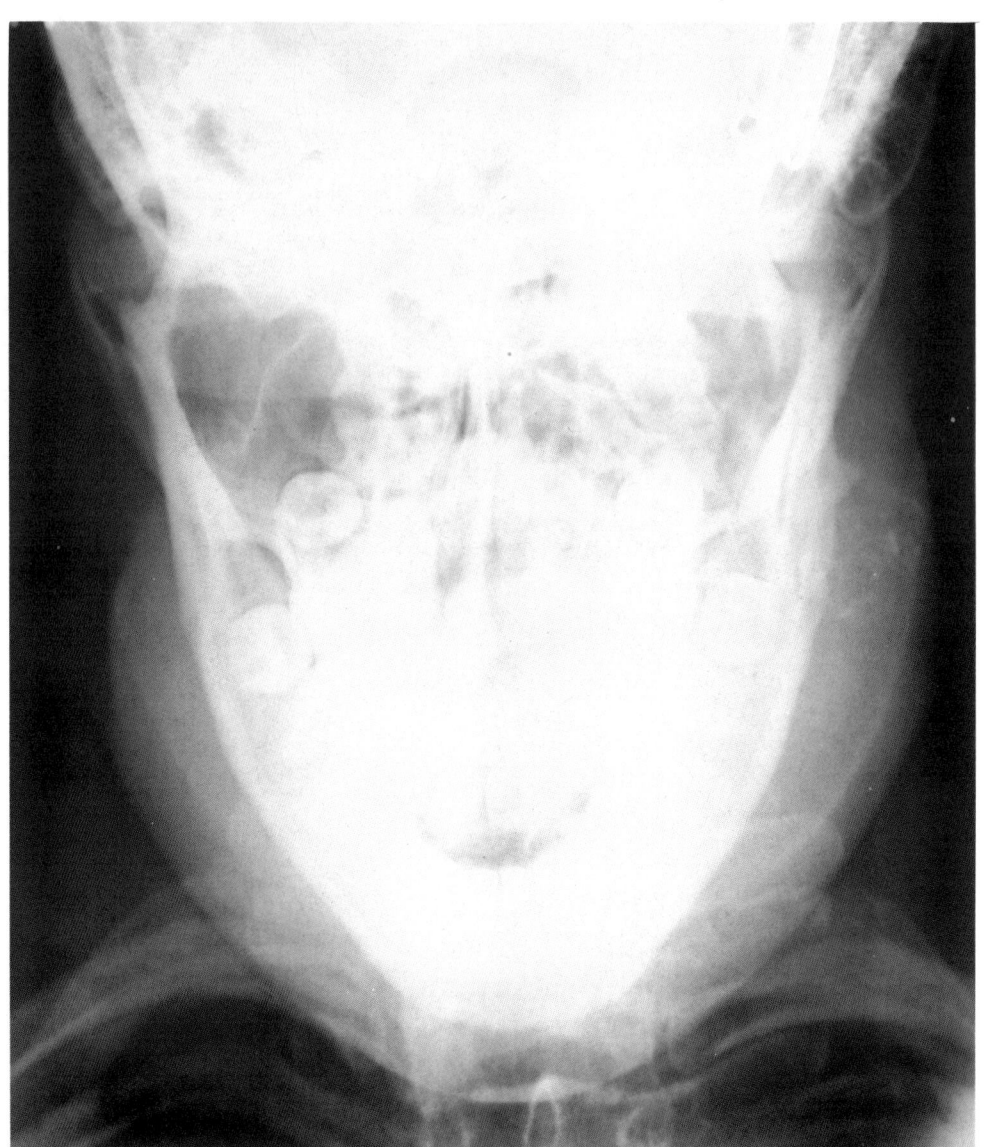

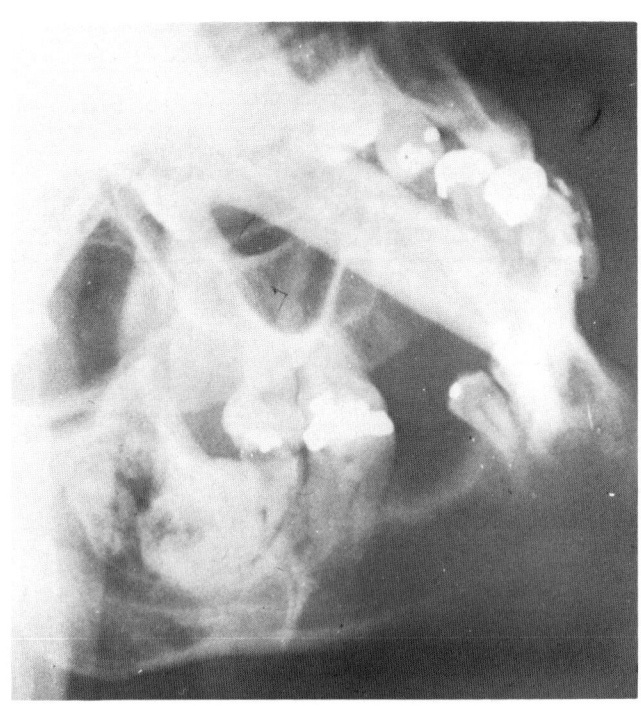

The Teeth   85

5.98 As the lesion matures, increasing amounts of mineralised dentine matrix are deposited, and it becomes increasingly radiopaque, as in this example in the mandibular molar region of a 40-year-old. The lesion is ovoid in shape with a clearly defined margin and is quite densely radiopaque anteriorly, although its posterior part contains a number of areas of radiolucency. OLM

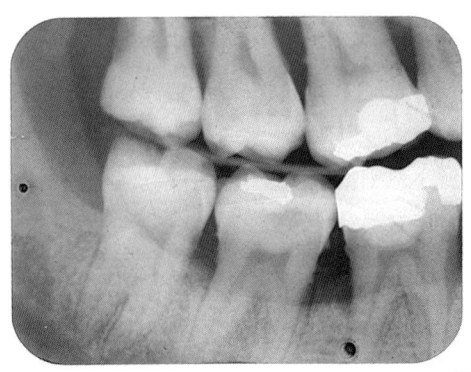

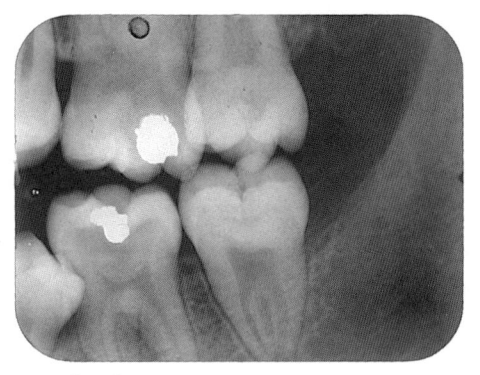

Dental caries
5.99 Dental caries results in the demineralisation of the teeth as a consequence of microbial activity, and consequently commonly occurs on those surfaces of the teeth where bacteria can colonise, namely in fissures, interstitial surfaces, cervical surfaces and on the cementum when it is exposed to the oral cavity. In fissure caries, there is often little radiological change in the enamel before the lesion has advanced to the dentine. In this example, there are lesions at different stages in all four molars. In both second molars, there is a small, radiolucent fissure lesion in the enamel, together with moderate involvement of the dentine. In |7, there is a pronounced radiopaque zone of reactive dentinal sclerosis at the advancing edge of the lesion. Note how the lesion has spread in the dentine along the amelo-dentinal junction. In |6, there is an extensive occlusal lesion in the dentine which has developed beneath a small, inadequate amalgam filling. Here again there are areas of sclerotic dentine (mesially, distally and pulpally) at the advancing front of the lesion. In |6, there is also a large dentinal lesion which has formed beneath another small, inadequate amalgam filling. There is evidence of marked, recurrent caries, with radiolucency of the enamel around the filling. The pulp is cariously exposed as indicated by the loss of continuity of the distal outline of the pulp, and there is dentinal sclerosis at the mesial boundary of the lesion. Note the disto-angularly impacted |5. BW

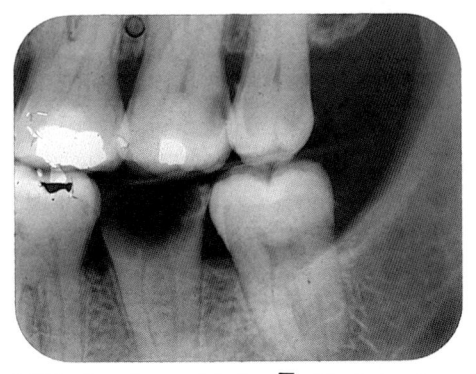

5.100 A typically cone-shaped dentine lesion 7|, with an ill defined margin, has formed beneath an inadequate occlusal amalgam filling, which obscures the recurrent lesion in the overlying enamel. Note the generalised loss of bone from the crests of the interdental septa, which is more marked in the maxilla, and the deposits of calculus cervically. BW

5.101 An advanced lesion |7 with destruction of most of its crown and exposure of both root canals. Note also the distal lesion |7. BW

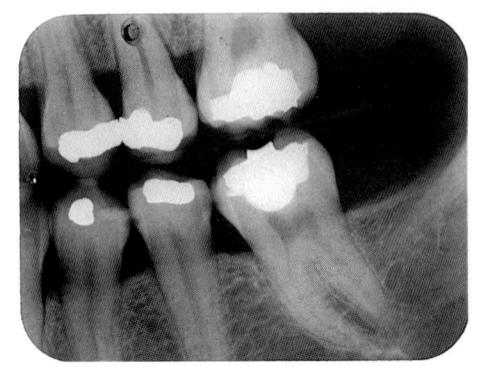

86 A Radiological Atlas of Diseases of the Teeth and Jaws

5.102 Early interstitial caries distally |4̄, mesially |5̄, distally |5 and mesially |6̄ resulting in triangular radiolucencies in the enamel just below the contact point with the apex of the triangle towards the amelodentinal junction. More advanced caries distally |5̄ involving enamel and dentine appears as a mushroom shaped radiolucency with the stalk towards the outer enamel surface. Although the dentine is involved, the deeper layers of enamel are still relatively radiopaque. BW.

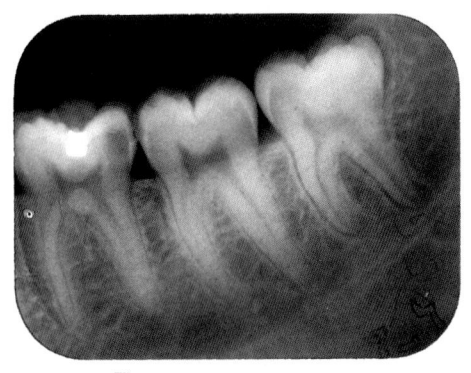

5.103 In |6̄, there is a small, radiolucent breach in the enamel surface distally, just below the contact point, leading to a larger, more ill defined area of radiolucency in the dentine. A small amalgam restoration is present occlusally. Note the early enamel caries mesially |7̄ and the incompletely developed partially erupted |8̄. P

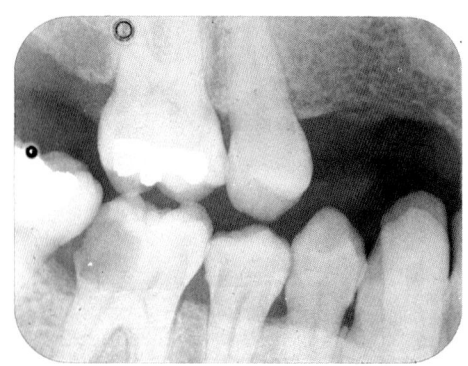

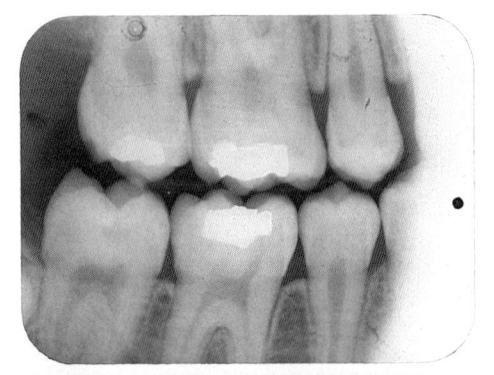

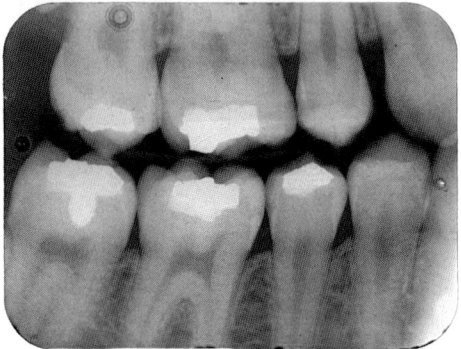

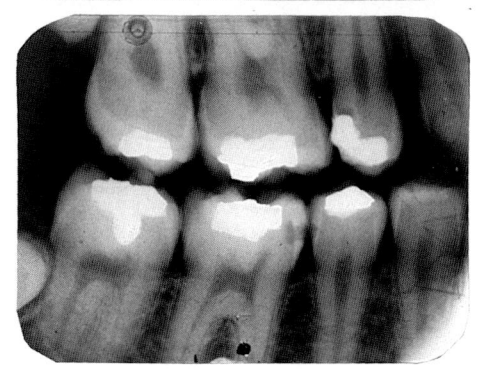

5.105 (top), 5.106 (middle) and 5.107 (bottom) Three radiographs of the same patient taken at yearly intervals to illustrate in particular the progressive development of lesions 5| distally, 6| mesially and 5̄| distally. In Fig. 5.107, an amalgam restoration has been inserted 5| distally, although caries still remains cervically. Note also the occlusal lesion 7̄| (Fig. 5.105). BW

5.104 An advanced lesion distally 6̄| with destruction of the enamel and exposure of the pulp chamber. BW

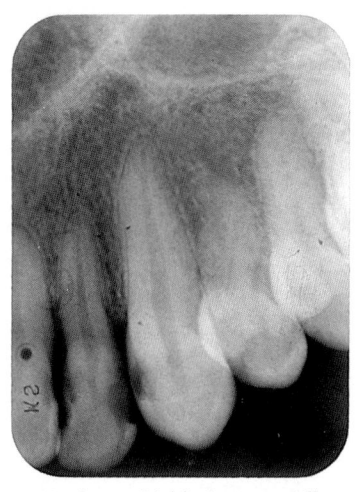

The Teeth 87

5.108 Interstitial lesions mesially and distally |2, and mesially |3. In the anterior teeth, such lesions have a typically craterform outline. Note again how the distal lesion |2 has spread laterally through the outer layers of the dentine towards the incisal edge. P

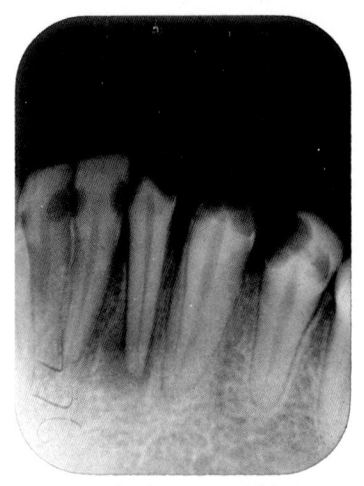

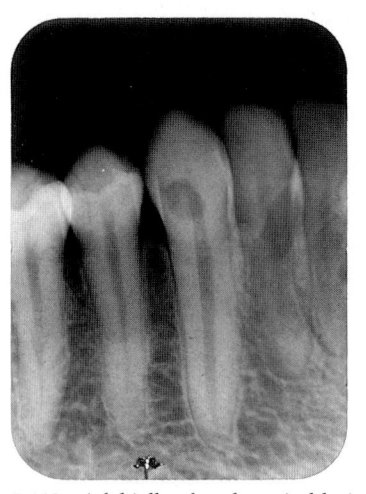

5.110 A labially placed cervical lesion 3|. In such lesions, the margin of the defect is usually clearly defined since the X-ray beam is parallel with the walls of the cavity. In this view, it is not possible to determine the relationship between the advancing edge of the lesion and the pulp chamber. P

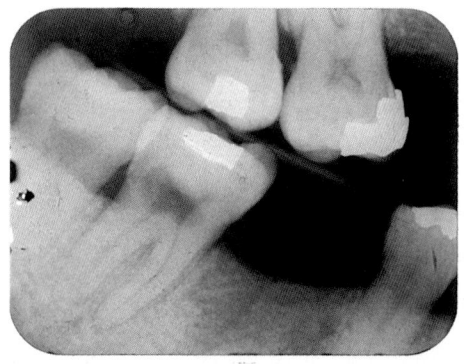

5.109 Multiple interstitial lesions in anterior mandibular teeth. In |2 and |3, there is loss of most of the crowns, and a clearly defined, periapical radiolucency is present |2. In |3 and |4, there are prominent radiopaque zones of reactive dentinal sclerosis around the lesions. P

5.111 A cervical lesion 7| causing a clearly defined, radiolucent defect partly superimposed on the pulp chamber. A similar appearance will be produced whether the lesion lies buccally or lingually. Note the triangularly shaped cervical radiolucency distal 7| and the calculus interdentally on the upper molars. BW

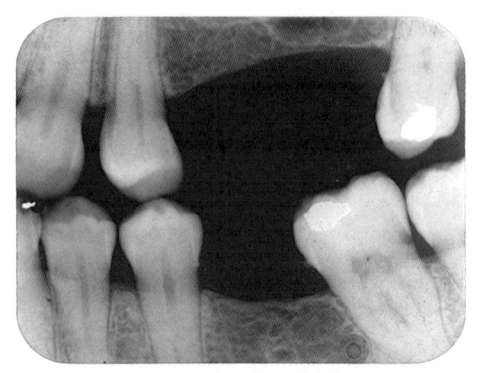

5.112 A cemental lesion which has extended into the dentine distally $\overline{7|}$ forming a punched out radiolucency in the region of the amelocemental junction. Compare this appearance with that of the cervical radiolucency $\overline{8|}$ mesially. Note the collar of cervical radiolucency $|\underline{4}$, which is wider than usual as a consequence of the loss of the crest of the surrounding alveolar bone. This appearance is produced by the contrast between on the one hand, the intrabony part of the root and the enamel covered crown, which are relatively radiopaque, and on the other hand, the cervical part of the root which is not invested in bone. BW

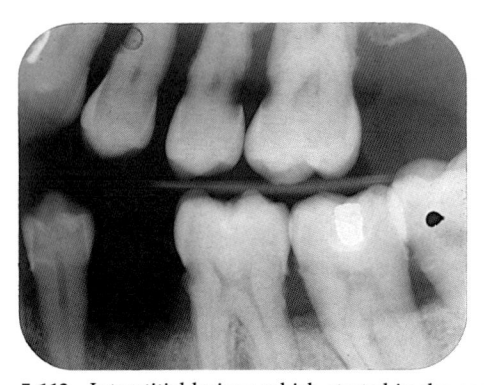

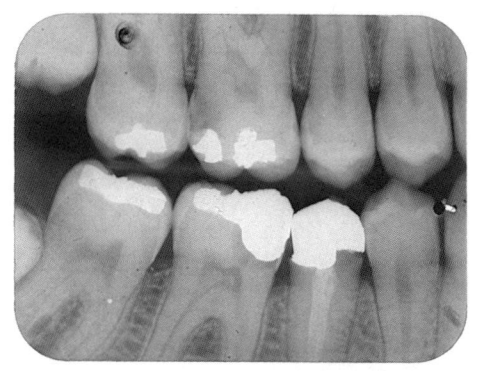

5.114 An extensive recurrent lesion $\underline{6|}$ distally beneath an inadequate amalgam restoration. Other recurrent lesions are present $\overline{5|}$ mesially and probably also $\overline{6|}$ mesially. Early lesions are present interstitially at most other contact points. Note the large pulp stones $\frac{6|}{6|}$. BW

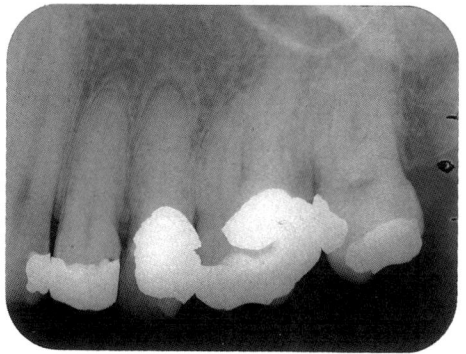

5.113 Interstitial lesions which started in the cementum cervically $|\underline{56}$ and $\overline{6|}$. The early lesion $\overline{6|}$ mesially forms a punched-out radiolucency, whereas the more advanced lesions $|\underline{6}$ mesially and $|\underline{5}$ distally form saucer-shaped radiolucencies with poorly defined margins. Note the basic difference in shape between these cementum lesions and lesions in the enamel (Figs 5.106 and 5.107). There is moderate loss of interdental bone and the presence of subgingival calculus indicative of chronic periodontitis. Cemental caries on the interstitial surfaces of the teeth is always preceded by alveolar bone loss, usually as a consequence of periodontal disease, thus exposing the cementum to the oral environment. BW

Acute periapical abscess

5.115 Periapical inflammatory conditions are usually a consequence of pulpal necrosis and/or infection. As a general rule, there are no significant radiological changes in acute apical inflammation arising *de novo*, since it takes approximately ten days for sufficient bone resorption to have taken place to show on a radiograph. However, if there is physical displacement of the tooth from its socket due to the accumulation of inflammatory exudate, changes may be apparent. In this example, there is widening of the radiolucent periodontal ligament space periapically $|\underline{5}$ due to occlusal displacement of the tooth, as shown by the projection of its cusps below the occlusal plane. There are large amalgam fillings in $|\underline{4567}$. P

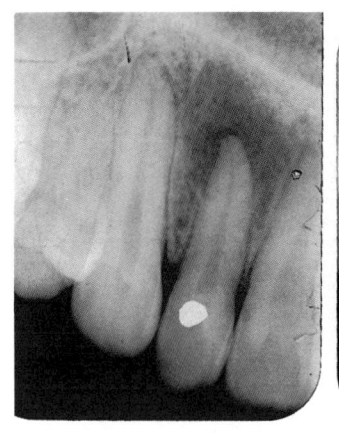

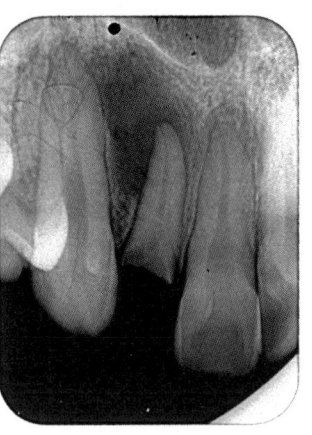

The Teeth 89

5.116 (left) and 5.117 (right) This acute periapical abscess has arisen in a pre-existing chronic abscess 2⌋, the latter having given rise to the poorly defined periapical radiolucency (Fig. 5.116). Note the palatal amalgam filling and loss of lamina dura apically. The tooth was put on open drainage, but the patient failed to attend until nine months later, when the crown had fractured off at the gingival margin (Fig. 5.117). The radiolucent area has now increased in size and the smaller circular area of more dense radiolucency distally to the apex 2⌋ indicates a perforation of the cortical bone. Note the superimposition of the radiolucent incisive foramen over the apex 1⌋, around which the lamina dura is continuous. P

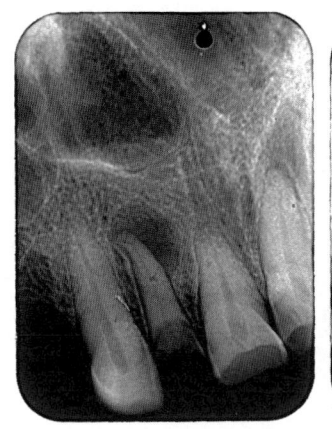

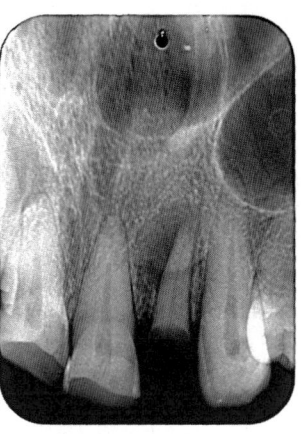

5.119 (left) and 5.120 (right) Advanced caries 2|2 in the same patient resulting in loss of their crowns and formation of periapical granulomas. These two examples illustrate the variable radiological appearance that such lesions may give. There is always an absence of the lamina dura around the affected part of the root, but whereas the radiolucency 2⌋ is clearly defined and surrounded by a thin, radiopaque lamina, that ⌊2, although of similar size, is less well defined. Within the radiolucent areas is a finer, less distinct, trabecular pattern due to the superimposition of the remaining overlying cortical and cancellous bone. It is probable that the lesion on 2⌋ is quiescent and that on ⌊2 is actively enlarging. Note the advanced attrition of the incisal edges 1⌋1. P

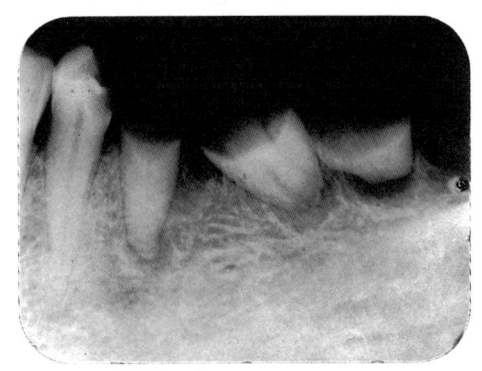

Periapical granuloma
5.118 Advanced caries ⌈5 78 has resulted in destruction of their crowns and only parts of the roots remain. On each root, there is a clearly defined periapical radiolucency, each surrounded by a radiopaque lamina, but no lamina dura surrounding the affected part of the root. The relatively superficial position of the root fragments ⌈78 indicates that they are being exfoliated. Note the infrabony pocket distally ⌈5 and the carious lesion distally ⌈4. P

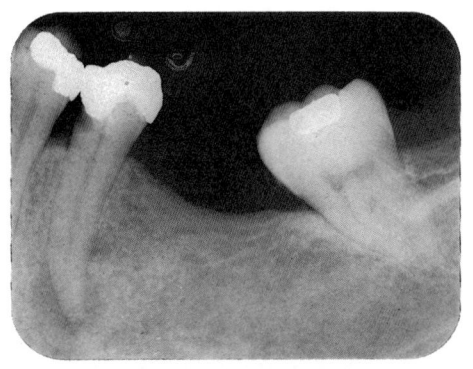

5.121 Two radiolucent areas associated with the root ⌈5. The larger one is periapical and has an indistinct outline. The smaller one is on the distal aspect of the root. The lamina dura is absent in relation to both lesions. There is a large amalgam filling with recurrent caries mesio-cervically. The large lesion is a periapical granuloma and the smaller one either an oblique extension of the lesion along the surface of the root or a separate granuloma arising from a lateral root canal. P

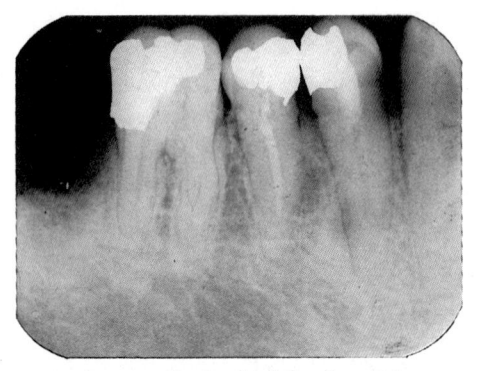

5.122 Two small, clearly defined, radiolucent areas situated mesially 5| and distally |4 due to granulomas developing on lateral root canals in these inadequately root-filled teeth with necrotic pulps. Both areas are surrounded by a thin, radiopaque lamina and there is loss of lamina dura. Note that the periapical tissues are normal. P

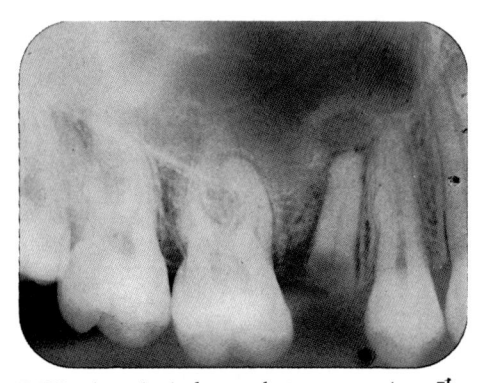

5.123 A periapical granuloma on a carious 5| root which has caused a nodular elevation of the floor of the antrum. To each side of the radiolucent granuloma, the thin cortical lamina of the antral floor is clearly displayed, and it is continuous with the more diffuse, radiopaque cortical thickening surrounding the antral surface of the lesion. This diffuse radiopacity is a consequence of reactive osteosclerosis. There is an absence of the lamina dura distally and apically 5|, with irregular destruction of the alveolar bone distally. Note the fine, radiolucent vascular channels lying in the bony wall of the antrum. P

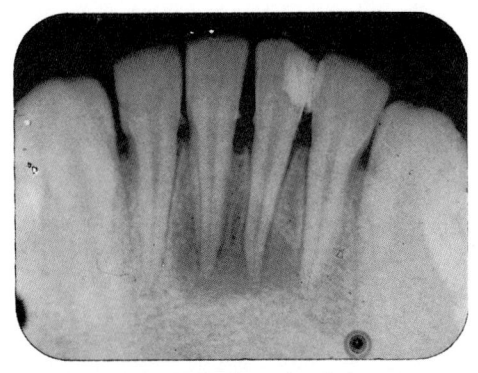

5.124 A triangularly shaped radiolucency associated with the roots of the lower incisors. The lesion originated on |1, which has a large distal cavity filled with radiopaque dressing material, and has spread to involve 1| and |2. The lamina dura is missing |1 and indistinct 1| apically, and the outline of the lesion is not clearly defined inferiorly. The finer, less distinct pattern of the remaining overlying cortical and cancellous bone, superimposed upon the radiolucent granuloma, is clearly shown. Note the spurs of calculus cervically. P

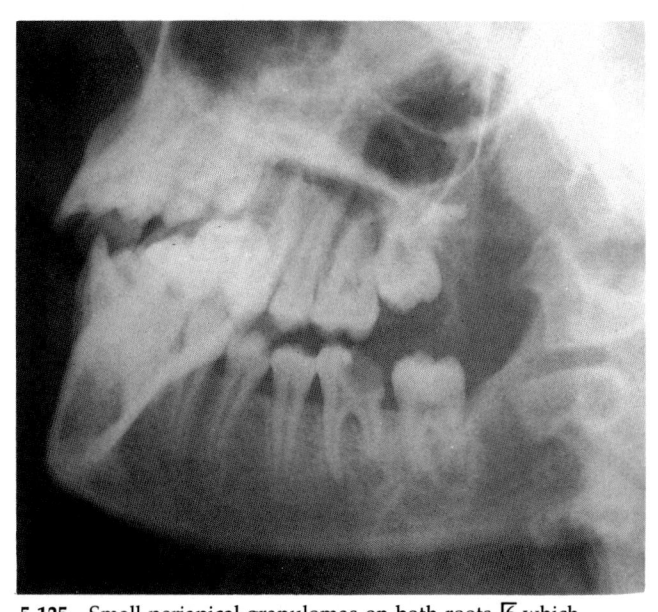

5.125 Small periapical granulomas on both roots |6 which has a large disto-occlusal carious cavity. The radiolucent lesions are surrounded by a thin, cortical lamina which is continuous with the lamina dura mesially and distally on both roots. Compare this with the similar appearance on both roots |7 apically which is due to the persistence of papillary tissue in these incompletely formed roots. The apical foramina |7 are still widely open. Note the rudimentary |8 which is at an early stage of development, and the absence of |8. OLM

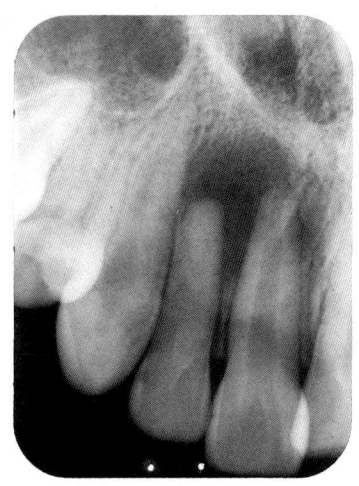

5.126 This radiolucent granuloma is associated with the apices 2|1, where there is no lamina dura. The periphery is not well defined, and the finer trabecular pattern of the overlying cortical and cancellous bone is clearly displayed. The lesion developed following trauma, and, as a consequence of pulpal necrosis 1|, there has been premature cessation of dentinogenesis in the root, which has a relatively wide canal. Disturbance of odontogenesis 2| has led to the formation of a flattened apex and progressive mineralisation of the root canal which is totally obliterated. P

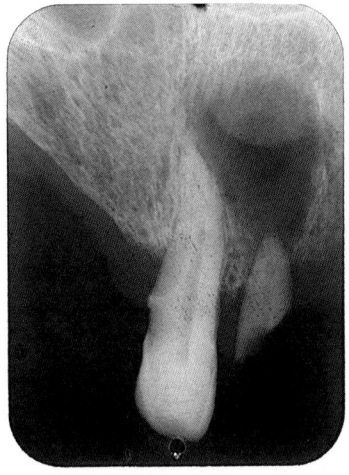

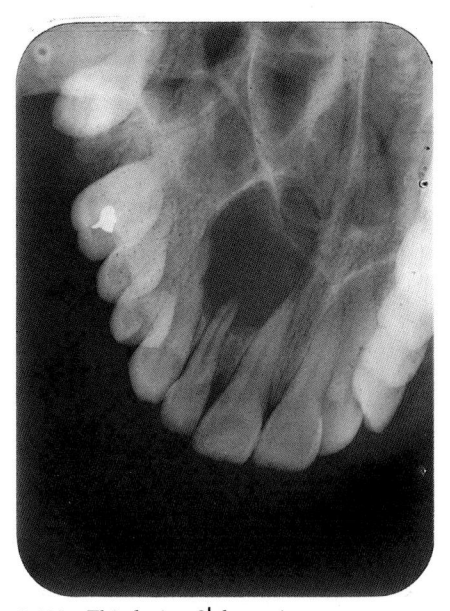

5.128 This lesion 2| has arisen as a consequence of pulpal necrosis from a deep palatal pit. The approximately circular radiolucent area is clearly defined and partly surrounded by a thin radiopaque lamina. The lamina dura is absent from the apical part of the root 2|, mesially 3| and distally 1|. Note the lateral border of the floor of the nose superimposed upon the radiolucent defect. UOO

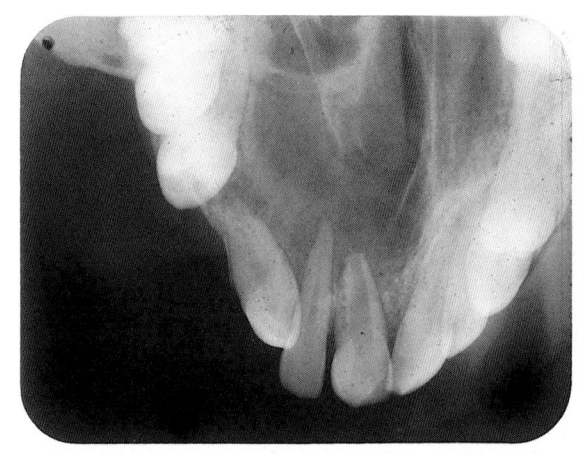

Dental (periapical) cyst

5.127 This lesion usually arises in a pre-existing periapical granuloma, and, since it enlarges by expansile growth, forms an approximately circular defect. In this lesion associated with 2| root fragment, there is a clearly defined, periapical radiolucency surrounded by a thin, radiopaque lamina and containing a circular, more radiolucent area centrally where the buccal cortical bone has been perforated. The lamina dura is absent apically. The radiopaque shadow with distinct, curved lower margin, which is superimposed on the upper part of the lesion, represents the soft tissue outline of the nose. P

5.129 A large cyst 1| which has arisen as a consequence of pulpal necrosis after fracture exposure. The large, poorly defined radiolucent area extends far back into the palate beyond the limits of the radiograph. The lamina dura is absent around the apical part of the roots 2|1. The anterior part of the lateral border of the floor of the nose is absent, indicating that the cyst has eroded into it. Note the oblique fracture of the mesial incisal edge, and the wide pulp chamber, root canal and apical foramen 1|, indicating that the necrosis occurred before tooth development was complete. UOO

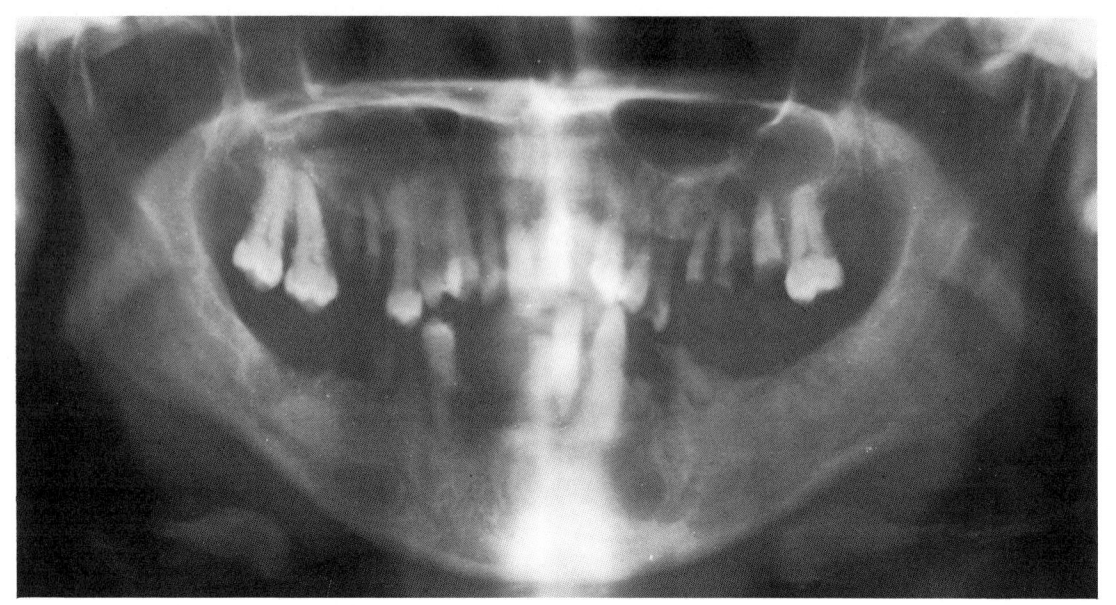

5.130 Dental cysts in both sides of the maxilla and in the left side of the mandible in a patient with gross dental neglect. Most of the teeth are carious and numerous roots are present. Associated with 6⌋ roots and ⌊7 roots are dental cysts, each of which has formed a circular radiolucent defect surrounded by a thin, radiopaque lamina of cortical bone. On both sides, the cyst projects into the floor of the antrum, although it is quite separate from it. In addition, there is a third dental cyst associated with ⌊4 root, although this lesion is not well displayed. The radiolucent defect in the right mandible appeared to be continuous with the inferior alveolar canal suggesting the possibility of a neoplasm of neural origin. However, this was found to be composed of granulomatous tissue containing large quantities of cholesterol crystals. PR

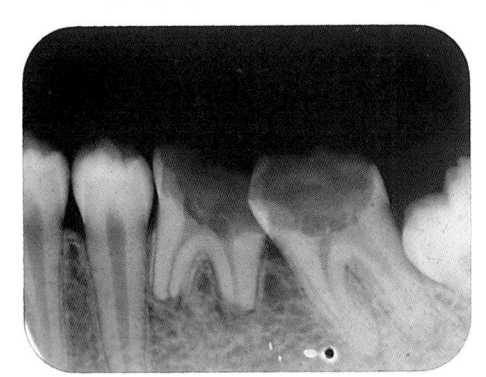

Root resorption
5.131 Root resorption usually starts on the external surface and may follow some local irritation such as trauma or inflammation, or be of unknown (idiopathic) origin. In this example, large carious cavities are present ⌊67 with exposure and necrosis of both pulps. There has been extensive resorption of the apical parts of both roots ⌊6 and reparative bone formation, so that only small areas of periapical radiolucency are present with absence of clearly defined lamina dura. There is a small radiolucent granuloma apically on the mesial root ⌊7. Note the crown of the partly erupted ⌊8. P

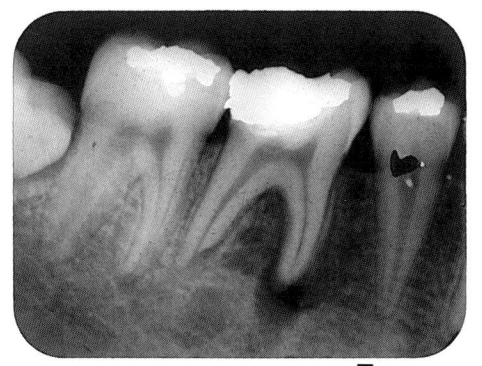

5.132 A large amalgam restoration 6⌋ obscuring an exposure of the distal pulp horn. The pulp has undergone necrosis and there is a clearly defined, periapical radiolucency, probably a granuloma, on the mesial root, with loss of the lamina dura apically and on the distal aspect of the root. There is resorption apically of both roots, more marked on the distal one. Note the pronounced clip mark overlying the pulp chamber 5⌋. P

The Teeth 93

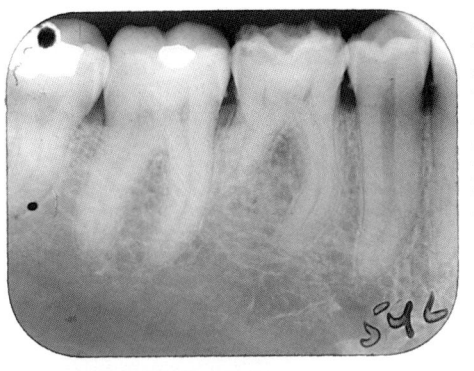

5.133 Idiopathic resorption of the distal root $\overline{6|}$, with reparative bone formation so that no radiolucent bone defect is present. There is enamel hypoplasia $\overline{6|}$ and partial obliteration of the pulp chamber and root canals due to mineralisation. P

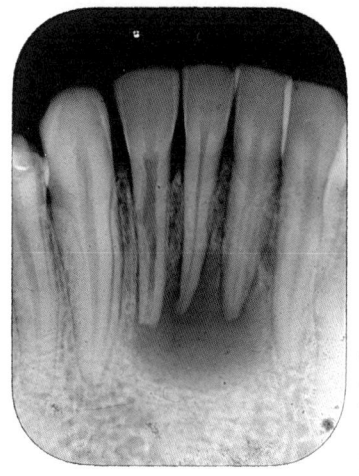

5.134 Trauma to the lower incisors has resulted in pulpal necrosis $\overline{21|}$ and development of a well circumscribed, clearly defined, periapical cyst involving the apices $\overline{21|1}$. In addition, $\overline{2|}$ has undergone irregular external resorption of the root. There is an apparent irregular enlargement of the cervical two-thirds of the root canal due to superimposition of the area of external resorption upon it. The continuity of the resorptive area with the root surface is confirmed by the extension of the radiolucent defect in the middle of the distal aspect of the root. There is also resorption of the apex $\overline{2|}$. It is often difficult on the basis of radiographic appearance to distinguish this pattern of resorption from idiopathic internal resorption, which occurs only very rarely. P

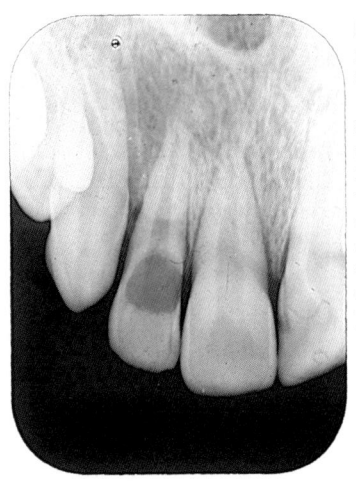

5.135 Idiopathic external resorption which started on the palatal aspect of the root $2|$, thus casting an approximately circular radiolucent shadow over the root canal. The retention of the normal outline of the root canal is often an important diagnostic feature in determining the external origin of the resorptive process. P

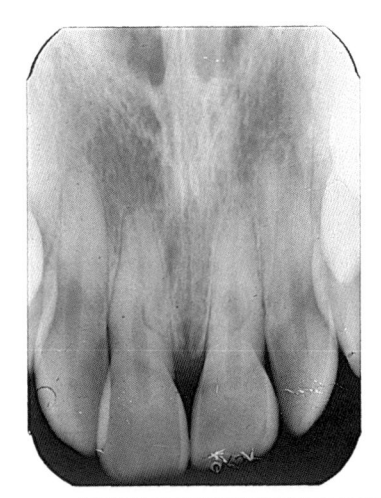

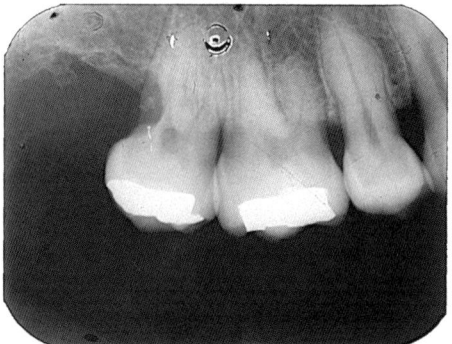

5.136 (top) and 5.137 (bottom) Idiopathic external resorption affecting a number of teeth in the same patient. This process typically starts in the cervical one-third of the root, and lesions are present $1|1$ and $7|$ distally. Simultaneously with the resorptive process, bony repair often occurs and radiopaque tissue is present within the defects of all three teeth. On $1|$, the lesion is mesially placed and its boundary from the normal tissue is outlined by a thin radiolucent line, whereas on $|1$ the circular lesion is of similar appearance, but is either labially or palatally placed and is superimposed over the midpoint of the root. In $7|$, the repair is less advanced and a broader band of radiolucency demarcates the saucer-shaped lesion from the adjacent dentine. The lesion may be confused with cementum caries and the clearly outlined margin, the extension of the lesion apically beyond the crest of the alveolar bone, and the presence of mineral within it are all important diagnostic features. Note the resorption apically on $6|$ root buccally. P

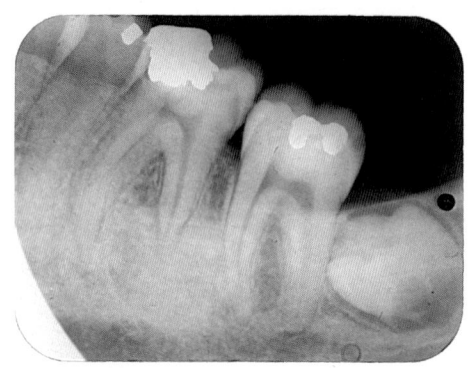

Periapical osteosclerosis

5.138 Periapical osteosclerosis may arise as a consequence of chronic pulpal inflammation. In this example, there is apical resorption of the distal root ⌐6 and an extensive area of radiopaque osteosclerosis, extending from the distal aspect ⌐5 to the mesial root ⌐7. The periodontal ligament space is still present apically around both roots ⌐6 and the periphery of the sclerotic area blends into the adjacent unaffected bone. Note the large amalgam mesio-occlusal filling ⌐6 and the mesio-angularly impacted developing ⌐8. P

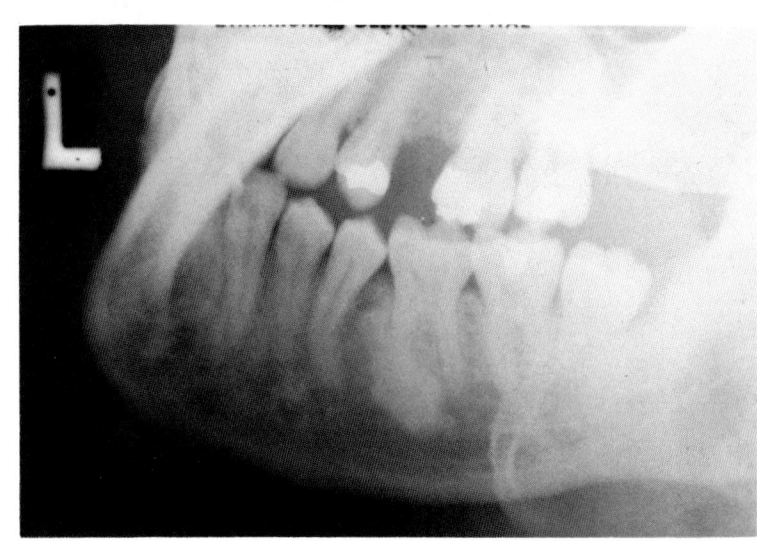

5.139 In this example, there is no obvious cause for the osteosclerosis around the mesial root ⌐6. The densely radiopaque area of sclerosis has an irregular periphery and blends into the surrounding normal bone. Its separation from the tooth is demonstrated by the persistence of a radiolucent periodontal ligament space of normal width around the root. Note the disto-angularly impacted ⌐8 with radiolucent pocket distal to the crown. OLM

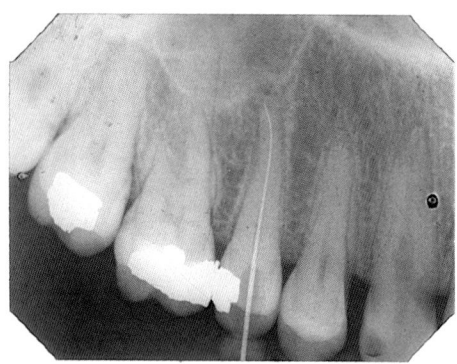

Root canal therapy

5.140 5⌐ became non-vital after unsuccessful treatment of a carious lesion with subsequent loss of the lamina dura and development of an apical radiolucency. Access to the root canal was obtained occlusally by removal of part of the amalgam restoration and a diagnostic plain broach (with an occlusally placed rubber stop) has been inserted to assess the length of the root canal prior to root filling. Note the close proximity of the floor of the antral cavity. P

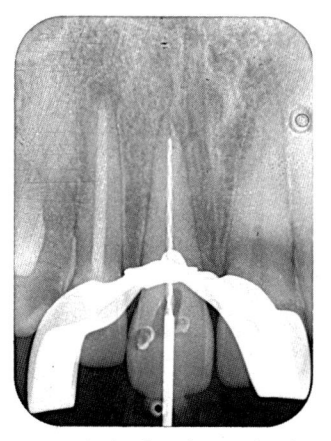

5.141 A check radiograph taken during root canal therapy demonstrates that the reamer has reached 1 mm short of the apex 1⌐ prior to root filling. There is a small radiolucent lesion mesio-apically, with loss of the lamina dura. Compare the corrugated appearance of the reamer with the smooth outline of the diagnostic broach (Fig. 5.140). The radiopaque rubber dam clip obscures most of the crowns of the adjacent teeth, but a distal, lined silicate filling and the palatal access cavity to the root canal 1⌐ are clearly shown. 2⌐, which has been root filled previously with a gutta percha point, has a small, residual apical radiolucency with absence of lamina dura. P

The Teeth 95

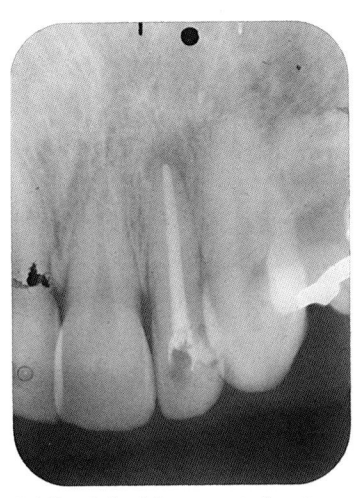

5.142 A freshly cemented gutta percha point in the root canal |2, prior to filling the palatal access cavity. There is a small, radiolucent, periapical granuloma with absence of lamina dura. P

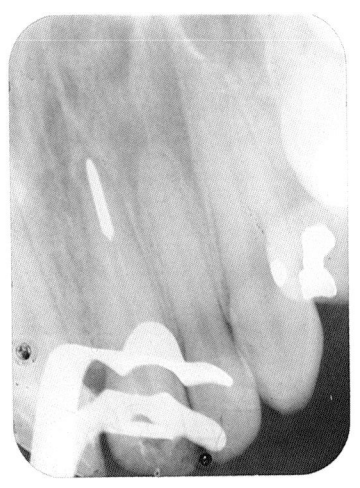

5.143 A sectional silver point, freshly cemented in the apical third of the root |1. Compare the greater radiopacity of this filling with that of the gutta percha (Fig. 5.142). The rubber dam clamp is still present on the crown. P

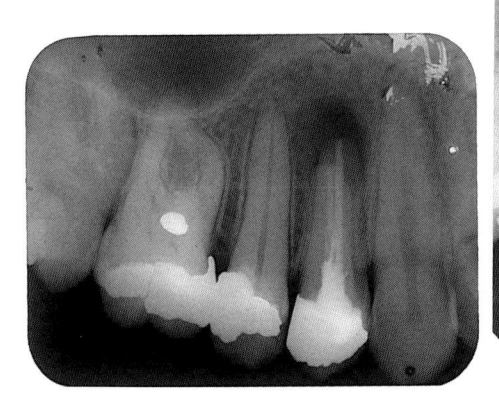

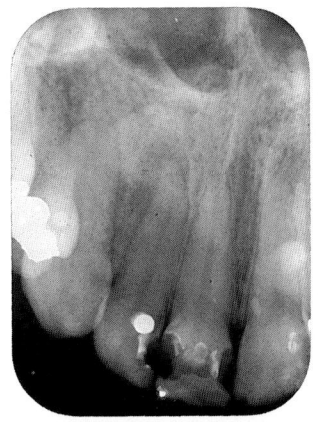

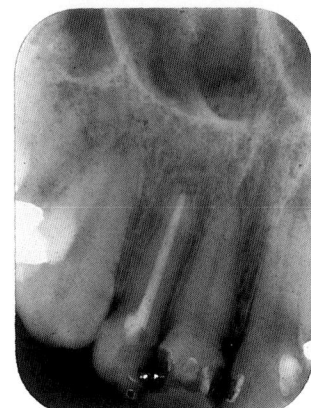

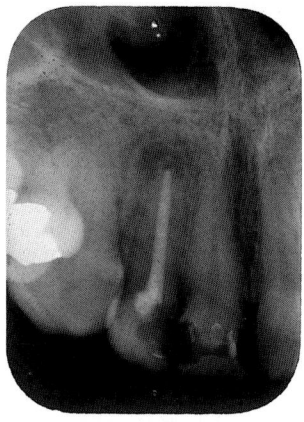

5.144 (upper left), 5.145 (above) and 5.146 (left) Sequential radiographs of 2| over a three-and-a-half year period. Prior to root canal therapy, there is loss of the lamina dura apically and an oval-shaped radiolucency with an ill defined margin, probably a periapical granuloma (Fig. 5.144). One year after root filling (Fig. 5.145), the radiolucency is smaller, and a further two-and-a-half years later (Fig. 5.146) bony repair is complete, with reformation of an intact lamina dura. P

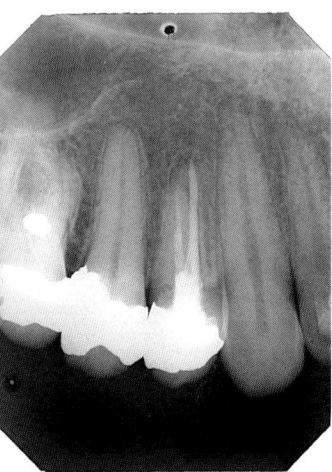

5.147 (far left) and 5.148 (left) A radiolucent periapical lesion 4|, probably a granuloma, with poorly defined outline and absence of lamina dura immediately after completion of root canal therapy (Fig. 5.147). Each root canal contains a separate gutta percha filling. After three years (Fig. 5.148), bone repair is complete and a normal trabecular pattern and continuous lamina dura now surround the apex. P

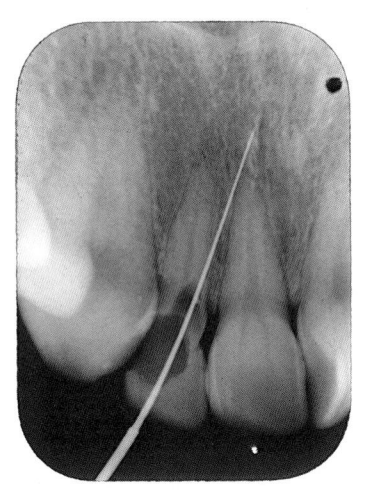

5.149 Root canal therapy was attempted 2⌋ following exposure of the pulp chamber in a distal cavity. As a consequence, access to the root canal was mesially inclined and a lateral perforation of the mesial aspect of the root has occurred. A plain broach has been introduced through the perforation into the surrounding bone. There is also a lateral root canal half way along the distal aspect of the root. P

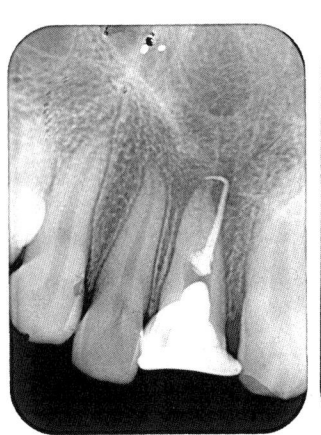

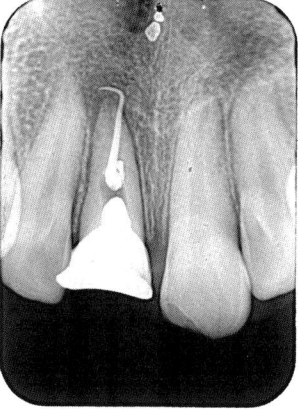

5.150 (left) and 5.151 (right) 1⌋ is inadequately root filled and has a lateral perforation of the root. There is a poorly defined, periapical radiolucency, probably a granuloma, with absence of lamina dura. The gutta percha point protrudes from the lateral perforation, its apical part being hooked and lying within the granuloma. A second radiograph (Fig. 5.151) taken with the X-ray source in a more medial position shows the hooked point more distally placed, indicating that the perforation is labial (parallax). Note the unusual design of the post crown! P

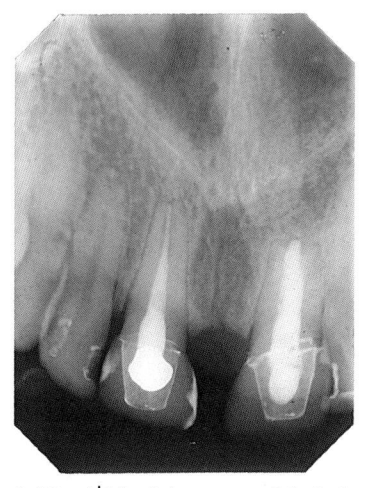

5.152 1|1 both have porcelain jacket crowns and root canal fillings. In 1⌋, the root canal is inadequately filled and radiolucent defects are apparent at each side of the gutta percha point. The periapical tissues are normal. In ⌊1, the root canal is properly filled and the tooth has been apicectomised as indicated by the flattened apical profile. Post-operative healing is complete, and an intact lamina dura and normal trabecular pattern surround the apex. In both teeth, the crown preparation is highlighted by the thin, radiopaque layer of cement, and in 1⌋ the greater density of the amalgam used to fill the access cavity to the root canal is apparent in the crown. Note the diastema 1|1 and the well defined anterior midline suture. P

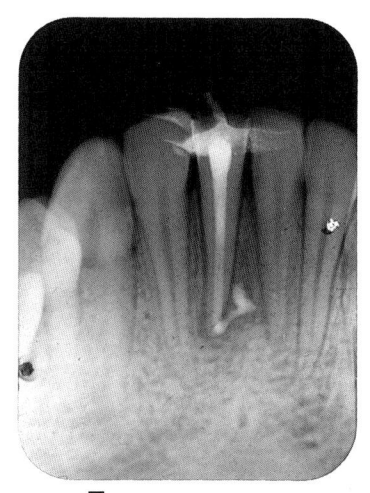

5.153 ⌈1 radiographed immediately after root filling with gutta percha showing excess cement extruded into the periapical tissues, where there is a small radiolucency. The increased radiopacity on the crowns 2̄1̄|1̄ is due to smearing of temporary dressing material. P

The Teeth 97

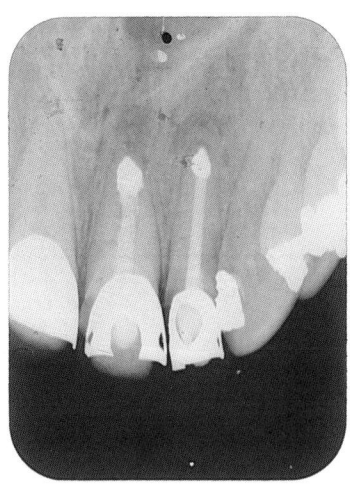

5.154 Apicectomies and retrograde amalgam root fillings |12 twelve months post-operatively. The periapical wound has fully healed, the apices of both teeth being encased in normal bone and surrounded by a thin, radiolucent periodontal ligament space and radiopaque lamina dura. The apically positioned amalgam fillings are well condensed and only an occasional particle of excess material can be seen. Both teeth have porcelain-faced gold crowns and contain gutta percha root fillings, that in |1 being not well condensed laterally. P

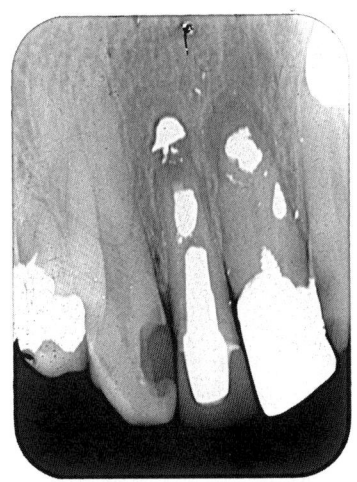

5.155 In this example, the retrograde amalgam root fillings 21| have been inadequately performed and excess material lies free in the periapical tissues, some six months post-operatively. The clearly defined periapical radiolucency 1| represents the healing apicectomy wound. 1| has a gold crown with screw-in post, 2| has a gold post and core with a jacket crown, and 3| has a large composite restoration mesially. P

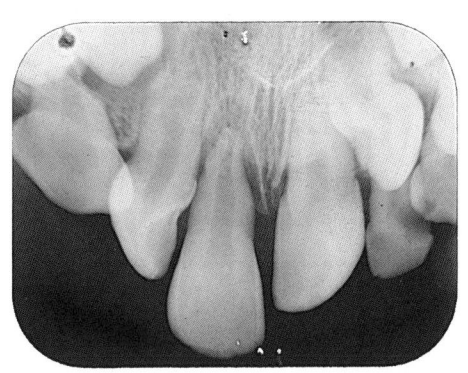

Subluxation of teeth
5.156 Subluxation 1| due to trauma one day previously in a child of eight. The tooth is displaced incisally from its socket, resulting in widening of the periodontal ligament space laterally and apically. The lamina dura is intact. P

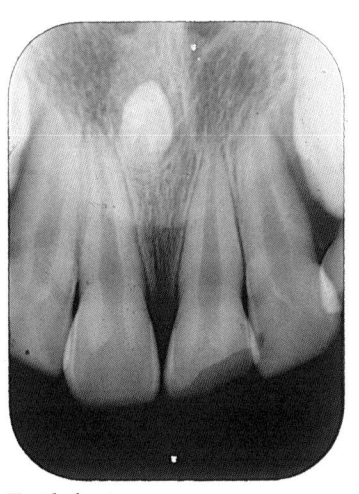

Tooth fracture
5.157 A recent oblique fracture through the crown |1, involving the distal portion of the incisal edge. The fracture extends into the dentine passing close to the coronal pulp chamber, and the incisal fragment is missing. Note the inverted, conical, supernumerary tooth (mesiodens) in the midline. P

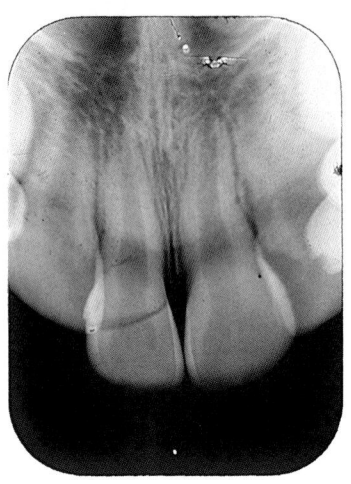

98 A Radiological Atlas of Diseases of the Teeth and Jaws

5.158 A recent, approximately horizontal fracture of the crown 1|, involving the coronal pulp chamber in a nine-year-old child. The incisal fragment is retained and on the mesial aspect the fracture line is subgingival. Note that root development is not yet complete in all the teeth. Note also the semilunar, radiopaque shadow of the nasal soft tissues superimposed upon the anterior teeth cervically. P

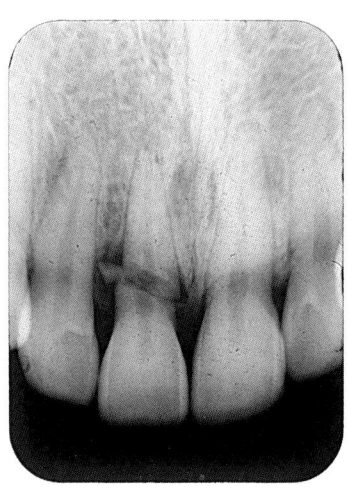

5.159 Comminuted oblique fracture of the coronal third of the root 1| with fragments visible within the fracture line. The crown of the tooth is slightly displaced distally. P

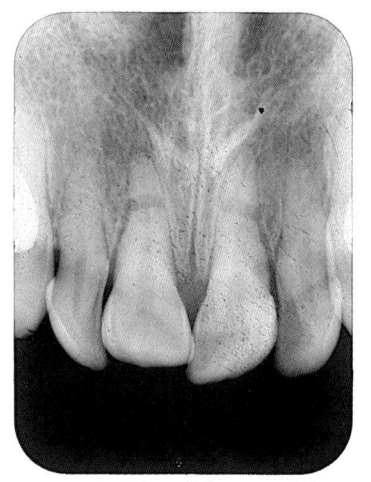

5.160 Bilateral horizontal fractures of the apical third of the roots 1|1, with displacement of the coronal fragments, as a consequence of which the fracture lines appear widened. P

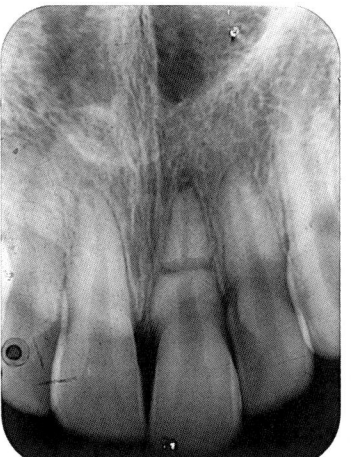

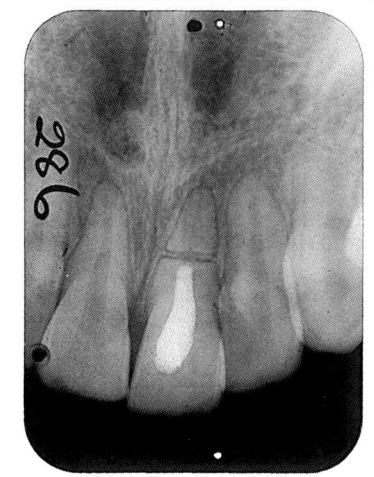

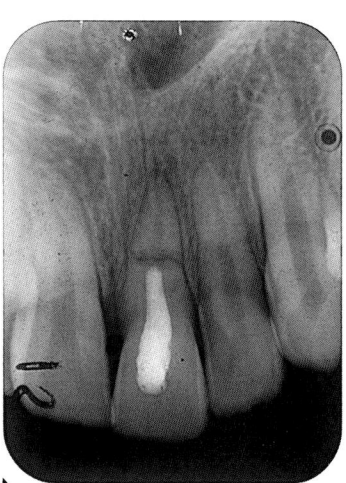

5.161 (upper left), 5.162 (above) and 5.163 (left) A horizontal fracture in the middle third of the root |1 in a 14-year-old child. There is slight displacement of the coronal fragment, but the crown is intact. One year after root filling of the coronal fragment (Fig. 5.162), the lamina dura remains intact. After a further year (Fig. 5.163), there is bone formation in the fracture line indicating healing. P

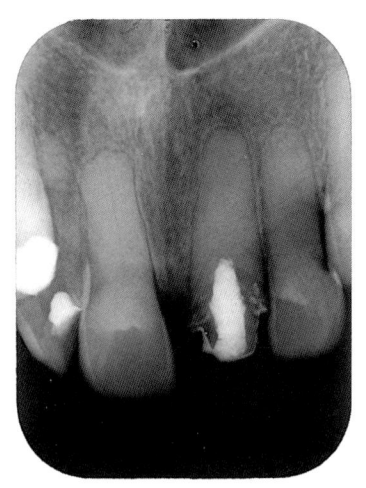

Pulpal sclerosis

5.164 Following a previous traumatic episode, there has been pulpal sclerosis 1|12 with obliteration of the pulp chambers and root canals of these teeth by deposition of atypical, reparative dentine. Such a pattern of sclerosis is not uncommon following severe trauma to a tooth which does not result in fracture. There has also been slight root resorption, the apices appearing blunted, but the lamina dura is still intact. Note the attempted root filling |1 which bears an acrylic jacket crown, and the crestal bone loss interdentally due to chronic periodontal disease. P

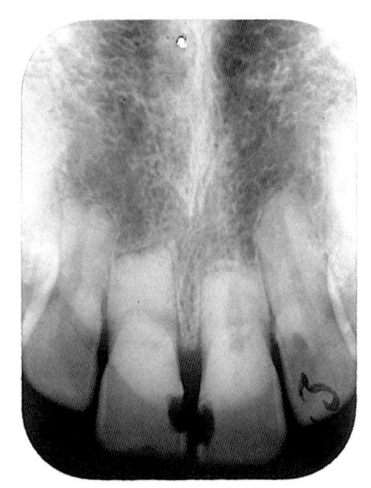

5.165 Varying degrees of pulpal sclerosis and apical root resorption 21|12 following trauma. The pulp chamber and root canal 1| are totally and |1 partially occluded. There is also apical resorption in all four incisors, being particularly advanced 1|1. Bony repair has accompanied the root resorption so that there is a normal lamina dura and periodontal ligament space around the roots. Note the unlined silicate fillings 1|1 mesially. P

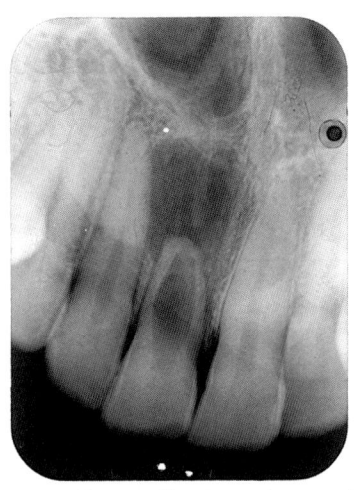

5.166 Trauma 1| prior to the completion of odontogenesis has led to disturbance of normal root development. There is a fracture through the dentine of the mesial angle of the incisal edge with loss of the incisal fragment. The root is short and there is an abnormally wide root canal, although the apical foramen appears normal. Subsequent to the trauma there has been pulpal necrosis, and there is now a clearly defined, oval, periapical radiolucency extending laterally over the roots of 2|1, indicative of a periapical cyst. Note the loss of lamina dura at the apex. P

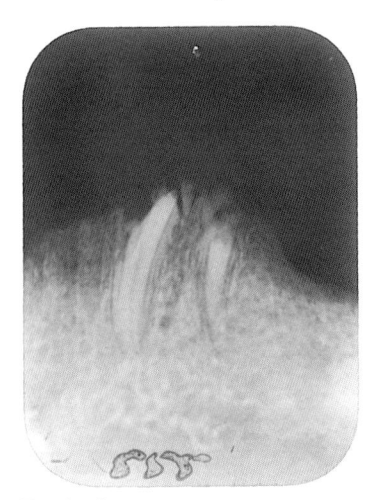

Retained roots

5.167 Two roots left in the premolar region of the mandible following attempted extractions. There is a markedly oblique fracture of the coronal aspect of the root |3 passing deeply into its socket mesially with a small retained fragment at the alveolar crest distally. The fracture surface is very irregular at the coronal aspect of the |4 root. Around both roots there is a normal periodontal ligament space and lamina dura. A root canal is clearly present in |3 root. P

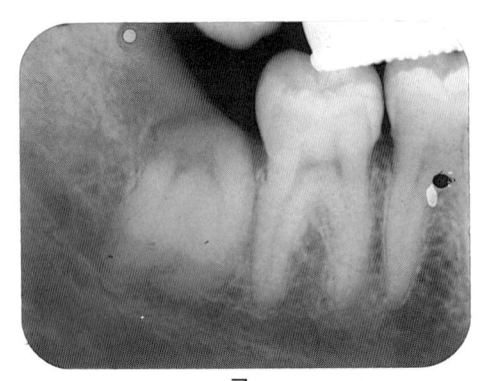

100   *A Radiological Atlas of Diseases of the Teeth and Jaws*

5.168 Retained roots 8| following fracture of the crown during attempted removal some weeks previously. The tooth was disto-angularly impacted and there is a marked distal curvature to the apex of its mesial root. A normal lamina dura and periodontal ligament space surround the roots, the image of which is superimposed upon, but does not impinge into, the inferior alveolar canal. The radiolucent canal runs uninterruptedly across both root apices. P

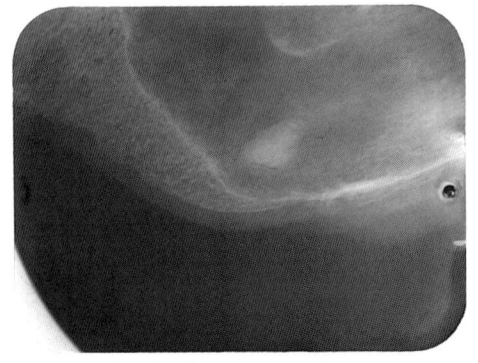

5.170 A deeply placed, retained root apex lying in an edentulous alveolus, many months after extraction of |6. Following tooth extraction, there has been alveolar resorption and apparent enlargement of the antrum into parts of the maxilla previously occupied by the teeth, so that the radiopaque lamina marking the floor of the antrum passes close to the surface of the edentulous ridge. The root is therefore superimposed upon the antrum, but not actually in it. Confirmation of its position is established by careful examination of the film, which reveals a normal periodontal ligament space and lamina dura around the apex. Note the inferior border of the zygomatic process above the root. P

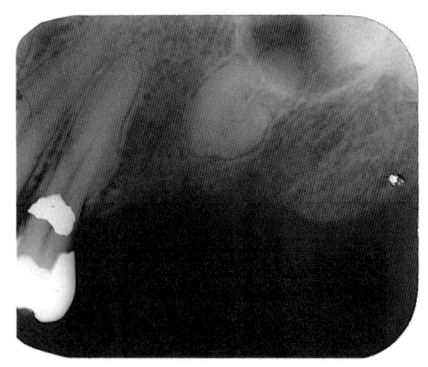

5.169 Retained, non-infected apices of all three roots |7 fractured off at the time of its extraction some years previously. The coronal part of the socket has fully healed and there has been complete bony remodelling. The apical fragments are surrounded by a thin, radiopaque cortical lamina and radiolucent periodontal ligament space: their root canals are obliterated, as is that in the apical part of the root |5. The antral cavity is superimposed upon the apical part of the palatal root |7. Note the radiopacity overlying the antrum, formed by the root of the zygomatic process. P

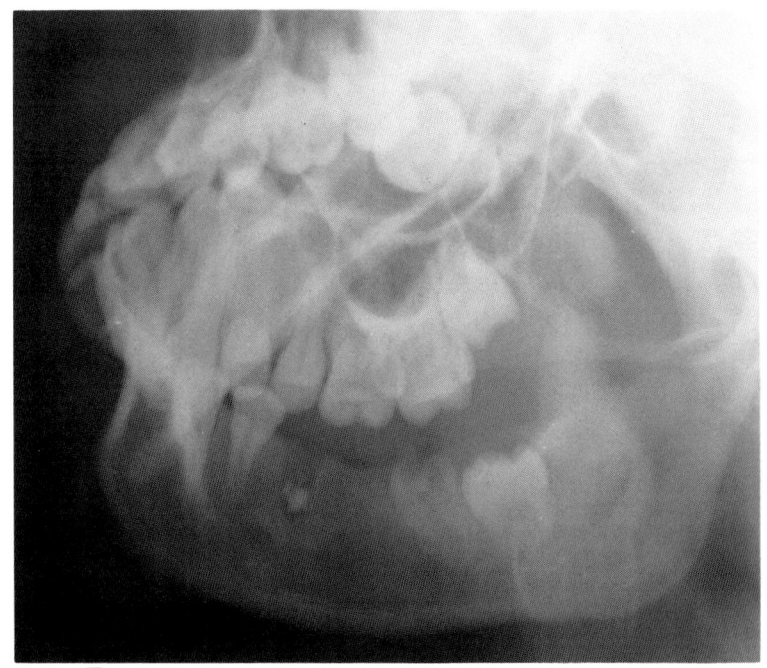

5.171 |7 has fractured cervically during attempted extraction a few weeks previously, and its roots are retained. |5 was extracted at the same visit, and the radiopaque outline of the socket is becoming indistinct. Several fragments of tooth debris are present. Note the circular radiolucency of the mental foramen just anterior to |5 socket, the unerupted, incompletely formed |8, and the supernumerary tooth (paramolar) between |67. OLM

The Teeth 101

5.172 Recent attempted extraction ⌊6 has resulted in fracture of its distal root at the level of the alveolar crest and its retention in the distal socket. The radiolucent mesial root socket is surrounded by a continuous, radiopaque lamina dura and the oral aspect of the socket contains some radiopaque zinc oxide dressing material. A radiopaque area of osteosclerosis surrounds the apex of the distal root. Note the thin linear radiopacity running obliquely across the roots ⌊78 due to the superimposition of the external oblique ridge of the mandible. OLM

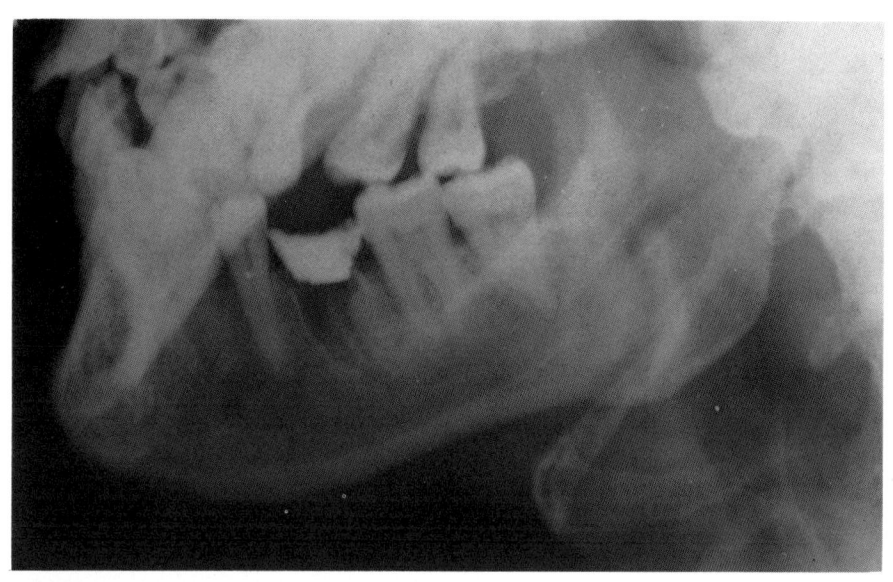

5.173 Attempted extraction ⌊6 in a 14-year-old, complicated by fracture of the crown cervically with retention of both roots and of one blade of the forceps. Note the dense radiopacity of the metallic forceps blade superimposed upon the mesial root. OLM

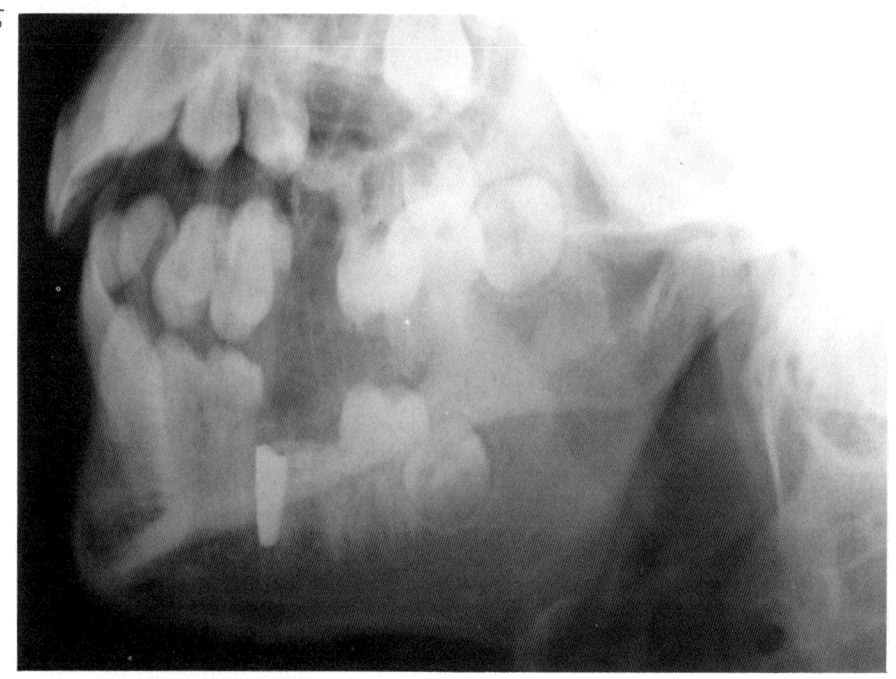

5.174 Small root fragments may be difficult to locate at operation, and stainless steel wires incorporated into a radiolucent localising plate may be helpful in establishing their exact position prior to surgery. This small, radiopaque root fragment is not surrounded by a lamina dura, suggesting the presence of inflammation. P

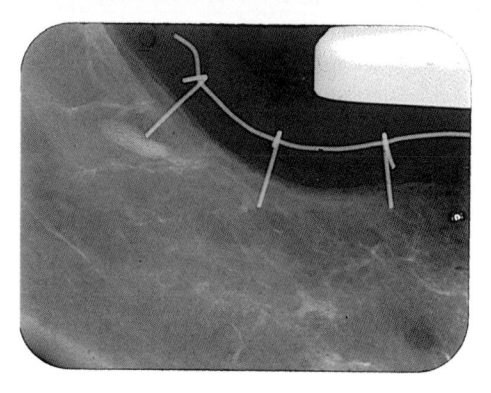

102 A Radiological Atlas of Diseases of the Teeth and Jaws

5.175 During attempted removal of a horizontally impacted 8̅|, the tooth was displaced into the lingual soft tissues so that its image is superimposed upon the ramus of the mandible. The radiolucent socket is clearly demonstrated and the displaced tooth inverted. The crown was partially divided prior to displacement, as indicated by the irregular area of radiolucency running across its cervical part. The radiopaque tip of the bur was broken in the process and has become free from the tooth following its displacement. The lingual position of the tooth may be confirmed on an occlusal radiograph. OLM

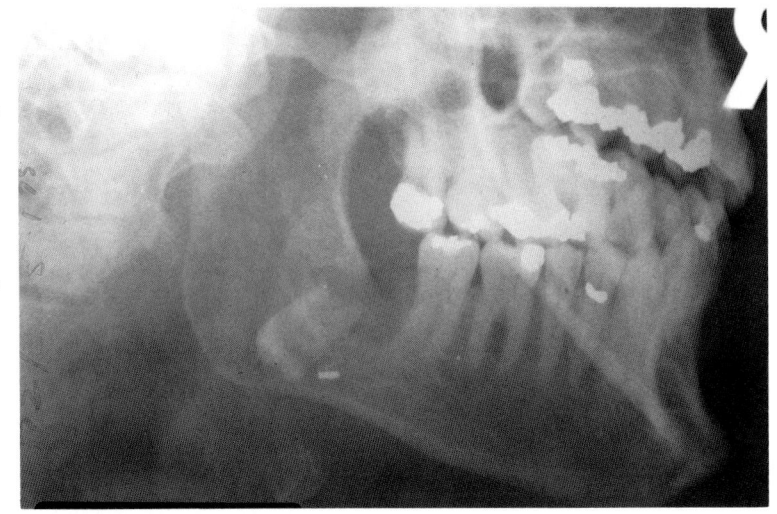

5.176 Attempted surgical extraction (in a 14-year-old) of |6̅ roots, which are inclined mesially and exhibit marked apical curvature distally, particularly on the mesial root. There has been excessive and inaccurately directed removal of bone between |6̅7̅, where there is a large area of radiolucency which at its mesio-inferior corner penetrates the cortical bone at the inferior border of the mandible. OLM

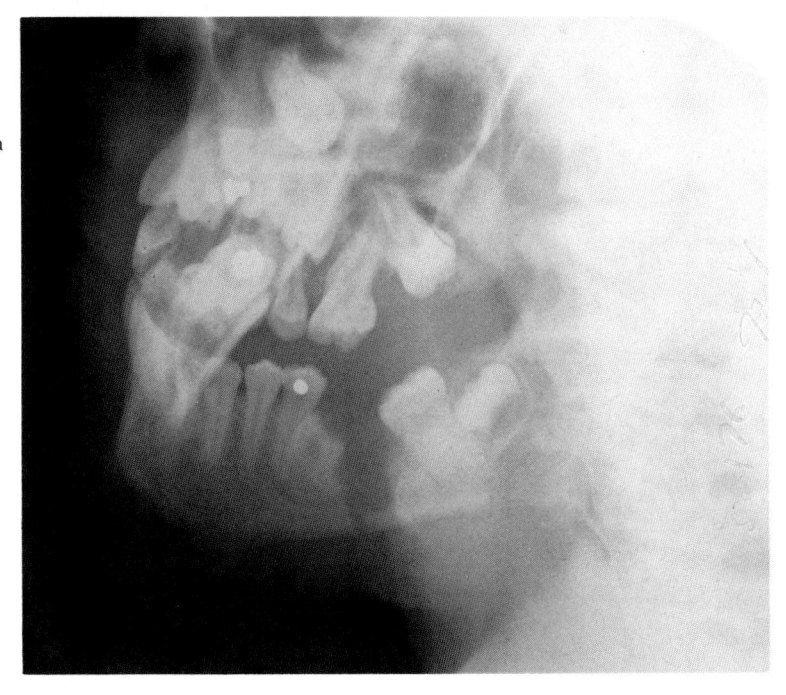

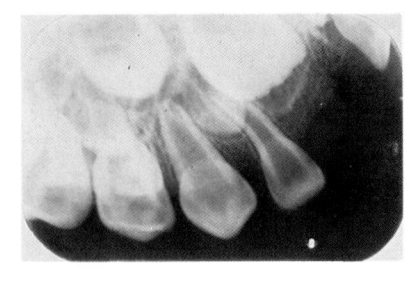

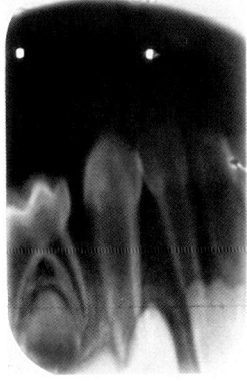

Hereditary hypophosphataemia (Vitamin D-resistant rickets)

5.177 (far left) and 5.178 (left) In this disorder, the teeth of the primary dentition have enlarged pulp chambers due to defective formation of the circumpulpal dentine. Characteristically, prominent cuspal extensions of the pulp chamber up to or close to the amelo-dentinal junction are present, as in this example, particularly in $\frac{C}{DC}|$. As a consequence, pulpal infection and periapical lesions are common. P

Chapter 6

The Periodontium

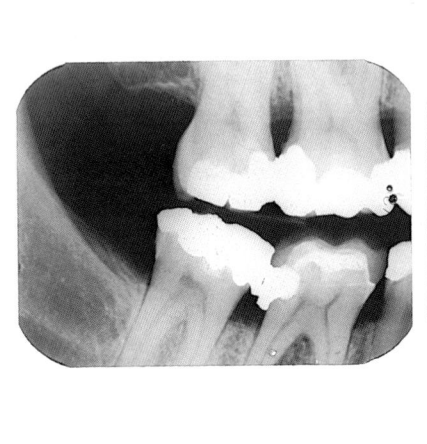

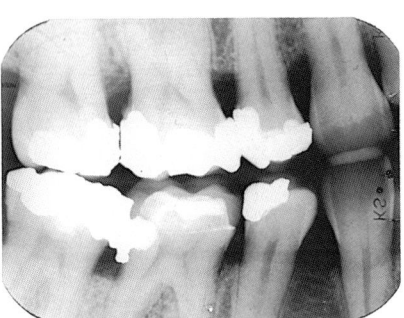

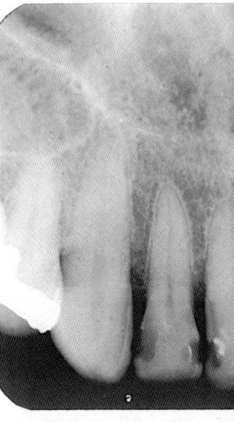

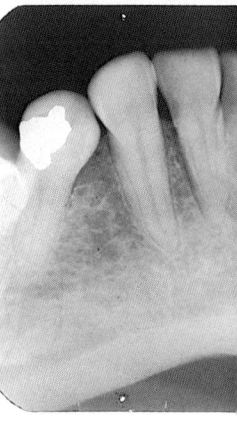

104 *A Radiological Atlas of Diseases of the Teeth and Jaws*

The Periodontium 105

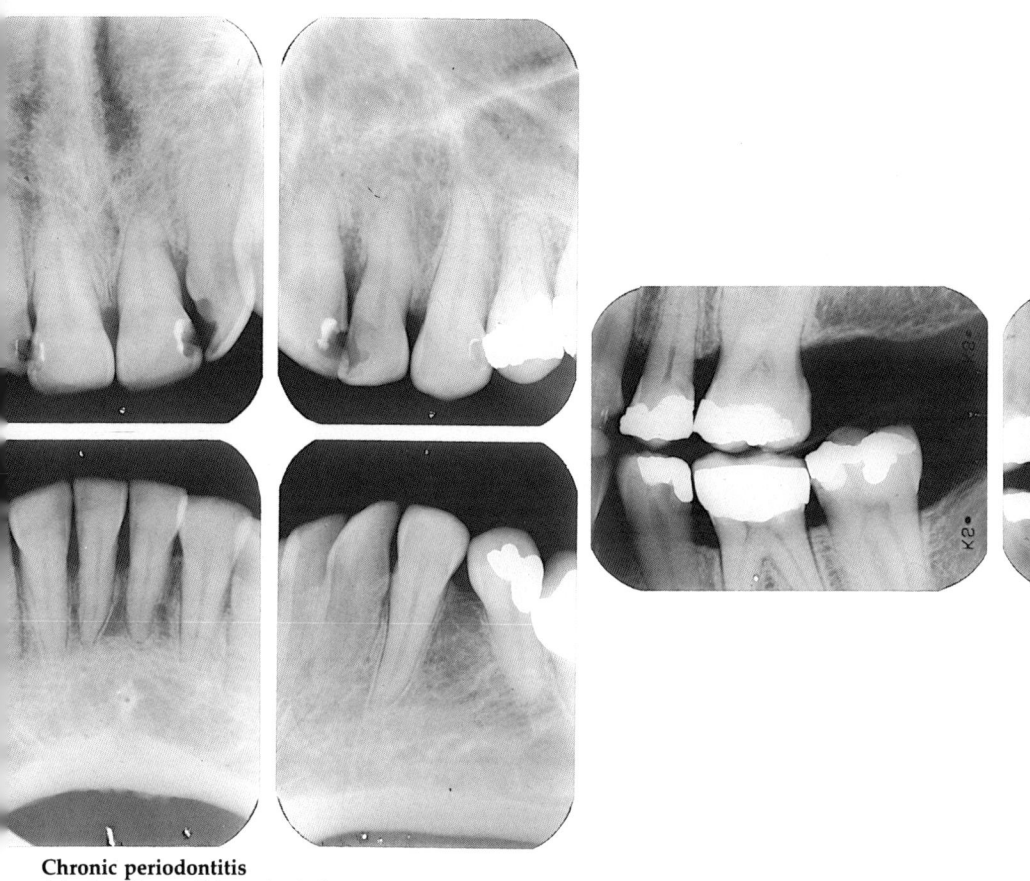

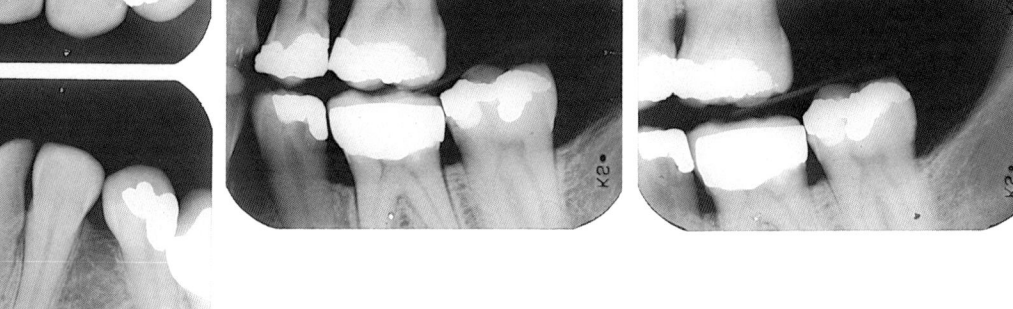

Chronic periodontitis
6.1 In this condition, the inflammatory process is accompanied by a progressive destruction of the alveolar bone starting from the crest, usually affecting all the dentition. In this early stage in a 35-year-old, there is loss of the cortical outline of the crests of the interdental septa, rather more marked on the right side than on the left. Prominent overhanging margins are present on the amalgam restorations 7| mesially and 6| distally, the latter of which also bears a porcelain crown. Note the recurrent caries distally |5 and the porcelain to gold crown |6. P & BW

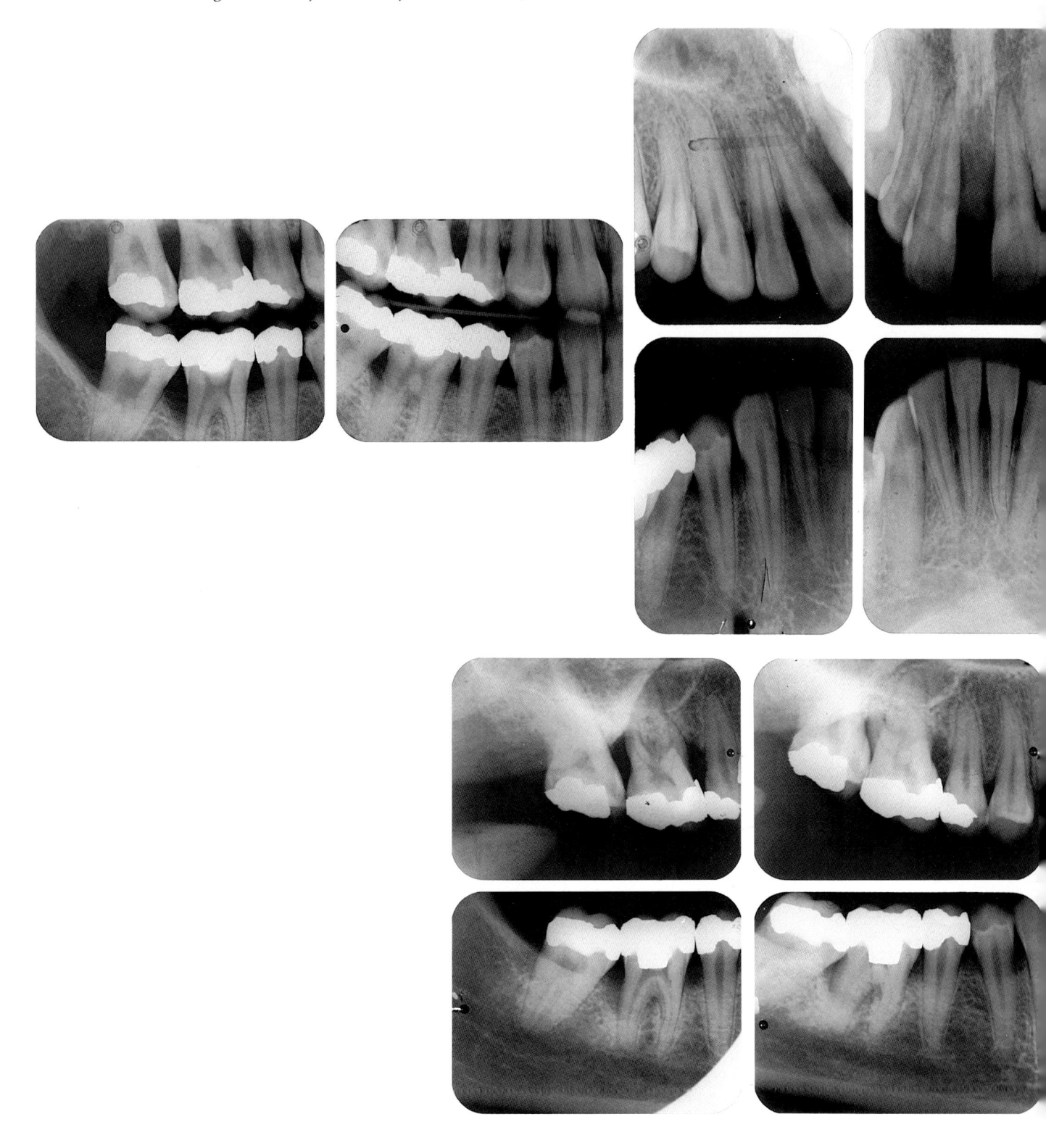

106 *A Radiological Atlas of Diseases of the Teeth and Jaws*

The Periodontium 107

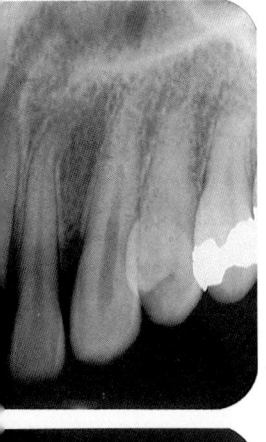

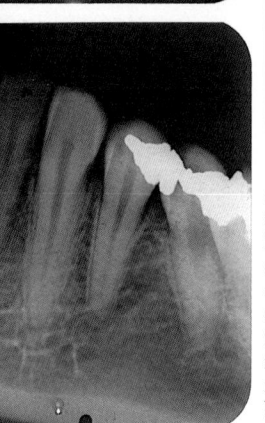

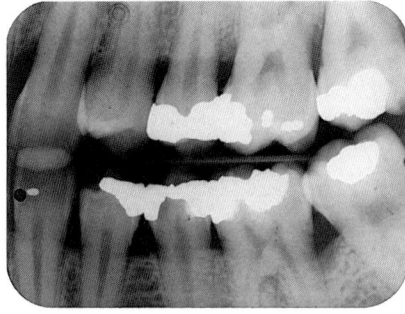

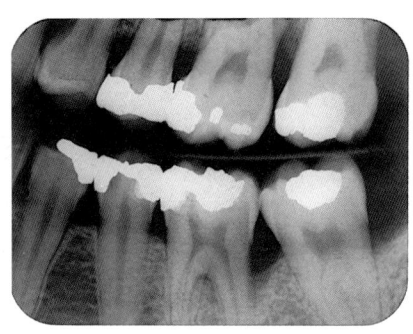

6.2 An intermediate stage, in which there is generalised irregular destruction of bone at the crests of the interdental septa, which show a loss of their cortical outline together with craterform radiolucency. The bone destruction is more advanced between the maxillary central incisors, where there is also a diastema, and in the four molar quadrants, where in the lower jaw there are infrabony pockets $\overline{76|67}$. In addition, there is some radiolucency inter-radicularly $\overline{|6}$, indicating early bifurcation involvement. P & BW

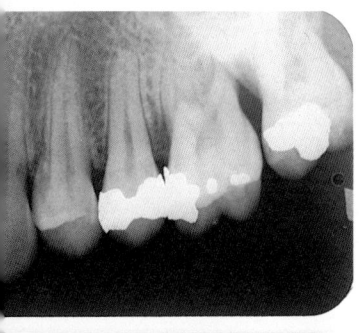

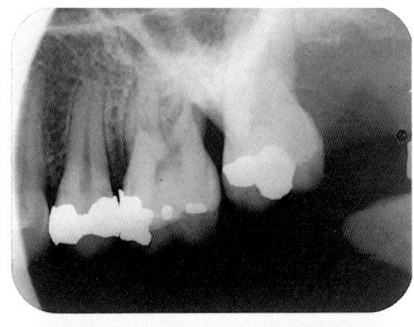

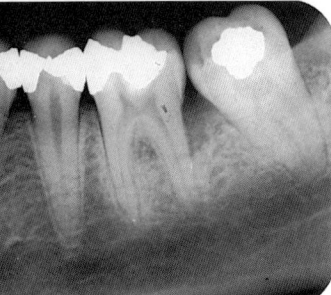

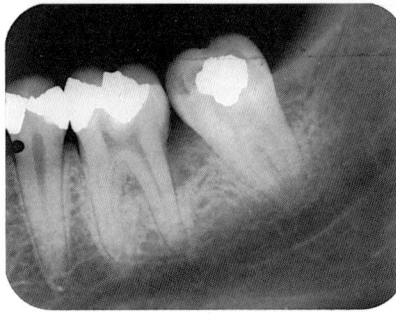

6.3 Bitewing radiographs should be used posteriorly to assess the extent of bone loss in chronic periodontitis. These periapical views of the same patient as Fig. 6.2 illustrate how an exaggerated picture of the bone loss may be obtained due to the angulation of the film relative to the X-ray tube, and how the image of the zygomatic process and arch may be projected over and obscure the roots of the maxillary molars, making interpretation difficult. P

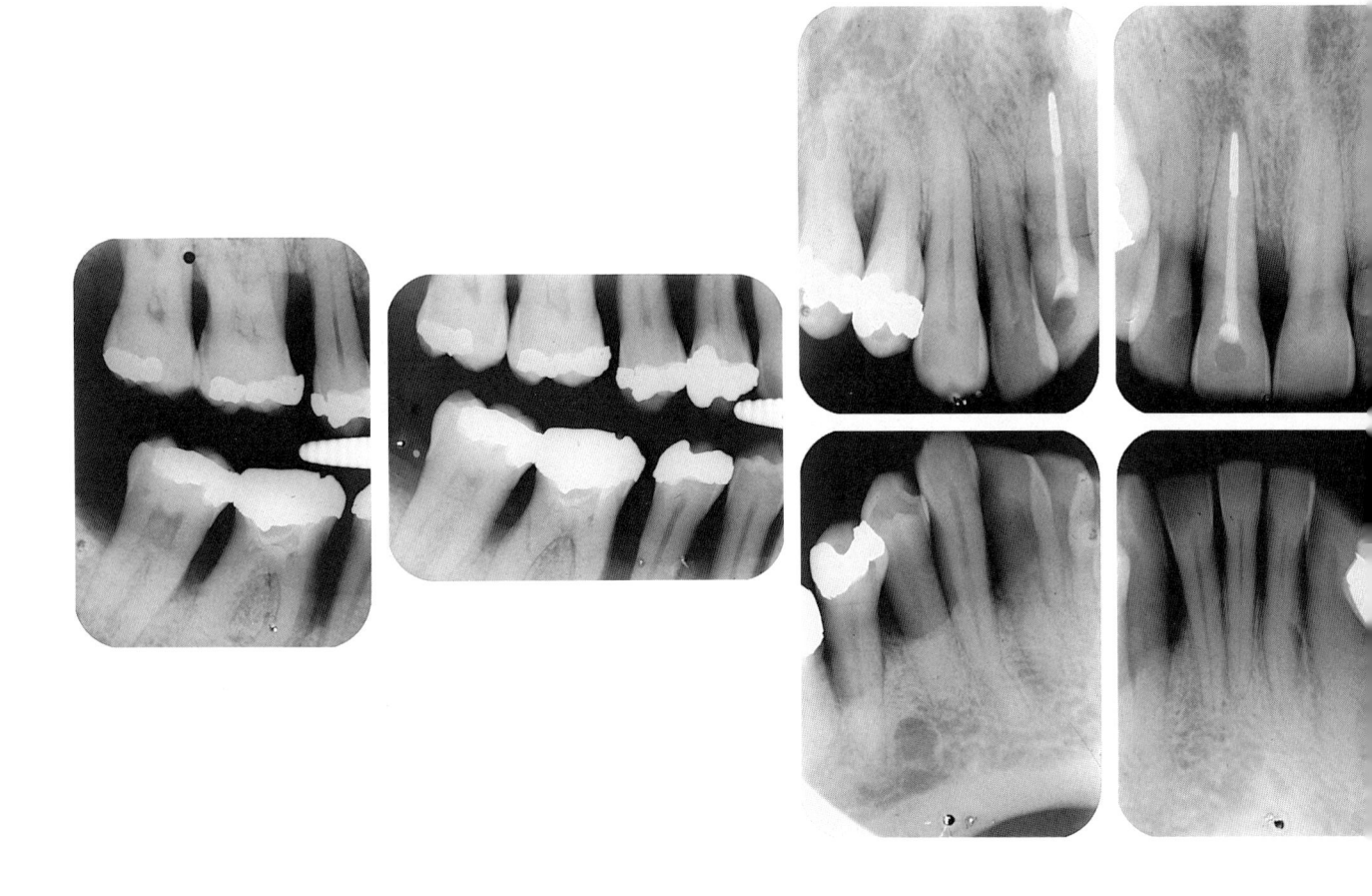

108 *A Radiological Atlas of Diseases of the Teeth and Jaws*

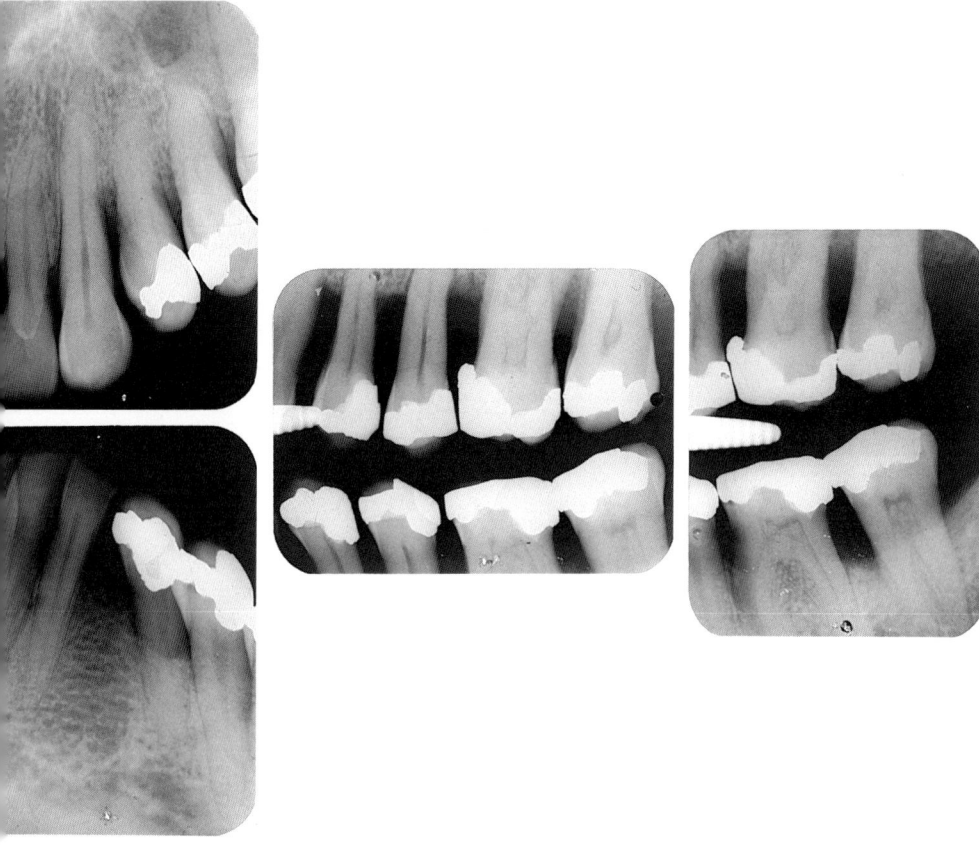

6.4 An advanced stage, which is particularly marked bilaterally in the molar regions. The bone loss is so advanced that its full extent is not evident on the conventional bitewing films, but is revealed when the film was held vertically. Note the root filling 1| with a sectional silver point apically and the overhanging amalgam restoration mesio-cervically |6. The right mental foramen is unusually clearly demonstrated between the apices 54|.
P & BW

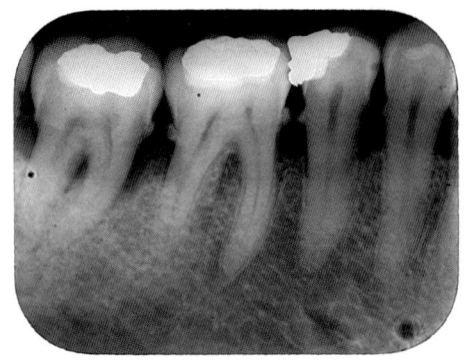

110   *A Radiological Atlas of Diseases of the Teeth and Jaws*

6.5 Heavy deposits of supragingival calculus forming projecting, radiopaque spurs from the cervical surfaces of the mandibular premolar and molar teeth. There is loss of the cortical outline of the interdental crests together with irregular radiolucent destruction of the bone. Note the radiolucency inter-radicularly $\overline{76|}$, where there is early bifurcation involvement. P

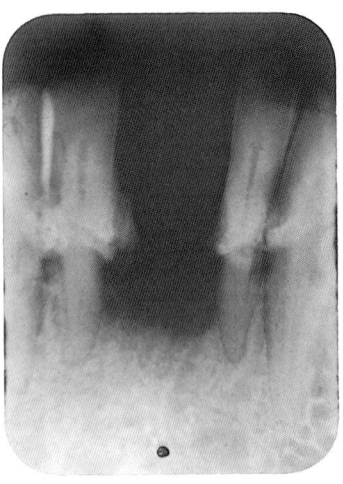

6.6 Heavy deposits of supragingival calculus cervically on the interstitial and lingual surfaces of the mandibular anterior teeth, except $\overline{1|1}$ which are missing. The deposits are of varying radiopacity and in part are layered, suggesting the formation of successive increments. There is advanced loss of the alveolar bone and absence of cortical lamina, particularly in the edentulous part of the ridge. P

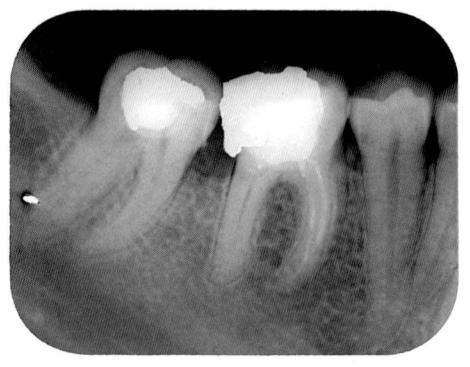

6.7 An area of localised periodontitis associated with the overhanging cervical margin on the large amalgam restoration $\overline{6|}$ distally. The underlying alveolar crest has a craterform radiolucency with loss of cortical outline, and a small spur of radiopaque calculus projects from the mesio-cervical surface $\overline{7|}$. There are fillings in two separate canals of the mesial root and in the pulp chamber $\overline{6|}$. P

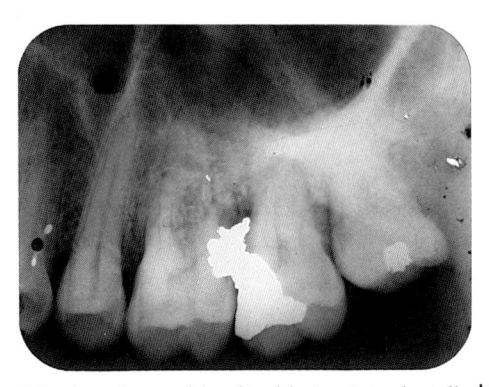

6.8 An advanced localised lesion interdentally $\underline{|67}$ associated with a gross excess of amalgam cervically on the mesio-occlusal filling $\underline{|7}$. There is bone destruction up to the apical third of the root $\underline{|7}$, although it is much less advanced in the other interdental spaces. P

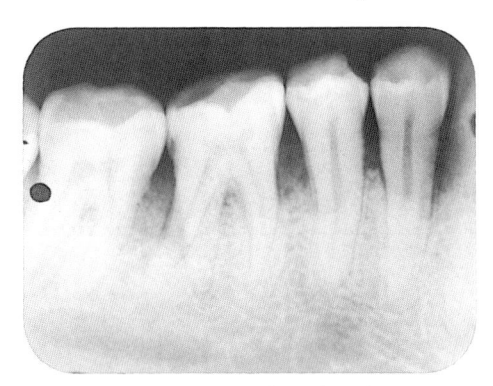

6.9 In this example, the bone loss has progressed at approximately the same rate around all the teeth (horizontal bone loss) and only the apical half of the roots remain supported by bone. There are irregularly radiolucent defects in all the interdental crests with loss of the cortical laminae. The bone loss is a little more advanced interdentally $\overline{76|}$, in association with the extra root of the three rooted molar, which exhibits early trifurcation involvement. Note the marked occlusal attrition. P

The Periodontium 111

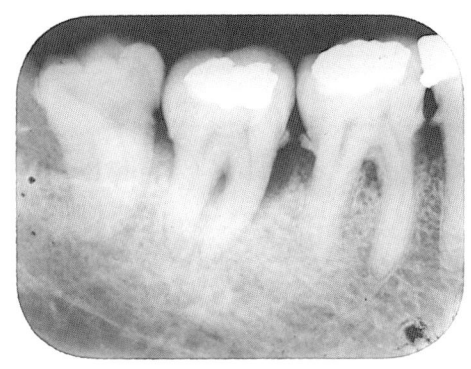

6.10 A different view of the same patient illustrated in Fig. 6.5, with bone destruction interdentally and bifurcation involvement in the right mandibular molar region. The bone loss has progressed interdentally 76| at different rates on the two root surfaces, forming two infrabony pockets separated by a residual spur of bone at the interdental crest. There are heavy deposits of calculus cervically. Note the shadow of the oblique ridge of the mandible running downwards and forwards across the crown 8|. P

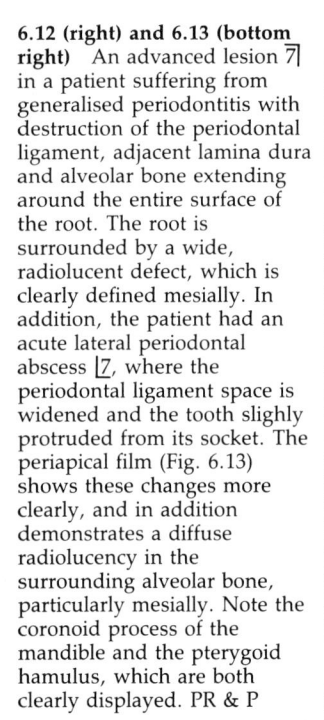

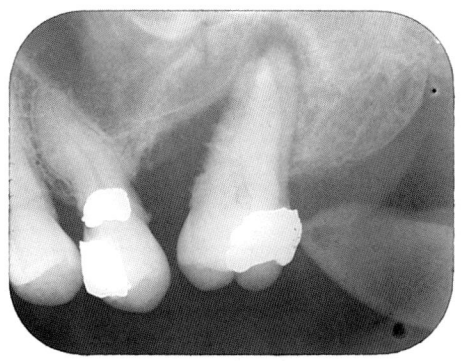

6.11 An advanced lesion with bone loss reaching to the apex of the involved molar. Radiolucent areas of bone destruction are present mesially, distally and apically, there being a deep, infrabony pocket mesially which is in close proximity to the thin cortical lamina of the antral floor. Projecting from the mesial root surface are numerous radiopaque spurs of calculus. Calculus is also present disto-cervically |5. Note the shadow of the thick mucoperiosteum covering the tuberosity, and of the coronoid process of the mandible in the lower right corner. P

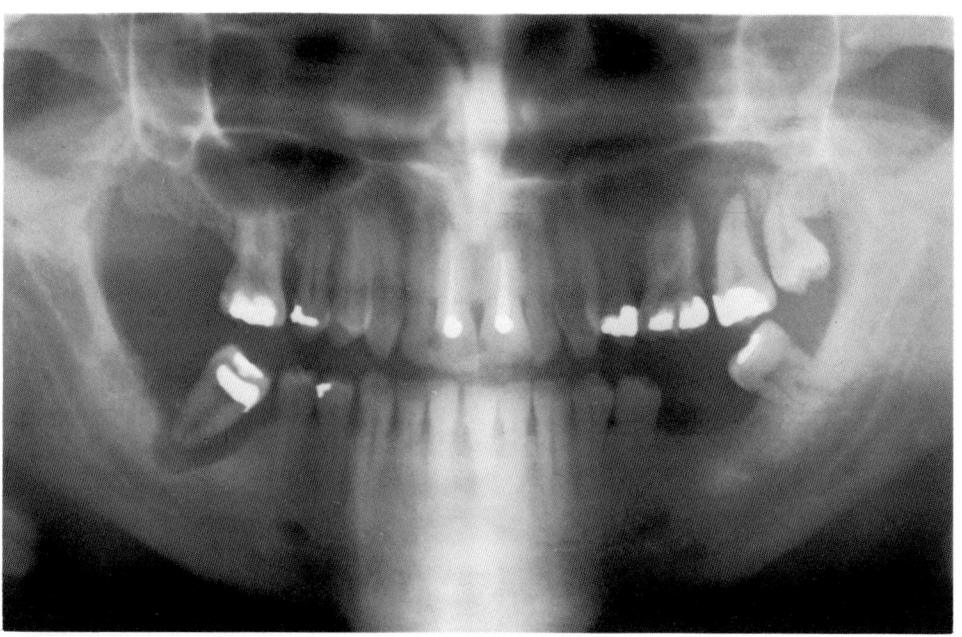

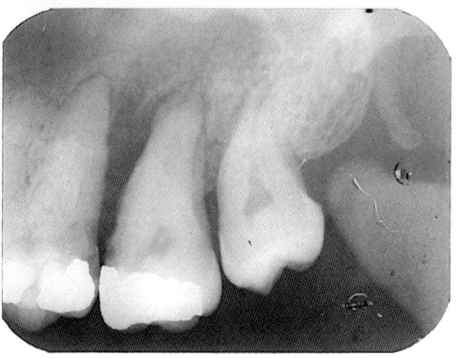

6.12 (right) and 6.13 (bottom right) An advanced lesion 7| in a patient suffering from generalised periodontitis with destruction of the periodontal ligament, adjacent lamina dura and alveolar bone extending around the entire surface of the root. The root is surrounded by a wide, radiolucent defect, which is clearly defined mesially. In addition, the patient had an acute lateral periodontal abscess |7, where the periodontal ligament space is widened and the tooth slightly protruded from its socket. The periapical film (Fig. 6.13) shows these changes more clearly, and in addition demonstrates a diffuse radiolucency in the surrounding alveolar bone, particularly mesially. Note the coronoid process of the mandible and the pterygoid hamulus, which are both clearly displayed. PR & P

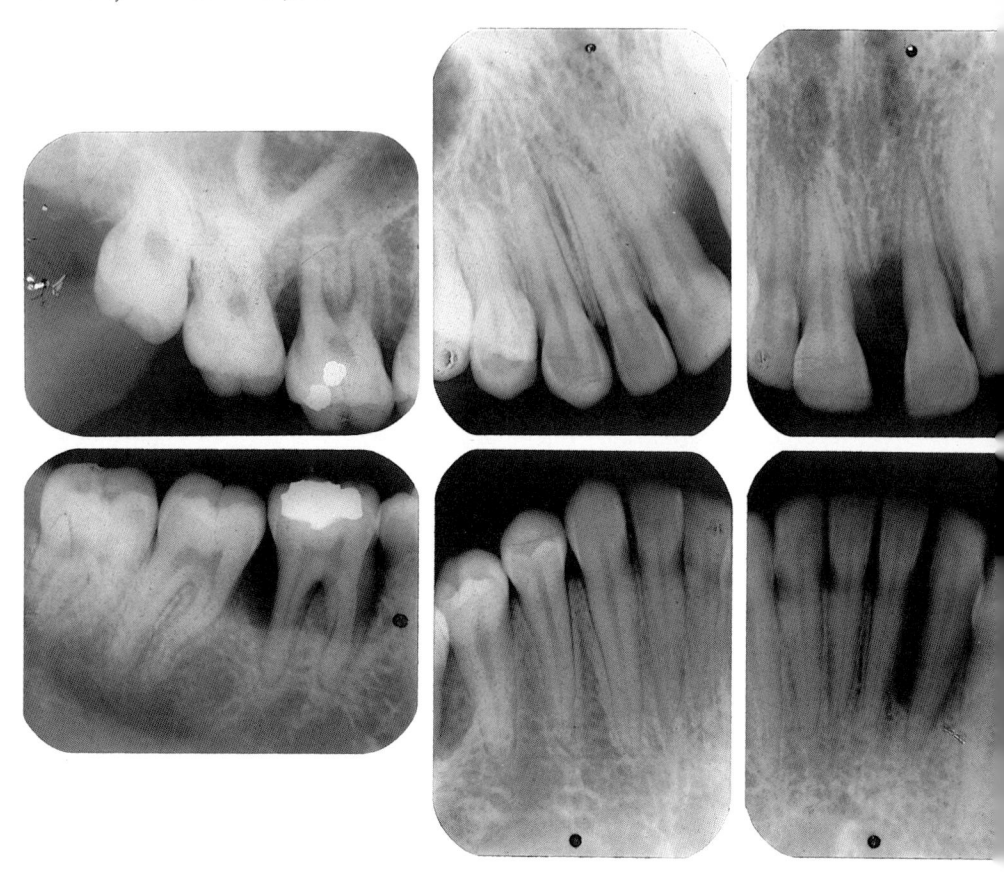

112 *A Radiological Atlas of Diseases of the Teeth and Jaws*

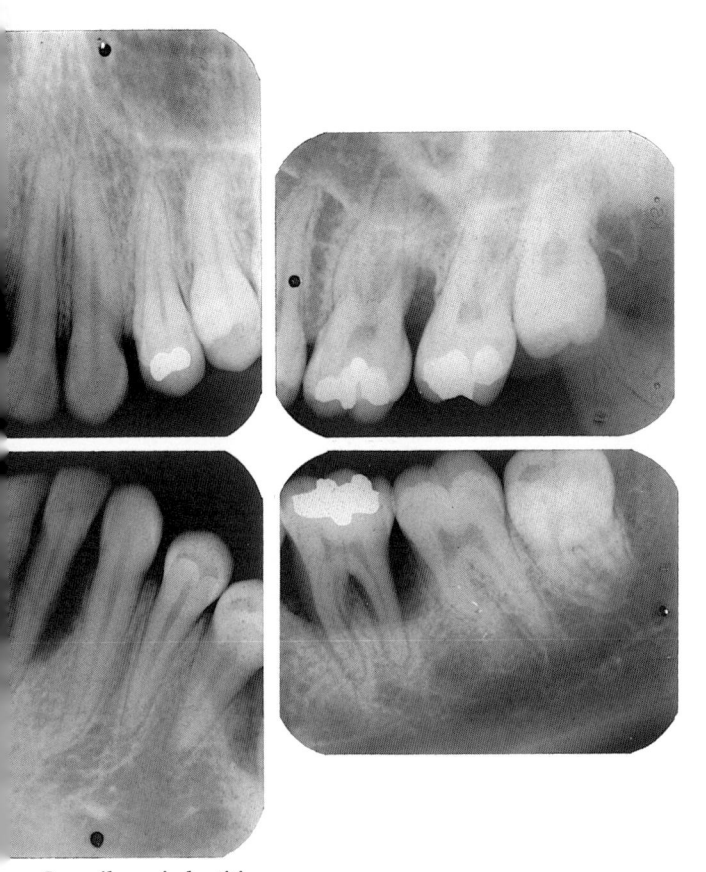

Juvenile periodontitis (periodontosis)

6.14 In this young adult, there is advanced bone destruction restricted to the incisor and first molar teeth, with little evidence of bone loss around the other teeth. The radiolucent area of bone loss $\overline{2|}$ has progressed almost to its apex, and that around the molar roots involves their furcations. This distribution of lesions is typical of the disorder, although other teeth may also be involved. P

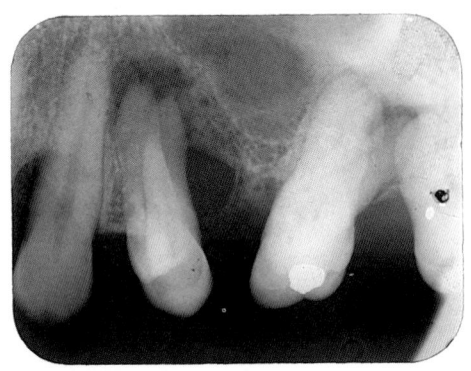

Lateral periodontal cyst
6.15 Overlying the roots of |4 is an ovoid radiolucency, around much of which there is a thin cortical lamina. The lamina dura distally and apically is absent, and the two roots are clearly displayed. The absence of bony trabeculae overlying the more occlusal part of the lesion indicates that the cortical plate of the alveolus has been perforated. Note the proximity of the lesion to the thin cortical lamina of the antral floor. P

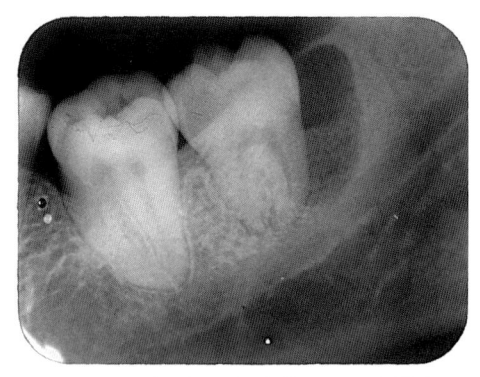

6.16 A cyst distal to the fully erupted |8, forming an ovoid radiolucency surrounded by a thin radiopaque lamina. It reaches down to the roof of the inferior alveolar canal and overlaps part of the distal root, although the apices are not involved. The more apparent radiolucency occlusally indicates that there is marked thinning of one of the cortical plates. P

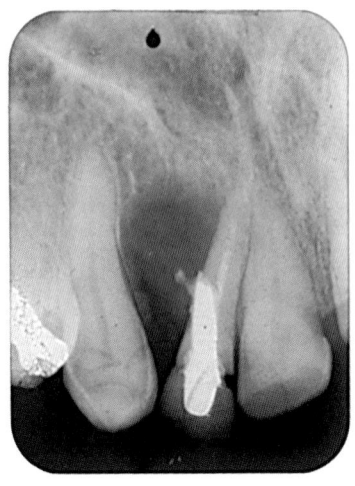

6.17 An infected lesion which has arisen as a result of a lateral perforation of the root 2|. A pear-shaped radiolucent defect is present in the interdental septum 32| with a poorly defined margin, extending from its crest inferiorly towards the apices superiorly. There is loss of the lamina dura mesially 3| and distally 2|, and displacement of both tooth apices away from the lesion. The tip of the metal post is projecting through the perforation and some radiopaque cement is lying within the adjacent soft tissues. The root filling is deficient apically and is poorly condensed. Note the similarity of this lesion to the globulo-maxillary cyst (Fig 7.20). P

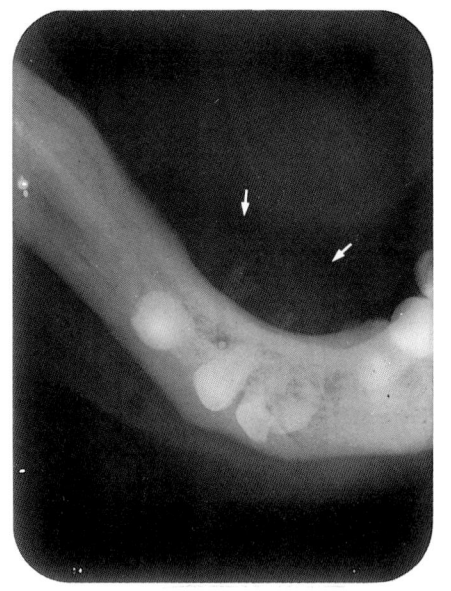

Fibrous epulis
6.18 Such soft tissue lesions do not normally show well on radiographs, but may be better demonstrated by reduced exposure. However, a proportion contain areas of mineralisation. The soft tissue outline (arrows) of this lesion on the lingual aspect of the lower anterior teeth extends from 5| to |2, describing a smooth curve. It contains several irregularly shaped mineralisations which are faintly radiopaque, many of them running at right angles to the surface of the mandible. LTO

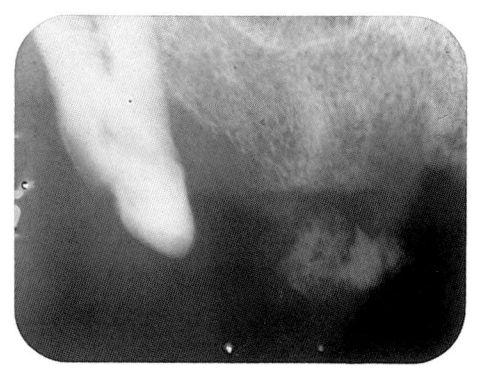

The Periodontium   115

6.19 Another inflammatory hyperplasia, the soft tissue outline of which is present in the maxillary right molar region, containing numerous radiopaque trabeculae of metaplastic bone towards its centre. There is no obvious continuity between the metaplastic bone and the underlying maxillary bone, the two being separated by radiolucent soft tissue, although there is a poorly defined area of radiolucency in the alveolus suggesting some bone resorption has occurred. The metaplastic bone lacks the fine trabeculation characteristic of normal bone. 8| is extensively carious with loss of its distal cusps, and a deep infrabony pocket is present mesially. P

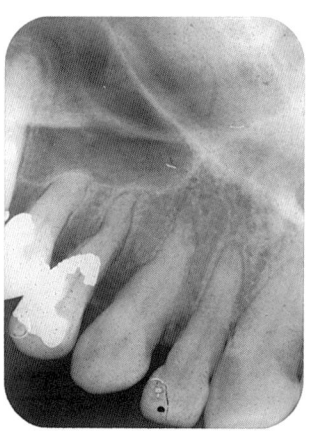

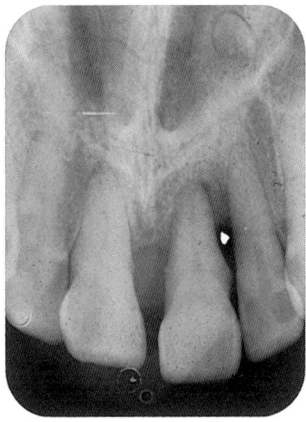

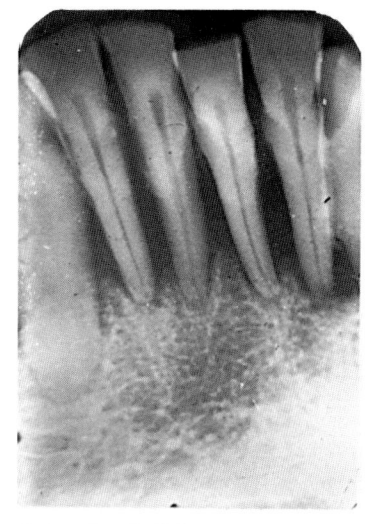

Avitaminosis C (scurvy)
6.22 In this condition, there may be early involvement of the periodontium leading to its rapid destruction. In this elderly patient, there is advanced loss of the interdental bone around the mandibular incisors, and the periodontal ligament space and lamina dura persist only in the periapical region of the teeth. Deposits of calculus are present on the cervical parts of the roots of the teeth projecting laterally and forming more densely radiopaque regions where they are superimposed upon the roots. P

Occlusal traumatism
6.20 (left) and 6.21 (right) Secondary occlusal traumatism in a patient with chronic periodontitis. There is generalised loss of bone from the crests of the interdental septa, which are blunted and exhibit irregular radiolucencies. The bone loss is particularly advanced |1. Around most teeth, the radiolucent periodontal ligament space is widened, so that it stands out more clearly than usual. This has arisen from the excessive movement of the teeth in their sockets, consequent upon the occlusal trauma. P

Chapter 7

The Facial Bones

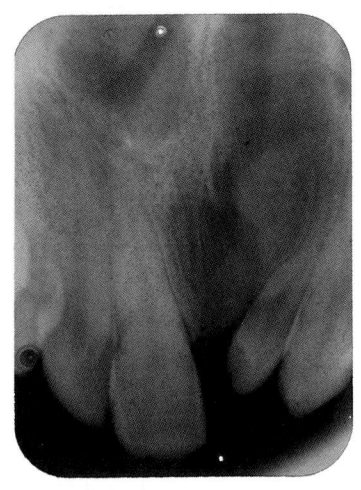

Cleft palate

7.1 A unilateral cleft extending through the left anterior alveolus. The poorly defined radiolucent defect runs between 1| and the malformed |2, which has a conical crown and a twisted root, the apex of which is curved mesially. The radiopaque lamina outlining the floor of the nose is absent on the affected side, indicating that the cleft extends into it. P

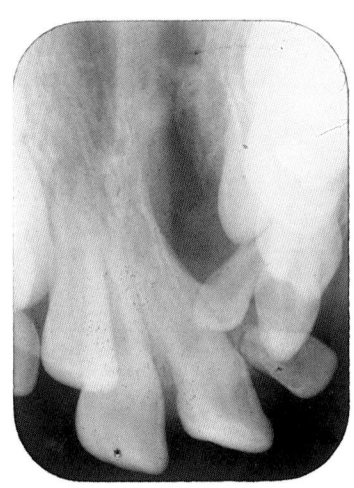

7.2 A unilateral, radiolucent cleft running between |B and |C, and which is continuous with the radiolucency of the nasal cavity, as indicated by the discontinuity of the lamina of the floor of the nose. To its mesial side, |1 is slightly retroclined, as indicated by its foreshortening, |2 is missing and |B is retained. Distally, two conical supernumerary teeth are present in a palatal position relative to the |CDE6. P

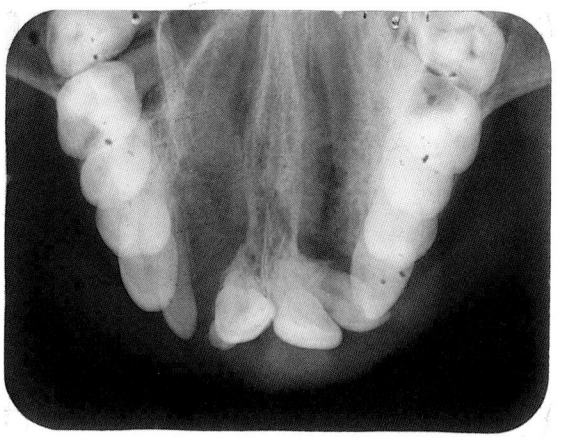

7.3 A bilateral cleft distal to 1| and |2, in which the central block of the premaxilla contains 1|12 and a small supernumerary tooth labially 1|. The premaxilla is continuous with the nasal septum, the outline of which is wider and more clearly visible than normal because of the palatal cleft. A conical supernumerary tooth is present distal to the cleft on the right. The lateral limits of the cleft running across the palate are often difficult to determine, but are probably indicated in this example by the radiolucent channels running antero-posteriorly to each side of the nasal septum. Note the artefacts overlying the occlusal surfaces of the teeth caused by damage to the emulsion of the film from the patient biting on it too firmly. USO

120   *A Radiological Atlas of Diseases of the Teeth and Jaws*

7.4 The majority of patients with cleft palate have underdevelopment of the maxilla producing a characteristic soft tissue outline. The tip of the nose is depressed and blunted and the upper lip retruded, so giving prominence to the lower lip. Note the prominence of the soft palate which forms an approximately vertical, radiopaque image, just posterior to the molar teeth. LC

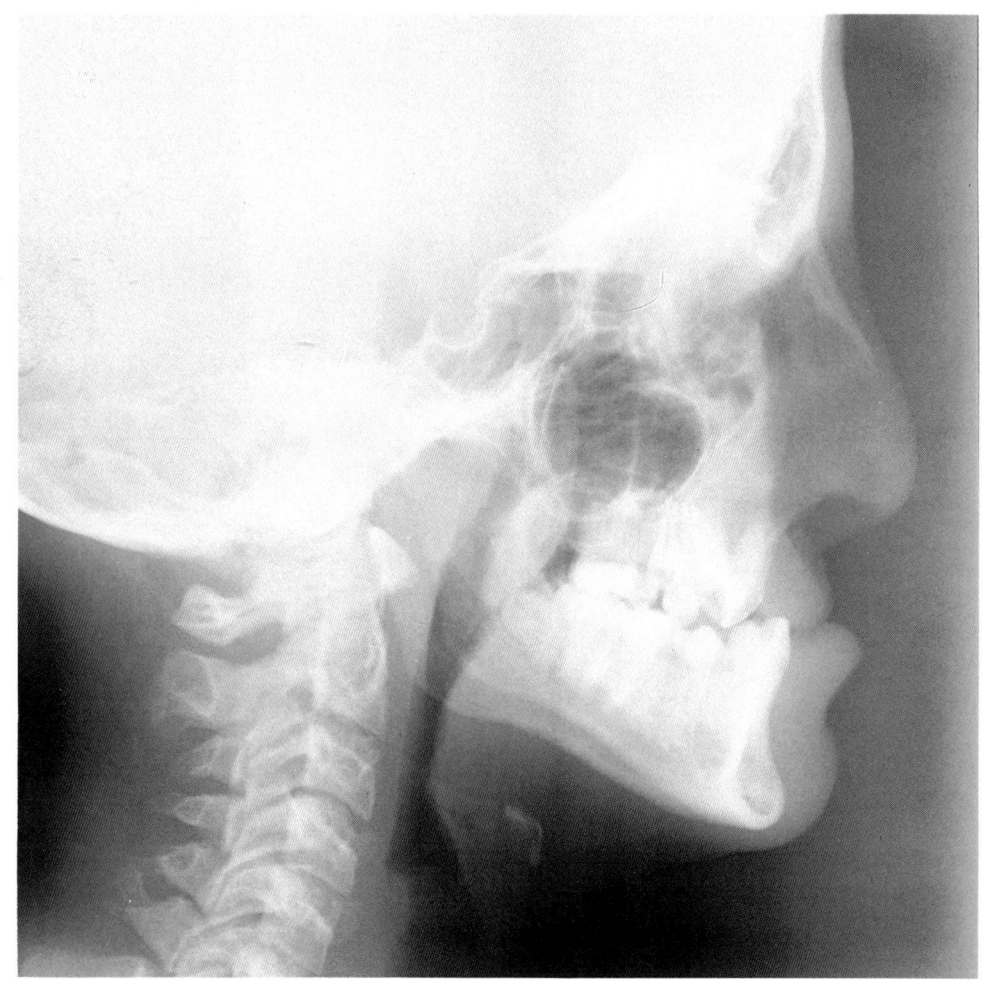

Torus mandibularis
7.5 This developmental abnormality consists of bilateral bony exostoses lingually to the mandibular premolar teeth. They are composed of dense cortical bone and are clearly displayed on this occlusal film, in which the genial tubercle can also be seen in the midline lingually. On a periapical film, they may be projected over the apices of the mandibular premolars, thus simulating an area of osteosclerosis. Note the unidentified, radiopaque fragments superimposed on the anterior margin of the tongue in the midline. LTO

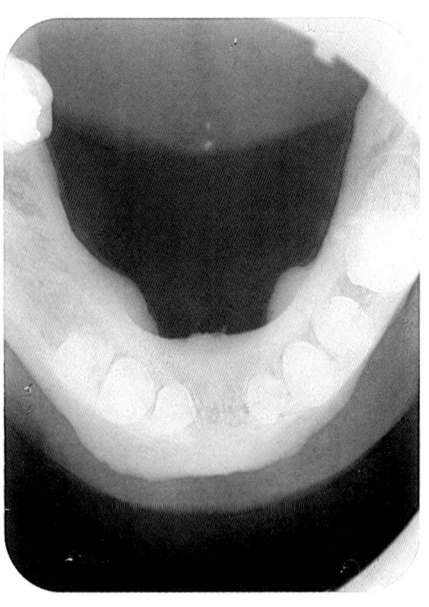

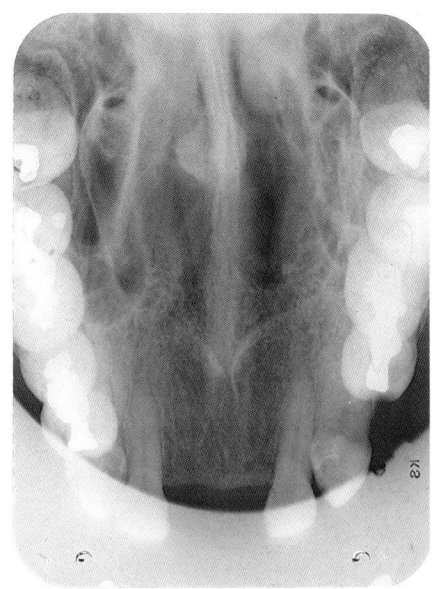

Torus palatinus
7.6 This developmental abnormality arises in the midline of the hard palate and forms a dense bony mass projecting into the mouth. In this example, a uniformly dense radiopaque mass is present on both sides of the nasal septum, although mostly on the right side. It has a smooth, clearly defined outline. USO

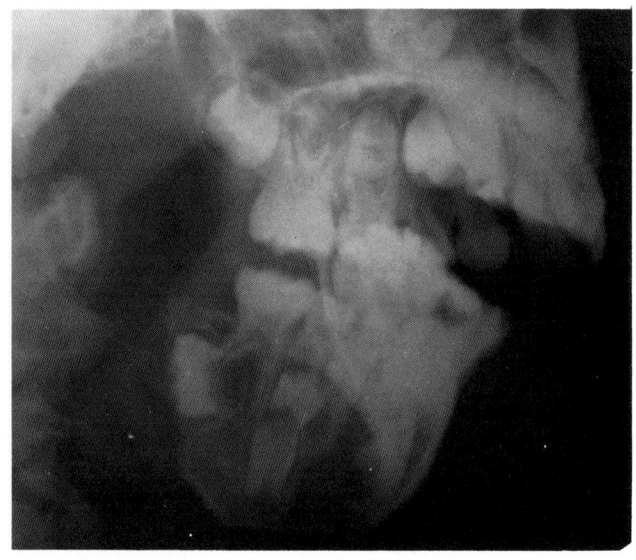

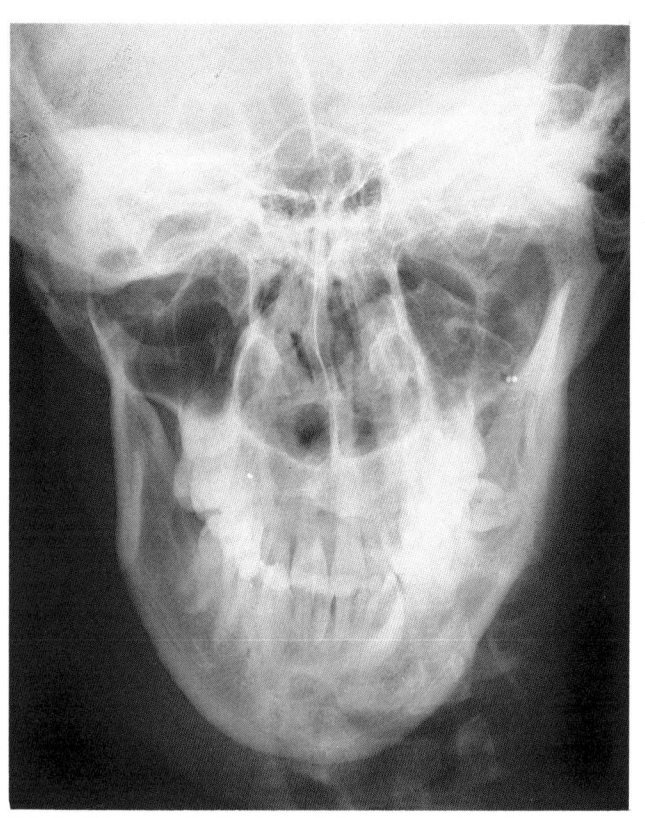

7.8 In this example, the defect is less severe, there being hypoplasia of the right mandibular ramus and condyle. The affected ramus is more medially placed, and the condylar head and coronoid process less well developed than on the normal side. There is deviation of the point of the chin to the affected side, although the mandibular and maxillary incisors are in normal relationship. The patient was also partially deaf on the right side and the pinna deformed. PA

First arch syndrome
7.7 In this condition, the development of any of the derivatives of the first branchial arch may be abnormal. On the affected side of this seven-year-old, there is complete absence of the condyle and ramus of the mandible resulting in pronounced micrognathia. E D| have erupted normally, but 6| is missing, and the developing 7| is displaced forwards, its crown lying horizontally and pointing posteriorly. 5| is also displaced anteriorly, lying beneath the unerupted 4|. In addition, the external auditory meatus is absent, but this is not clearly demonstrated in this film. OLM

Mandibulo-facial dysostosis (Treacher–Collins syndrome) 7.9 (top) and 7.10 (bottom) This developmental anomaly largely affects structures derived from the first branchial arch and groove. The maxilla and mandible are both underdeveloped, the latter markedly so, producing a receding chin (Fig. 7.9). There is also underdevelopment of the supra-orbital ridges, the zygomatic bones and zygomatic arches, all of which are difficult to identify. There is malocclusion with proclination of the maxillary and mandibular incisors, and crowding of the teeth (Fig. 7.10). The inferior border of the mandible is concave with pronounced antegonial notching and, in this example, the right maxillary antrum is less well developed. The pinna of the ear on the right side is underdeveloped and abnormally shaped. LC & PR

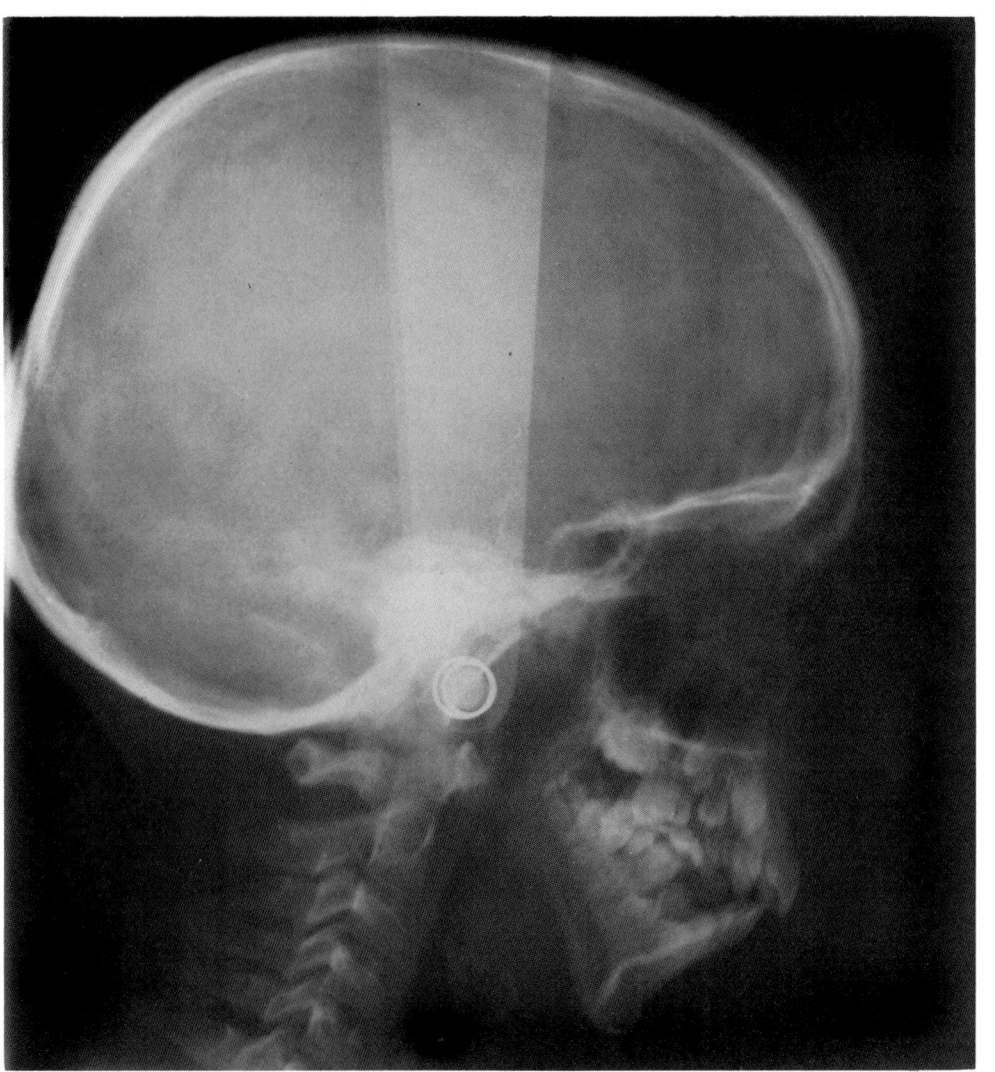

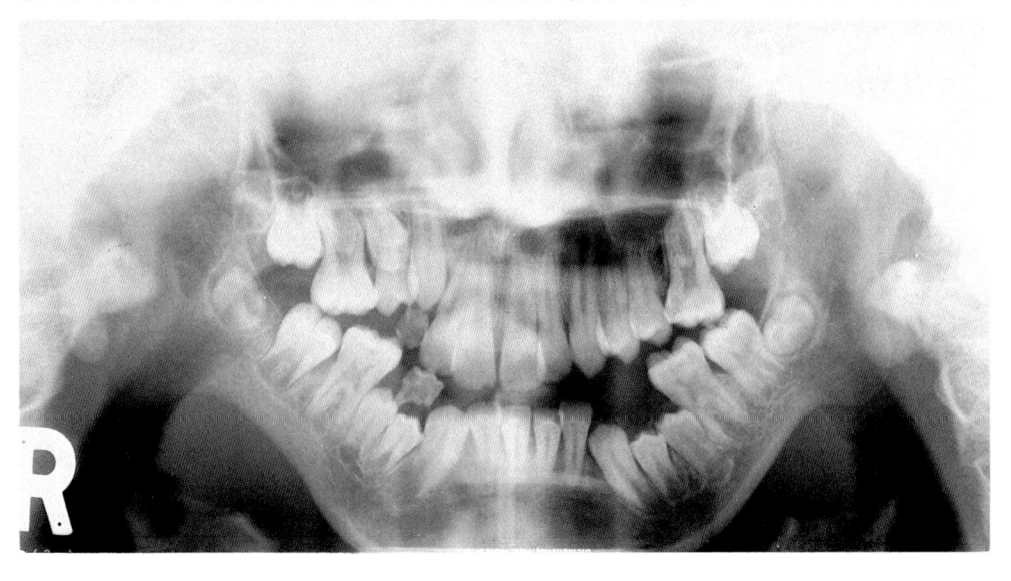

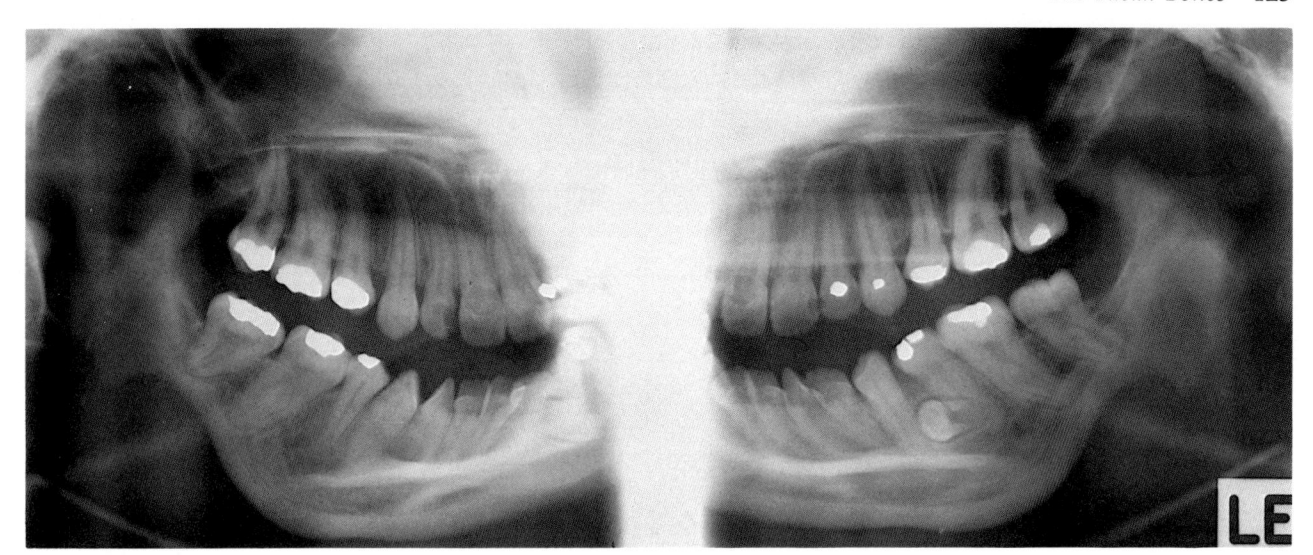

7.11 A severe example of mandibulo-facial dysostosis, showing marked underdevelopment of both rami of the mandible with absence of the condyles, extreme bowing of the inferior border of the mandible, with pronounced antegonial notches and absence of the zygomatic complexes bilaterally. Note the unerupted, incompletely developed, supplemental premolar in the left mandible. PR

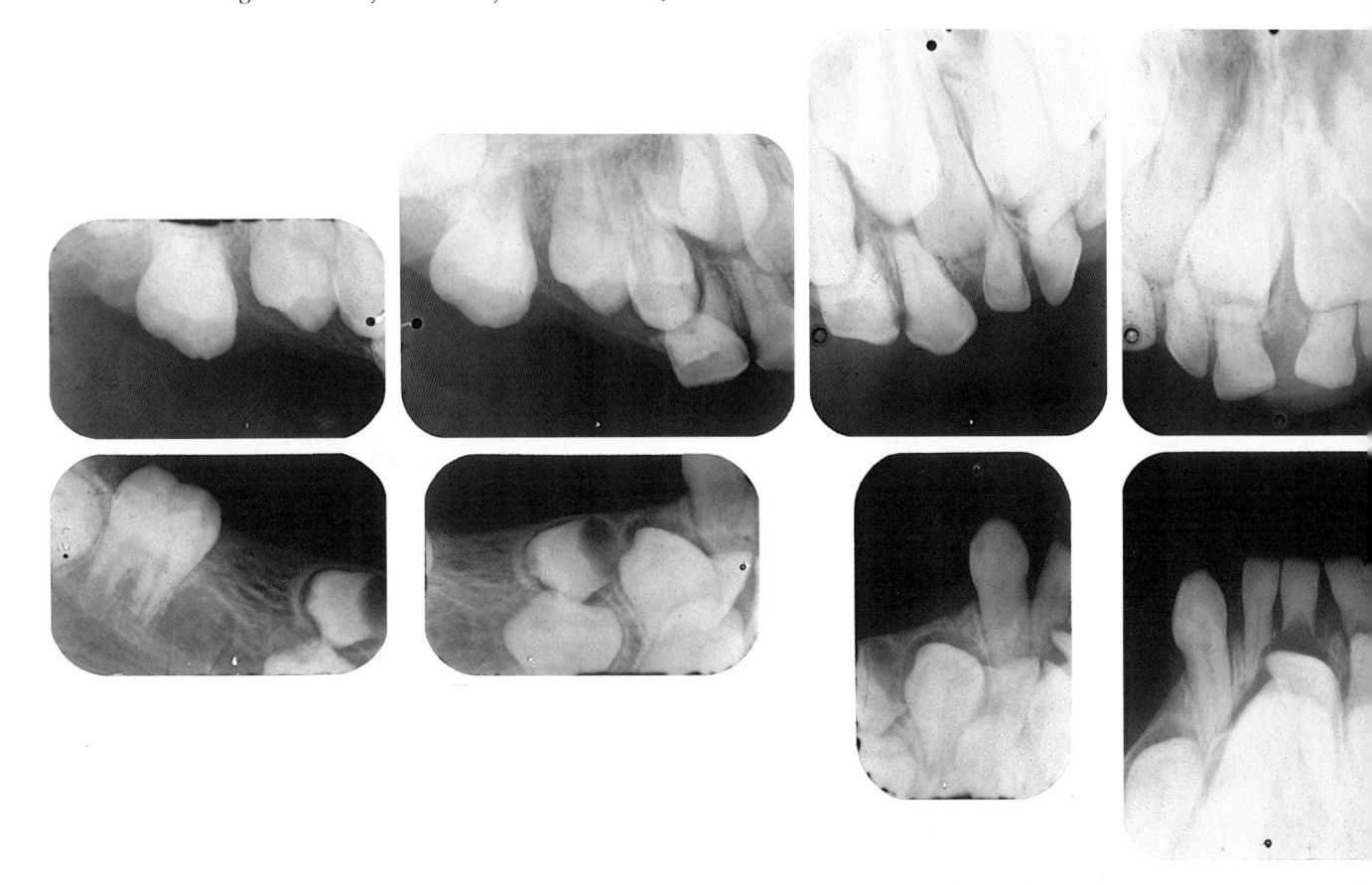

124 A Radiological Atlas of Diseases of the Teeth and Jaws

The Facial Bones 125

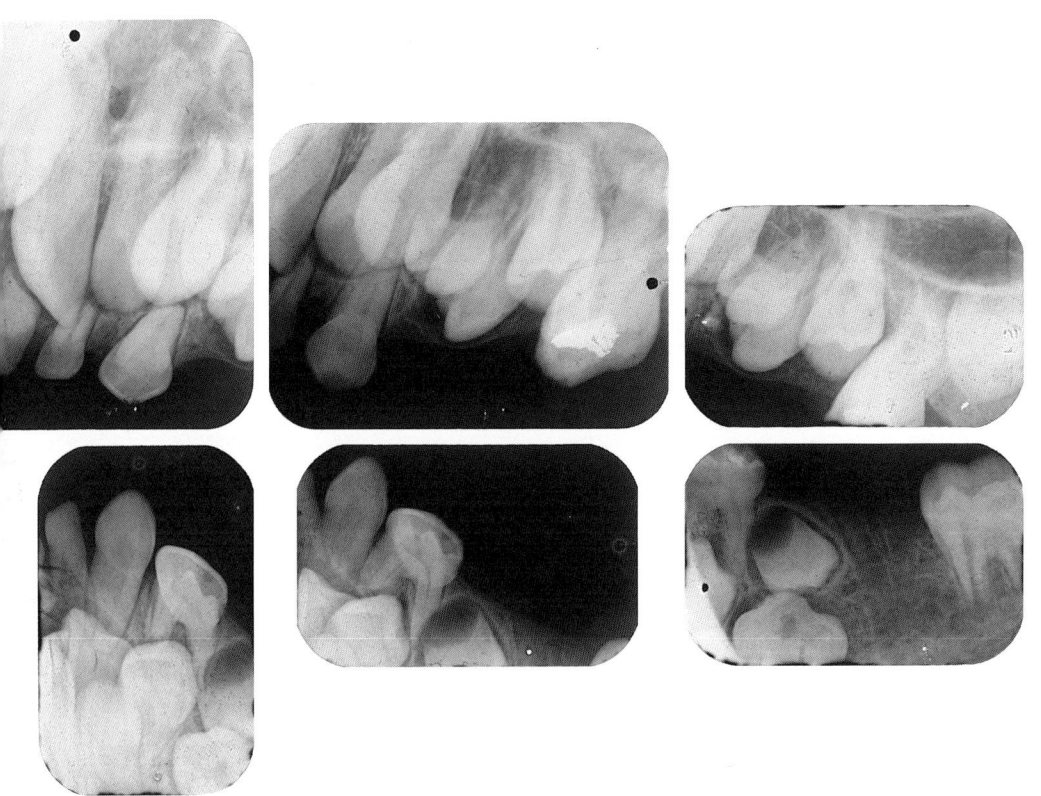

Cleido-cranial dysostosis
7.12 (above) 7.13 (right) In this disorder, there is delayed eruption of the permanent teeth, so that multiple, unerupted teeth, often including supernumeraries, are present, together with retention of the primary dentition. In this 14-year-old, all these features are present. There are several unerupted supernumerary teeth, which can be identified because their stage of development is behind that of the normal dentition. In addition to the dental abnormalities, many skeletal anomalies may be present, including the absence of the clavicles and the presence of Wormian bones, frontal bossing and maxillary retrognathism. In this case (Fig. 7.13), there is increased interorbital separation (hypertelorism), and several Wormian bones within the sagittal suture system of the vault of the skull, as indicated by the complex suture pattern. P & PA

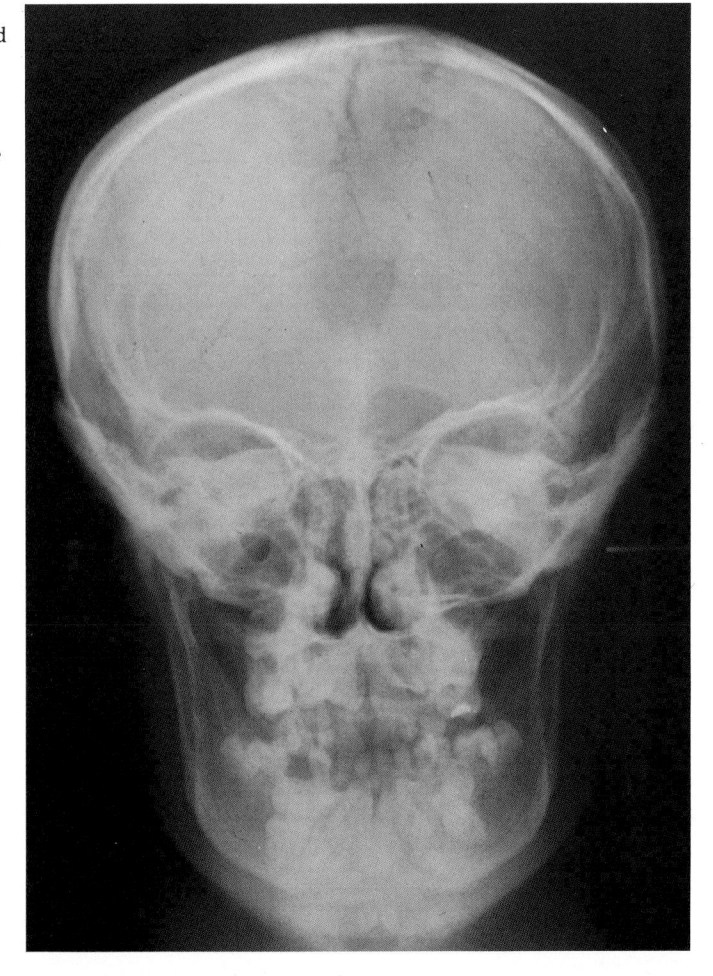

7.14 Many of the permanent teeth fail to erupt, even after many years, as demonstrated in this twenty-eight year old. The erupted teeth are:
$$\frac{7\ DS\ 2\ |\ 3S56}{6\ \ \ \ \ |1|12CD56}\ .\ PR$$

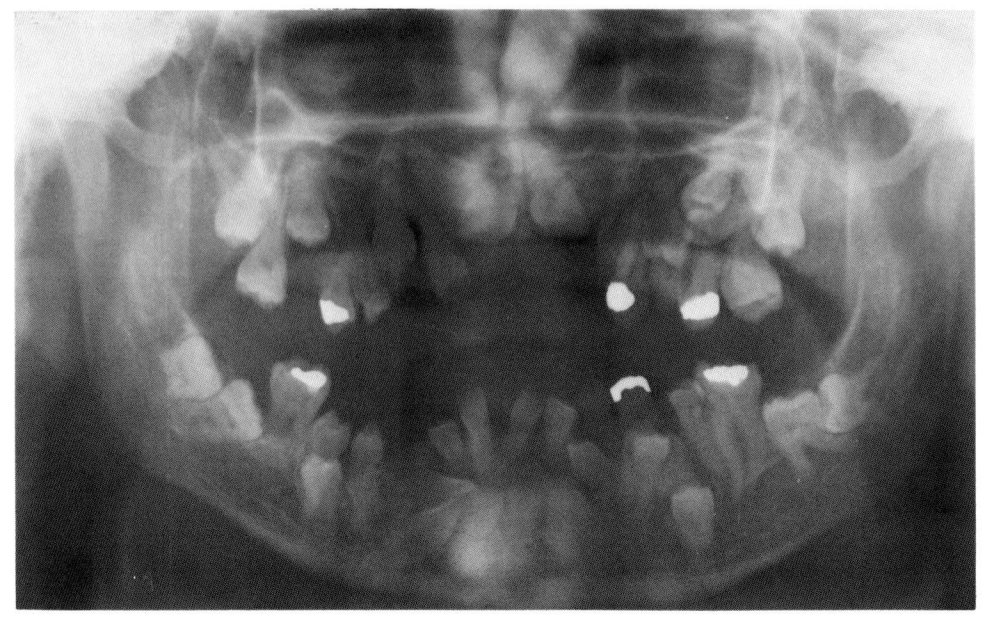

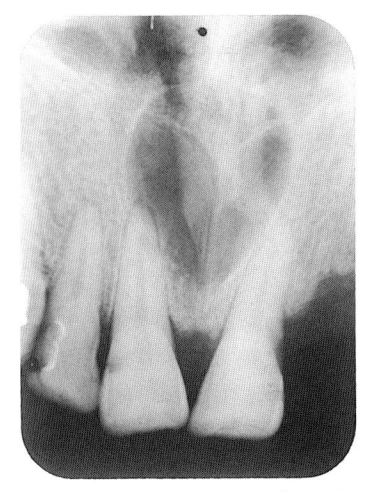

Nasopalatine (incisive canal) cyst

7.15 These developmental cysts produce a radiolucent defect in the anterior part of the midline of the maxilla and may be circular, pear-shaped or bilobed in outline. This pear-shaped lesion is bounded by a thin, radiopaque lamina and has caused slight divergence of the roots 1|1. The lamina dura and periodontal ligament space are continuous apically 1|1, and there are no grossly abnormal features coronally. Note the radiopaque images of the anterior nasal spine and anterior border of the floor of the nose superimposed on the radiolucent lesion. P

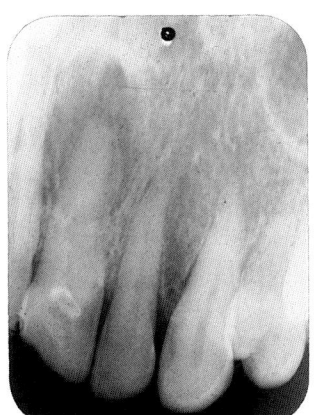

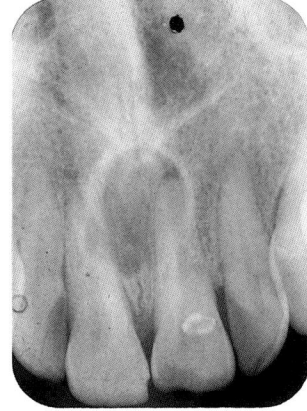

7.16 (left) and 7.17 (right) A small cyst may present difficulty in diagnosis for two reasons. Firstly, it is difficult to differentiate radiologically from a large incisive foramen, although a radiolucency greater than 6.0 mm in width laterally is likely to be cystic. Secondly, the area may be superimposed upon the roots 1|1, thus simulating a periapical lesion. In this example, the circular radiolucency, which is surrounded by a thin, radiopaque lamina, is superimposed upon the apical half of the root |1, although the periodontal ligament space and lamina dura are intact. A second film (Fig. 7.17), taken with the X-ray tube in the midline, reveals the palatal position of the lesion (parallax) between the roots of the two teeth. P

The Facial Bones 127

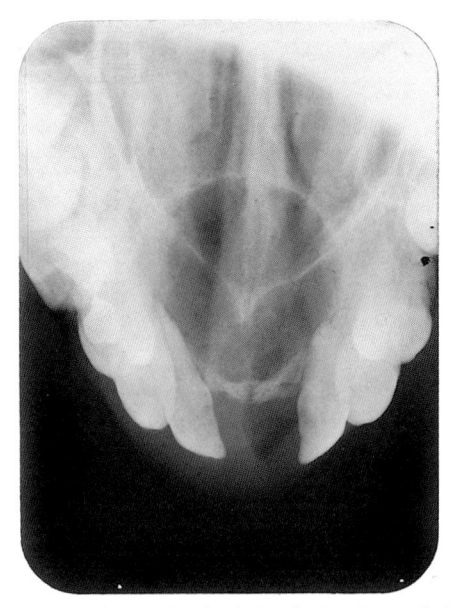

7.18 A large, clearly defined, circular, radiolucent lesion, bounded by a radiopaque lamina in the anterior midline of the maxilla in which 1|1 are absent. The teeth have been missing for several years, and the resulting gap is greatly reduced. In the absence of 1|1, the radiological differentiation between a nasopalatine cyst and a residual dental cyst may be difficult, but as a general rule a dental cyst would occur rather more to one side of the midline. Note the radiopaque images of the anterior nasal spine, anterior border of the floor of the nose, and anterior part of the nasal septum, which remain intact and are superimposed upon the lesion, and also the persistent anterior, midline suture. USO

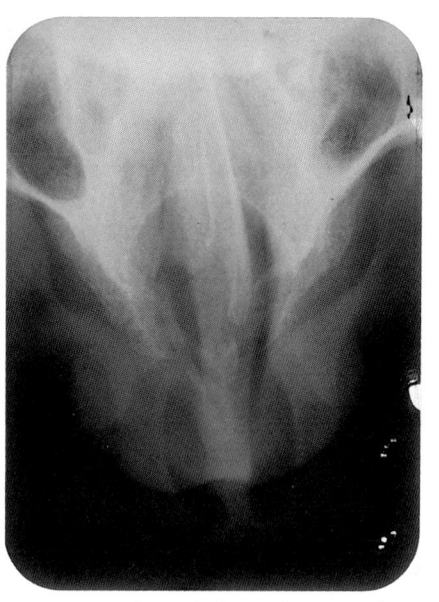

7.19 A circular, radiolucent lesion in the anterior midline of the palate of an edentulous patient. It is bounded by a thin, radiopaque lamina and has expanded the labial aspect of the ridge. Superimposed upon the lesion, the anterior part of the nasal septum is defective and a bilobed, radiolucent defect is present in the anterior part of the right side of the floor of the nose, indicating that the lesion has expanded into the nasal cavity. Note the shadow of the soft tissues of the nose. UTO

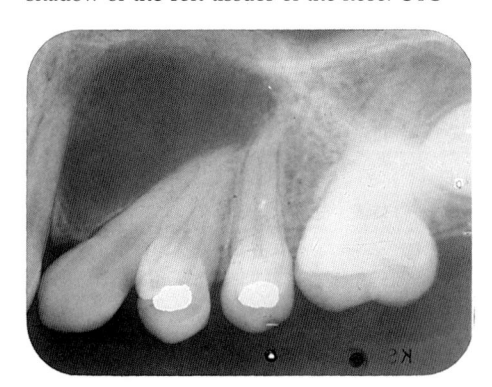

Globulomaxillary cyst
7.20 This cyst is believed to arise from proliferation of epithelial residues at the line of fusion of the globular and maxillary processes. Thus it typically arises between the maxillary second incisor and canine, as in this example, resulting in displacement of their roots mesially and distally, respectively. This radiolucent cyst has a clearly defined margin and is pear-shaped, the bell of the pear lying superior to the roots of the teeth. There is slight expansion upwards of the cortical lamina of the floor of the nose, and despite the size of the lesion the crestal bone interdentally |23 remains intact. |4 root has also been displaced distally. P

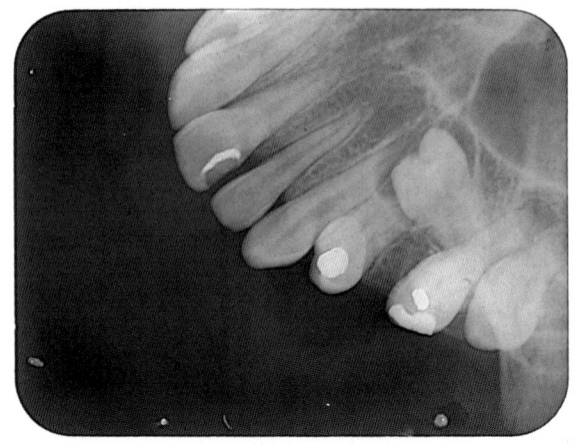

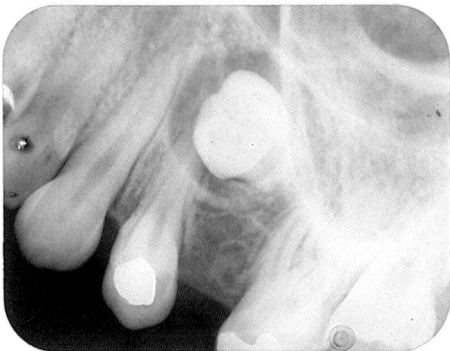

128   *A Radiological Atlas of Diseases of the Teeth and Jaws*

Dentigerous cyst

7.21 (top) and 7.22 (bottom)   The dentigerous cyst is an expansile lesion associated with the crown of an unerupted tooth, causing a radiolucent defect of increasing size. In a small lesion such as this one, radiological distinction from a large tooth follicle is impossible. The circular, radiolucent lesion is surrounded by a thin, radiopaque lamina and envelops symmetrically the crown of |5 up to its neck. The lesion lies palatally to |4 (parallax), which is not displaced and is separated by diastemas from the adjacent teeth. UOO & P

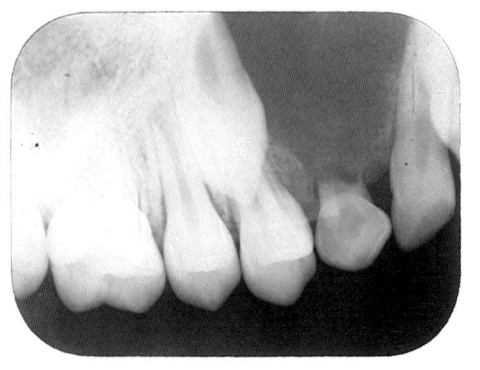

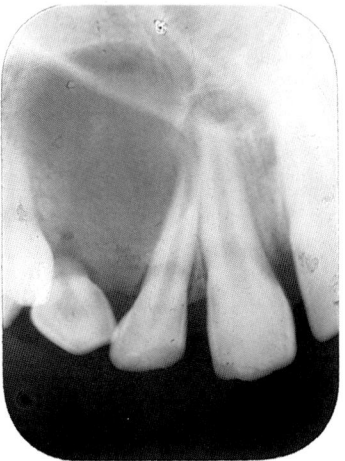

7.23 (top) and 7.24 (bottom)   In the maxilla, these lesions most commonly arise on canines, as in this example in a 12-year-old. The approximately circular radiolucent cyst arising on 3| is of uniform density and is circumscribed by a clearly defined, thin, radiopaque lamina. The unerupted tooth is vertically placed, lying in the posterior wall of the cyst. The root 4| and 2| are displaced distally and mesially, respectively, and C| is retained, although there is advanced root resorption. Note the intact radiopaque lamina of the anterior margin of the floor of the nose running obliquely across the lesion (Fig. 7.24). P

7.25   In this six-year-old, there is a large, radiolucent cyst associated with the crown of the developing, unerupted |1, which together with |2 has been displaced posteriorly. The approximately circular lesion has caused expansion of the buccal surface of the maxilla, where only a thin lamina (arrows) of bone remains. A| has exfoliated from above the normally erupting 1|, but the root of |A is displaced laterally showing no evidence of resorption, and the other primary teeth are still present. The circular area of darker radiolucency within the lesion and the absence of the lamina of the anterior margin of the bone of the floor of the nose indicate that it has been perforated. UTO

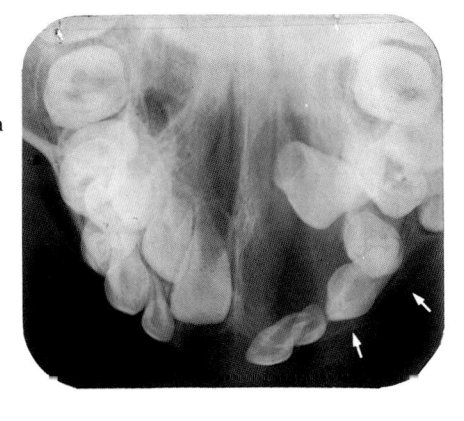

The Facial Bones 129

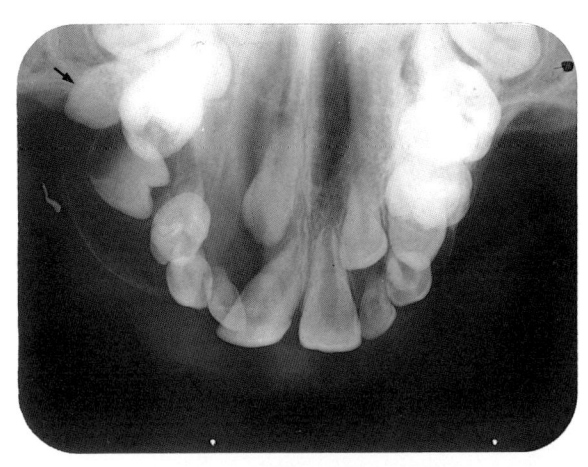

7.26 This large, well circumscribed, approximately circular, radiolucent cyst extends from the midline of the palate medially to the margin of the expanded alveolus laterally, where only a thin lamina of bone remains. The lesion has arisen in an eight-year-old, on the crown of an unerupted 3⎦ (arrow) which is displaced posteriorly. DCB1⎦ are erupted normally, although the root 1⎦ is displaced mesially. When compared with the unaffected side, 2⎦ and 4⎦ are unerupted and displaced medially and buccally, respectively. USO

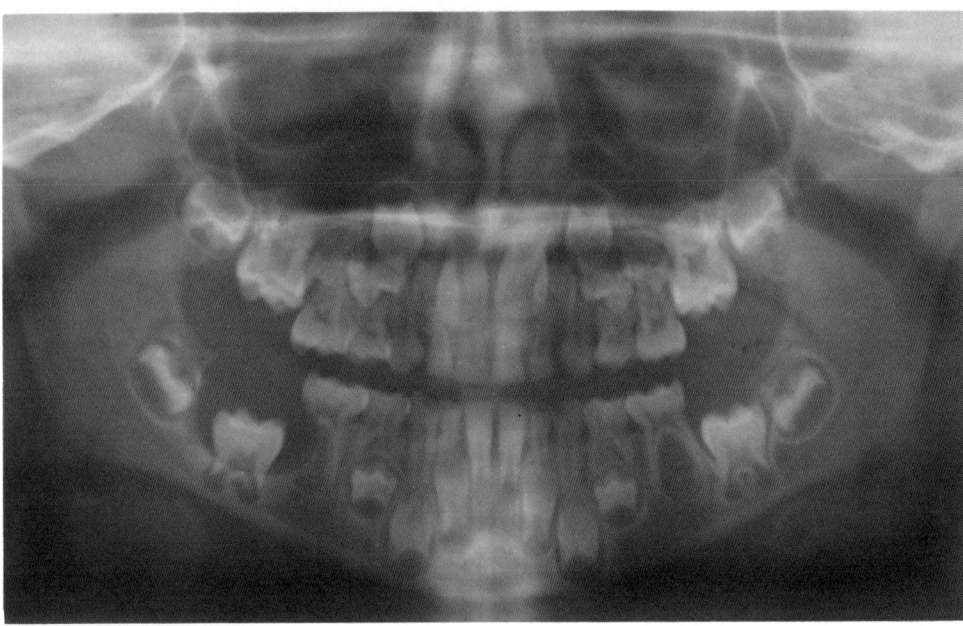

7.27 A small, circular, radiolucent cyst encompassing symmetrically the crown 6⎦ in a six-year-old. The crestal bone is perforated and the overlying soft tissues expanded, but the rest of the lesion is bounded by a thin, radiopaque lamina. The associated tooth is displaced inferiorly and only its crown projects into the cyst cavity. There has been resorption of the whole of the distal root E̅⎦. Note the failure of 5̅⎩5̅ to develop, although faintly radiolucent follicular spaces are present inter-radicularly E̅⎪E̅. PR

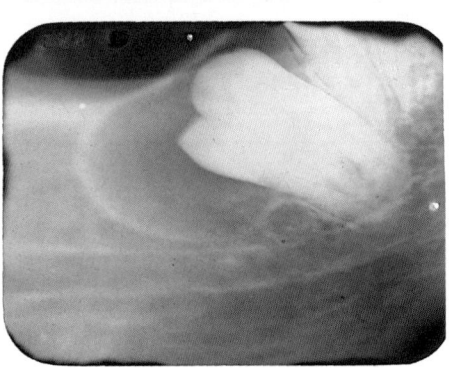

7.28 Another small cyst lying eccentrically around the crown of a disto-angularly impacted 8̅⎦. Because of the position of the tooth, the majority of the radiolucent cyst cavity lies postero-inferiorly. It is surrounded by a thin, radiopaque lamina and has caused expansion of the overlying alveolus. Note the inferior alveolar canal, which is normal. P

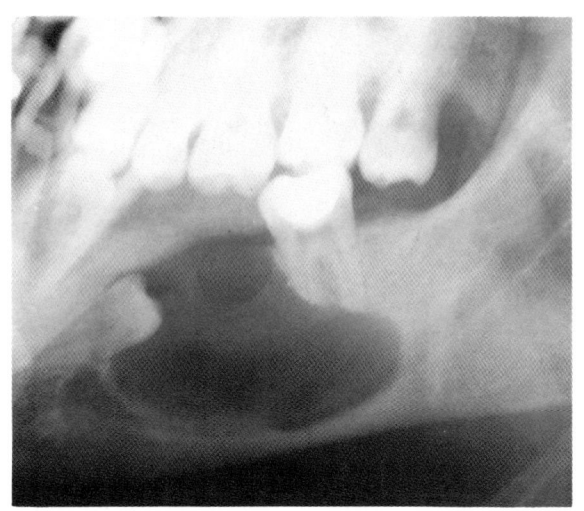

130   A Radiological Atlas of Diseases of the Teeth and Jaws

7.29   A cyst arising on the crown of an unerupted ⌊5 in a partially edentulous mandible. This tooth lies horizontally, its crown facing distally and projecting into the clearly defined radiolucency which reaches to the ⌊8 region posteriorly and to the inferior border of the mandible. The apices of both roots of ⌊7 are blunted and the mesial root shortened, indicating resorption has occurred. Clearly defined areas of darker radiolucency within the lesion indicate perforation of the buccal or lingual cortical plates. The inferior alveolar canal is displaced towards the inferior border of the mandible. OLM

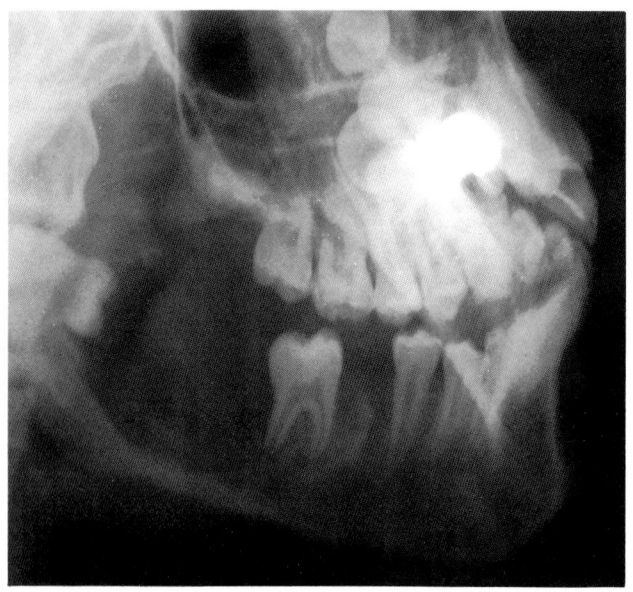

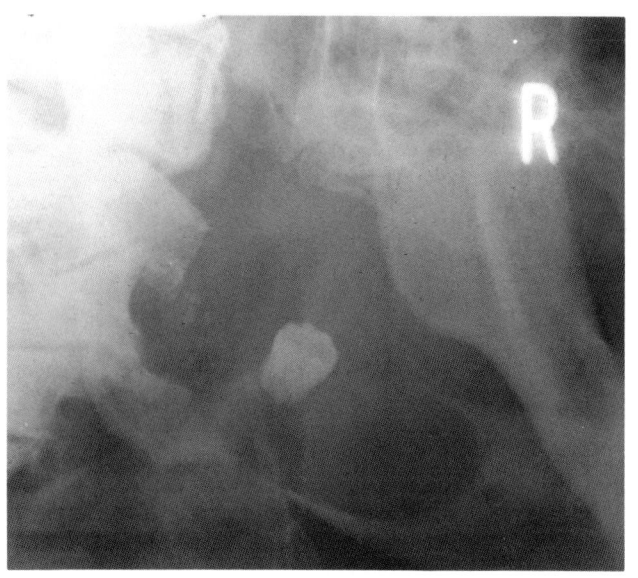

7.31 (above) and 7.32 (right)   A large cyst associated with an unerupted 8̄| in an otherwise edentulous mandible. The clearly defined radiolucency extends from the coronoid notch of the ramus posteriorly, to the 5̄| region anteriorly. The alveolar surface of the mandible and anterior aspect of the ramus up to the base of the coronoid process have been perforated, and only a thin layer of cortical bone remains inferiorly, although there is no evidence of pathological fracture. In the posterior part of the lesion, there are several radiopaque flakes, which are probably remnants of the cortical bone. The radiopaque images (Fig. 7.31) of the hyoid bone and of the bodies of the atlas and axis vertebrae overlie the cystic defect. There is buccal and lingual expansion of the ramus (Fig. 7.32), and 8̄| lies transversely on the buccal side of the cyst. OLM & PA

7.30   A large cyst associated with an unerupted 8̄|, which which has been displaced into the ramus of the mandible. The clearly defined radiolucency surrounds the crown of the tooth posteriorly and passes anteriorly to the distal aspect 7|, in which root formation is not yet complete. The U-shaped radiopaque image of the hyoid bone overlies the cystic defect. Note the undiagnosed, radiodense foreign body superimposed upon the upper teeth. OLM

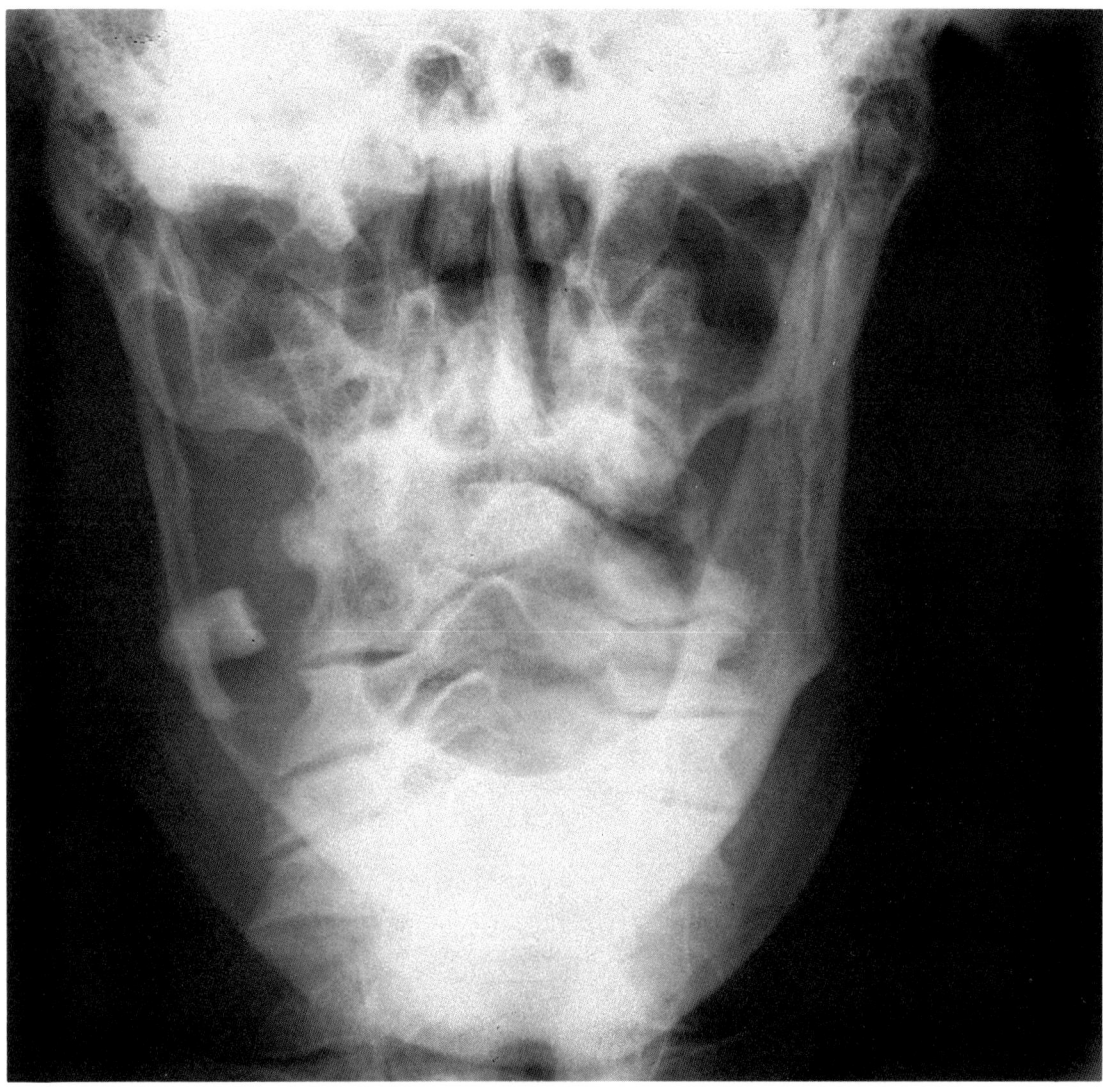

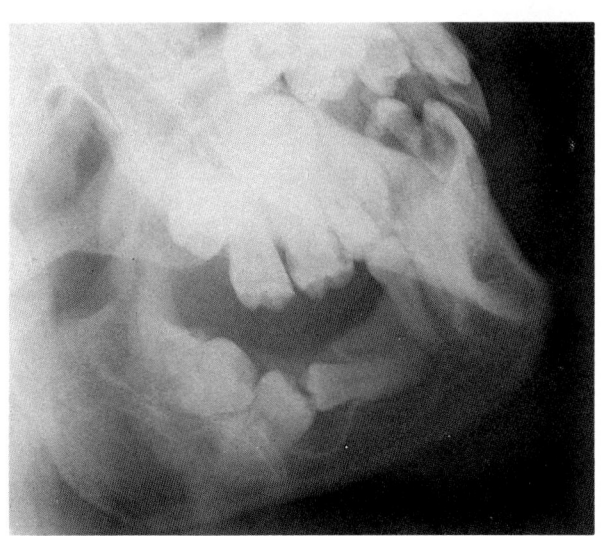

7.33 Rarely, more than one tooth may be associated with the same cyst. In this example, the crowns of $\overline{7|}$ and $\overline{5|}$, which are mesio-angularly and disto-angularly impacted, respectively, project into the radiolucent cyst cavity. A thin, radiopaque lamina surrounds the lesion inferiorly and anteriorly. $\overline{8|}$ is horizontally impacted, its crown surrounded by a radiolucent follicular space of normal size. $\overline{6|}$ is missing. OLM

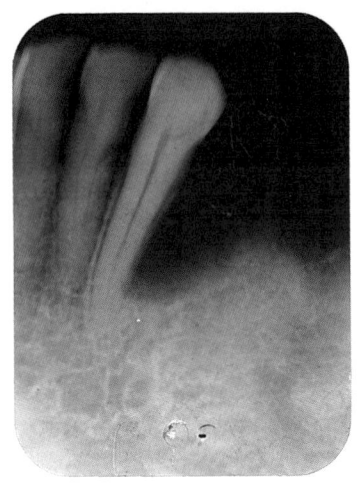

132 *A Radiological Atlas of Diseases of the Teeth and Jaws*

Odontogenic keratocyst
7.34 This lesion has a very varied radiological appearance and may simulate many other types of odontogenic cyst and tumour. In this example, there is an ovoid radiolucency distal to $\overline{3|}$, with a clearly defined lower margin and loss of the lamina dura and alveolar bone distally. P

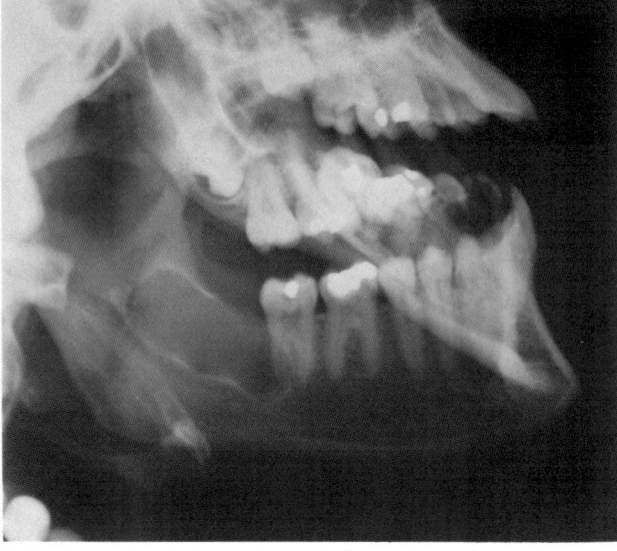

7.35 An oval radiolucent lesion in the molar region and ramus of the right side of the mandible. It has a slightly scalloped outline which is demarcated by a thin, radiopaque lamina, except superiorly distal to $\overline{7|}$. The anterior extremity of the lesion overlies the distal root $\overline{7|}$, and the inferior margin approximates the inferior alveolar canal. Note the absence of $\overline{8|}$ indicating the probable primordial origin of the cyst. OLM

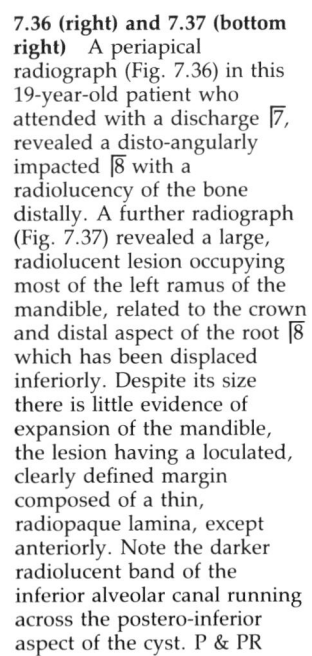

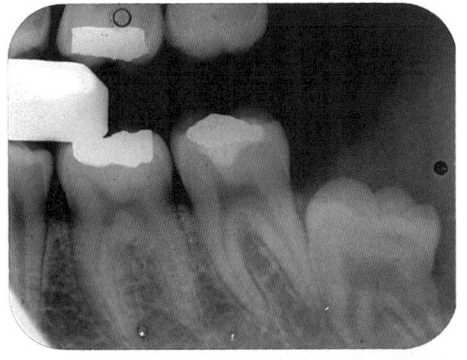

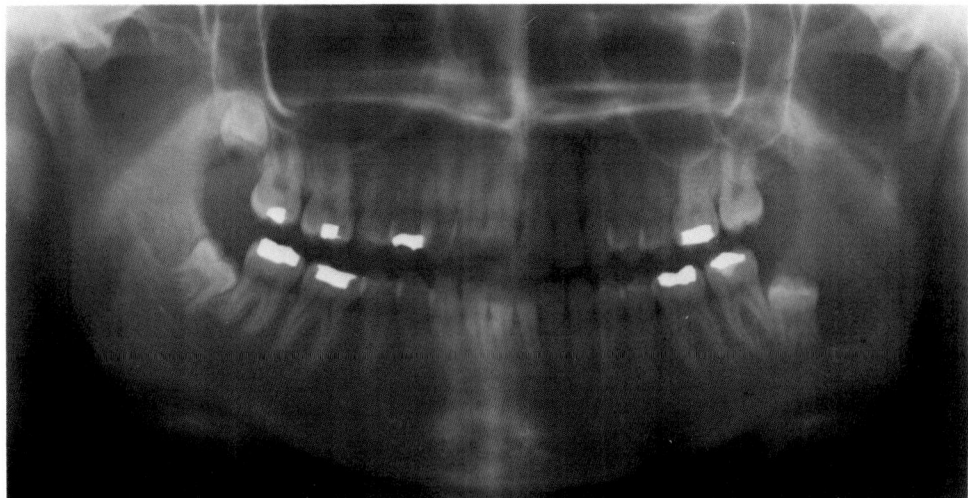

7.36 (right) and 7.37 (bottom right) A periapical radiograph (Fig. 7.36) in this 19-year-old patient who attended with a discharge $|\overline{7}$, revealed a disto-angularly impacted $|\overline{8}$ with a radiolucency of the bone distally. A further radiograph (Fig. 7.37) revealed a large, radiolucent lesion occupying most of the left ramus of the mandible, related to the crown and distal aspect of the root $|\overline{8}$ which has been displaced inferiorly. Despite its size there is little evidence of expansion of the mandible, the lesion having a loculated, clearly defined margin composed of a thin, radiopaque lamina, except anteriorly. Note the darker radiolucent band of the inferior alveolar canal running across the postero-inferior aspect of the cyst. P & PR

The Facial Bones 133

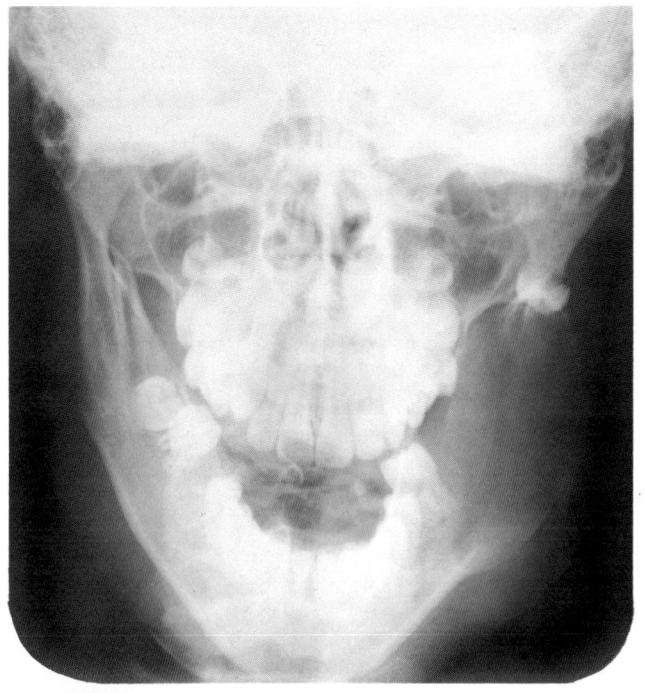

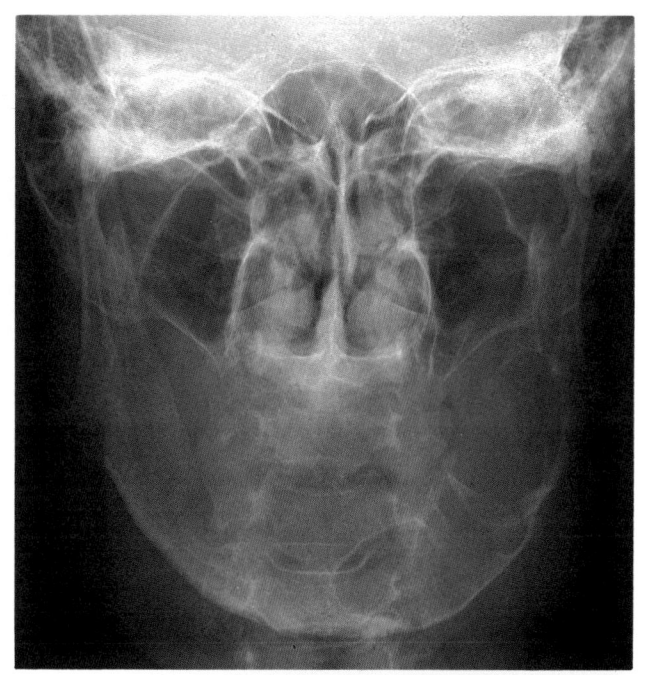

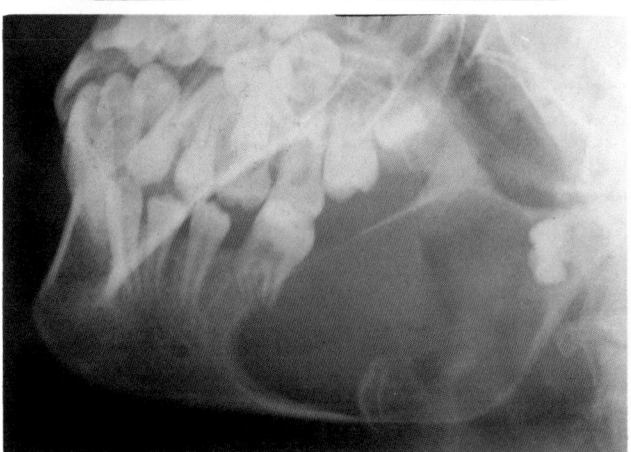

7.38 (top) and 7.39 (bottom) In this 13-year-old, there is a large, radiolucent lesion of the left ramus associated with an unerupted ⌐8, which has been displaced into the neck of the condyle. The ramus is expanded anteriorly, buccally and lingually with marked thinning of the cortical bone. The cyst has a smooth outline with a thin, radiopaque lamina. The relationship of the lesion to the crown of the tooth could be interpreted as that of a dentigerous cyst, but closer examination indicates that the cyst does not envelope the entire crown, suggesting that the tooth is outside the lesion. Further, the early stage of development ⌐8 associated with a cyst of this size, makes a diagnosis of dentigerous cyst unlikely. Note the inferior alveolar canal which has been displaced postero-inferiorly by the cyst. The shadow of the hyoid bone is superimposed upon the lesion inferiorly (Fig. 7.39). PA & OLM

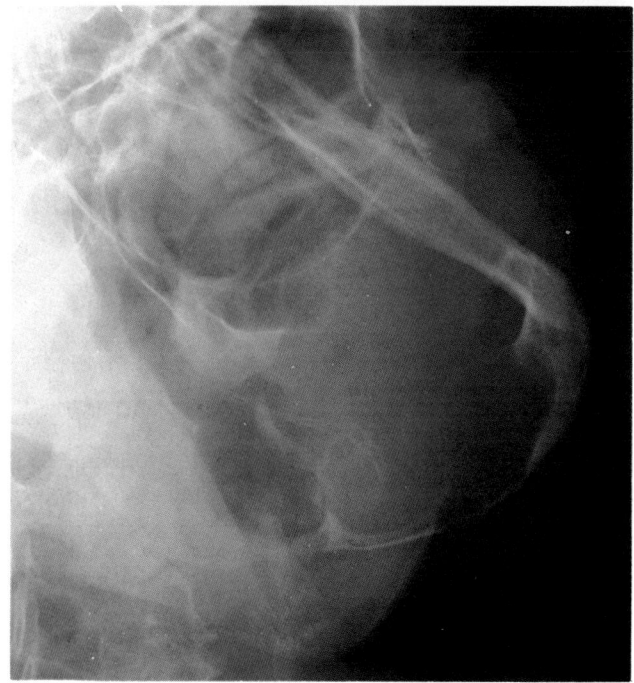

7.40 (top) and 7.41 (bottom) A large, multilocular, radiolucent lesion of the left body and ramus of an edentulous mandible, extending to the midline. All round the lesion there is thinning of the cortical bone, which has been eroded on the alveolar aspect, and despite its size there is only slight expansion of the lingual aspect of the mandible. Bony septa divide the lesion into locules, giving an appearance similar to that of ameloblastoma. Note the superimposition of the hyoid bone over the lesion (Fig. 7.41). PA & OLM

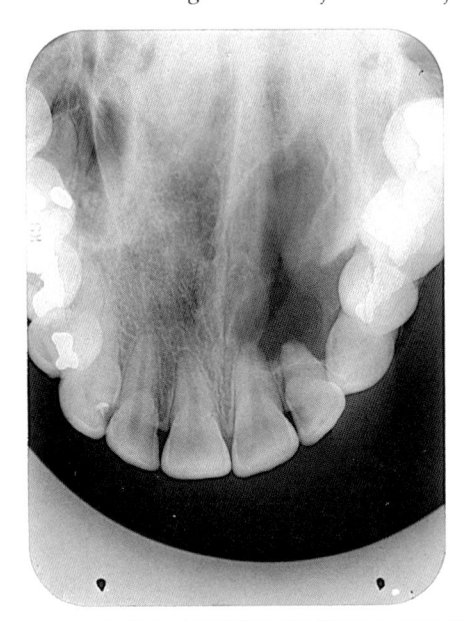

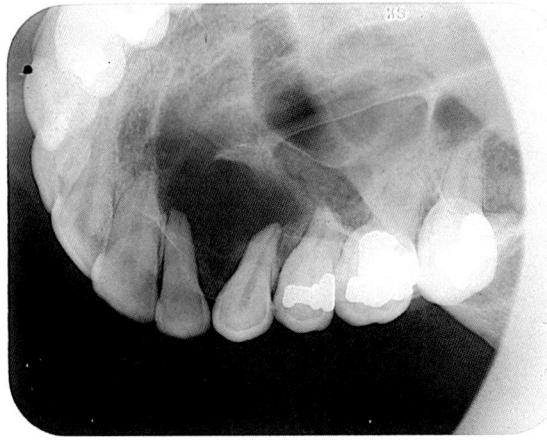

7.42 (top) and 7.43 (bottom) A radiolucent lesion of the left maxilla with a loculated outline partly surrounded by a radiopaque lamina. It extends from the midline of the palate to the alveolus from |1 to |6. There is displacement of the roots |2 and |3 mesially and distally, respectively. The variation in the degree of radiolucency of the lesion indicates a variable amount of thinning and possibly perforation of the cortical plates. The exact outline of the cyst is difficult to determine because of the superimposition of the images of the maxillary antrum, nasal cavity and zygomatic process. Note the resorption of the apical parts of the roots |12 and the absence of lamina dura disto-apically |2 and mesio-apically |3. USO & UOO

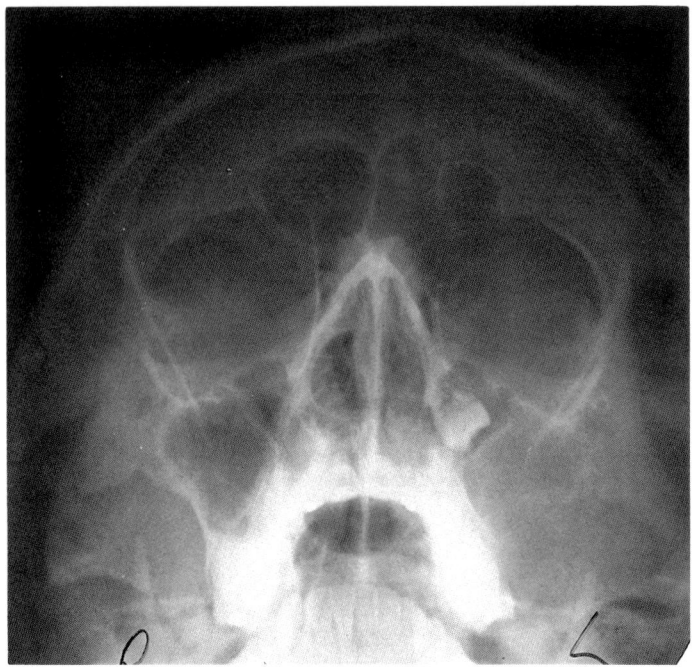

7.44 A large lesion of the left maxilla occupying the majority of the antrum and associated with an unerupted |8 which has been displaced into its roof. The full extent of the lesion is difficult to determine as its outline is indistinct, but the antrum is relatively radiopaque and there is destruction of its lateral wall. The radiopaque boundary of the roof of the antrum is clearly shown, together with the infra-orbital foramen. OM

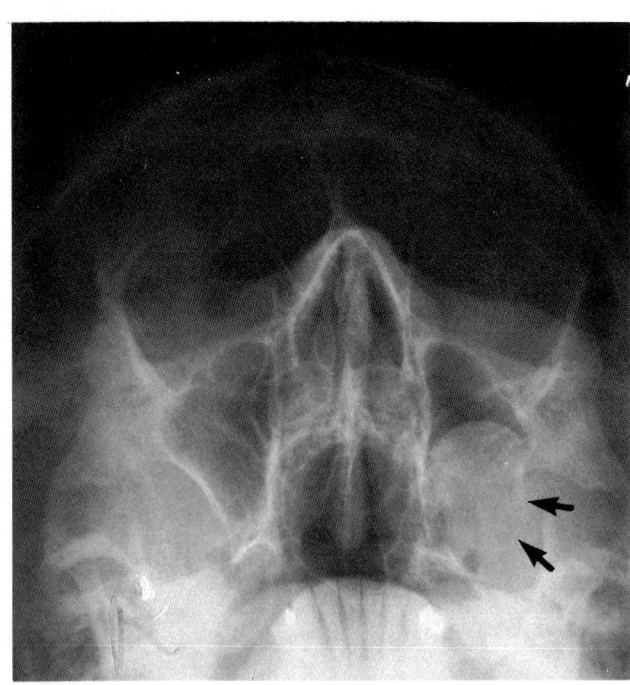

7.45 (top left) and 7.46 (bottom left) A cyst in the edentulous left maxilla which has expanded the lateral wall (arrows) and floor of the antrum, forming a relatively radiopaque, dome-shaped mass projecting into it. The overall radiopacity of the lesion, together with the thin, radiopaque lamina superiorly (Fig. 7.46), indicate that it is surrounded by a thin layer of bone and thus separate from the antral cavity. Note the two vertically running, radiolucent, pterygo-maxillary fissures (Fig. 7.46), each bounded by thin, radiopaque laminae, at the posterior aspect of the mass. The anterior one is projected from the opposite side of the jaw and is superimposed upon the mass, its superior end leading to the densely radiolucent pterygo-palatine foramen. OM & L

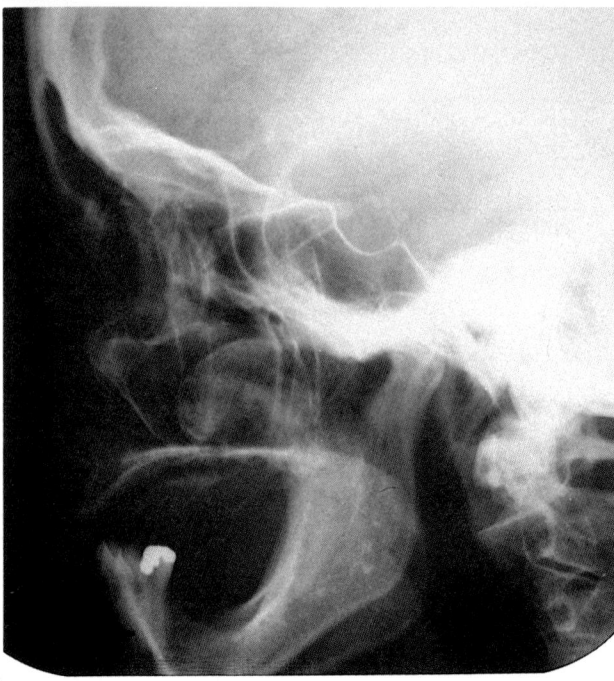

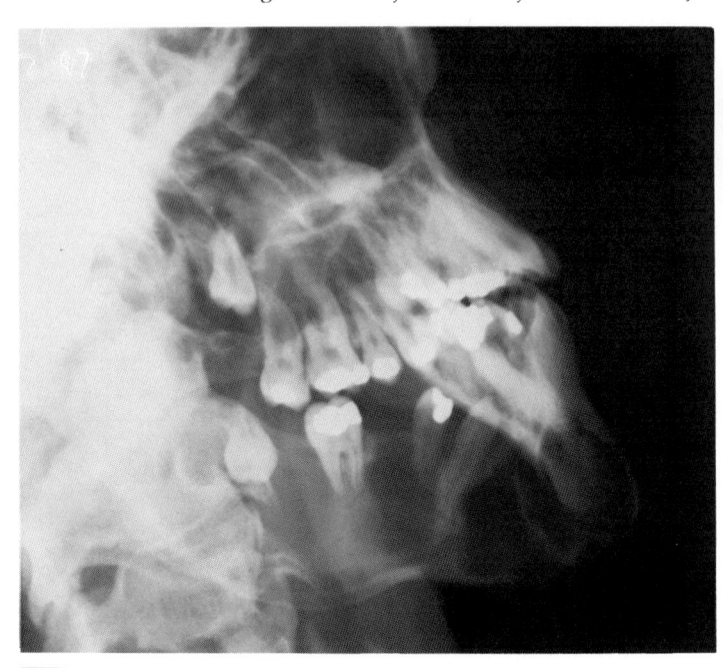

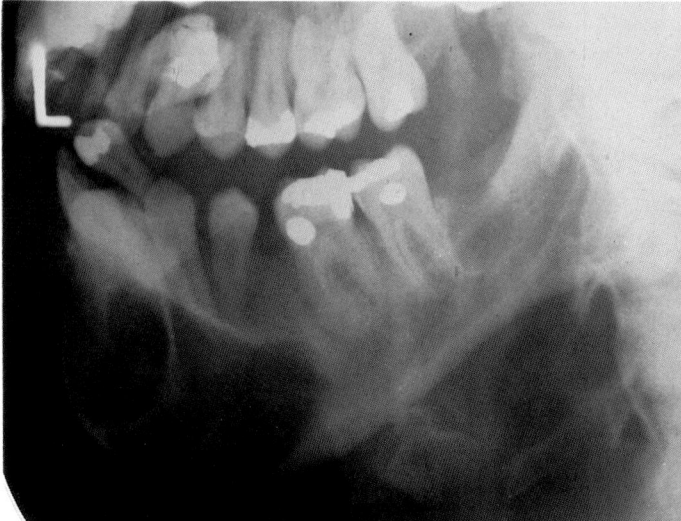

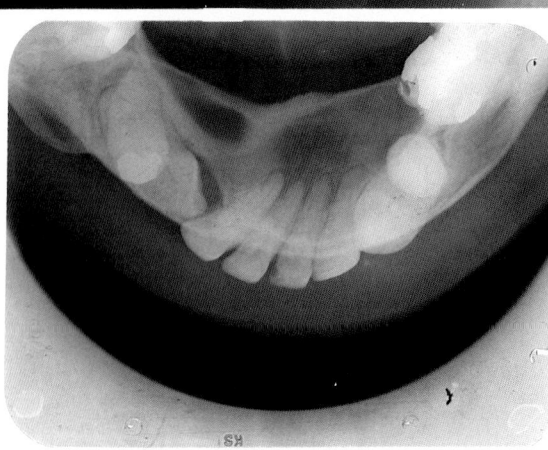

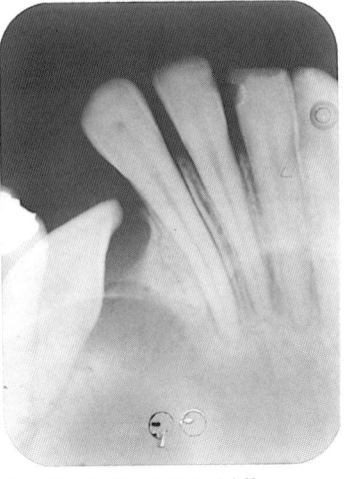

7.47 (top left), 7.48 (middle left), 7.49 (bottom left), 7.50 (above) and 7.51 (right) Multiple radiolucent lesions in the jaws of a patient with the Gorlin and Goltz syndrome. There are three separate cysts in the mandible, one in the right molar region and ramus (Fig. 7.47), one in the anterior part of the mandible extending from 3| to |6 (Figs 7.47 and 7.48) and one in the |8 region (Fig. 7.48). The mandible is expanded inferiorly in the right molar region and inferiorly and lingually (Fig. 7.49) in the anterior part. The cyst outlines are loculated with a clearly defined, radiopaque lamina. There is displacement of the associated teeth, 8| being inverted and unerupted (Fig. 7.47) and 3| incompletely erupted, the inferior aspect of its crown being surrounded by a large follicular space (Fig. 7.50). Note the normal periodontal ligament space and lamina dura around the roots of the anterior teeth, between which Hirschfeld's vascular canals are clearly displayed, and the postero-inferior displacement of the inferior alveolar canal (Fig. 7.47). Patients with this syndrome often have other skeletal abnormalities, including bifid ribs, bifid vertebral spines and areas of dystrophic mineralisation of the soft tissues, notably of the diaphragmatica sellae and falx cerebri (Fig. 7.51). OLM, LTO, P & PA

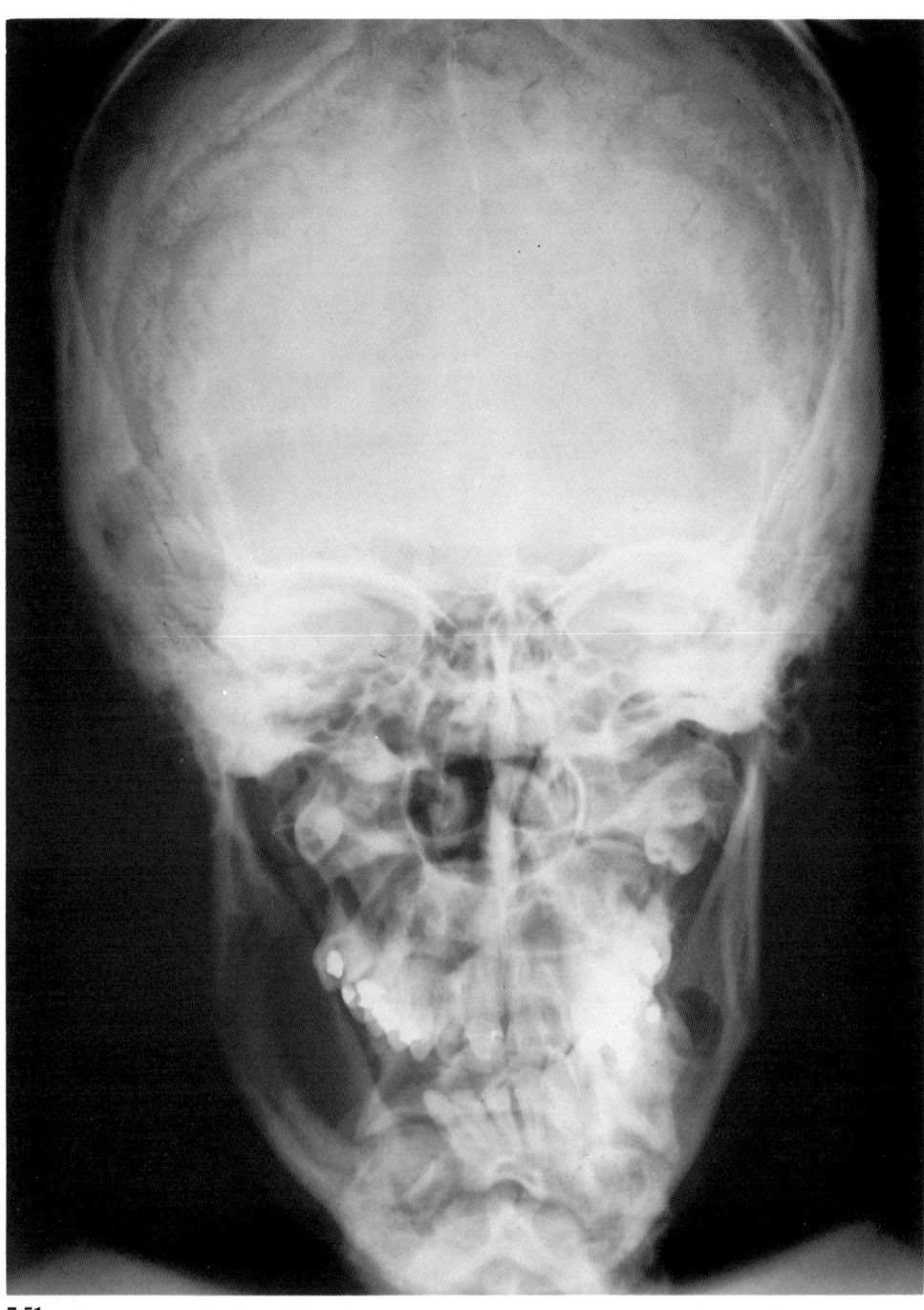

7.51

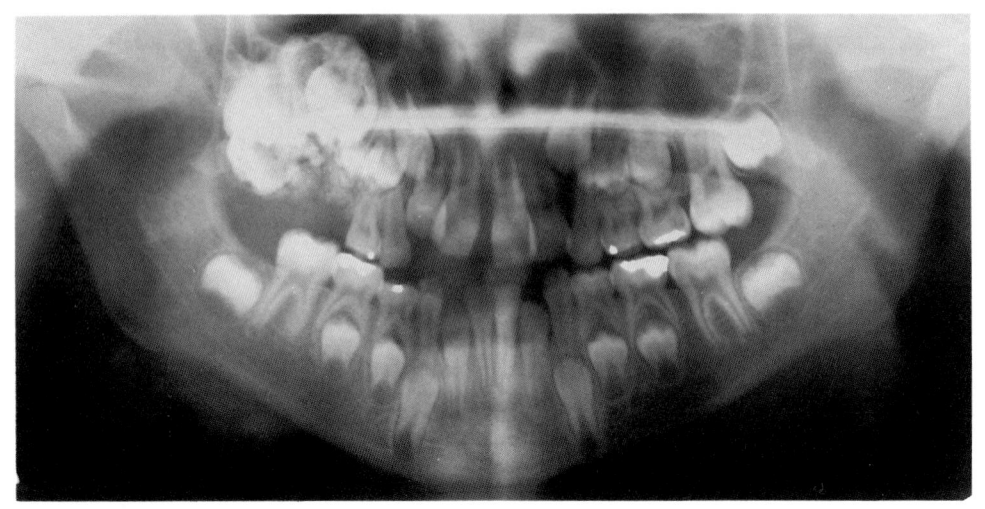

Ameloblastic fibro-odontome

7.52 In its early stages prior to deposition of mineralised tissue, this hamartomatous lesion is predominantly radiolucent, but as increasing numbers of centres of odontogenesis arise, more and more radiopacities develop within it. In this example in the right maxilla of an eight-year-old, the mass contains numerous small, rounded, radiopaque structures (some of which resemble denticles) and projects into the antrum, the floor of which is raised. It has a clearly defined margin, and around its antero-superior aspect there is a thin, radiopaque lamina of cortical bone and radiolucent capsular space. E| , 654| and 7| are unerupted and have been displaced by the mass, E| lying over its centre, 6| posteriorly, 7| inferiorly and 54| mesially. This lesion was followed over a number of years and as it matured it became more densely and more uniformly radiopaque without increasing in size. PR

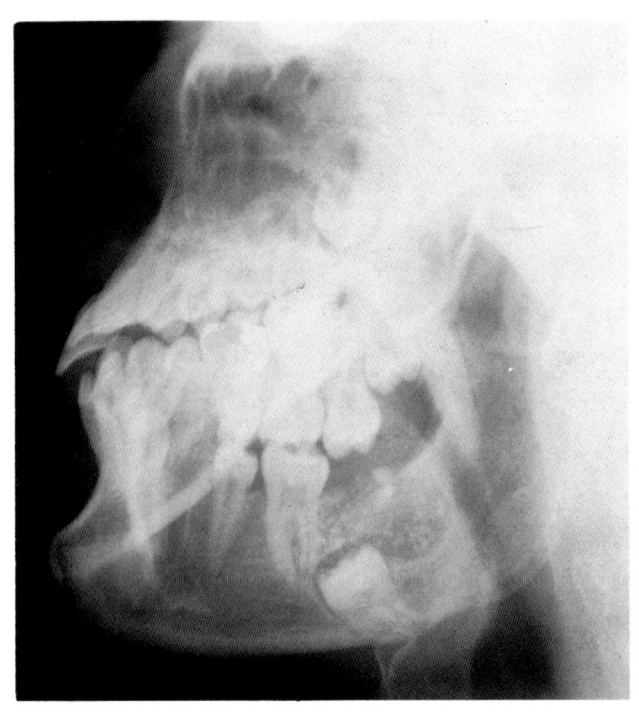

Odontoameloblastoma

7.53 A lesion at an intermediate stage of development in the |678 region of a 14-year-old. There is a well defined, ovoid radiolucency in the alveolar part of the bone which is expanded occlusally, and around which lies a thin, radiopaque lamina posteriorly, although its anterior margin is superimposed upon |6 roots and is not well demonstrated. It contains numerous, irregular radiopacities randomly scattered throughout the mass, some of them, particularly superiorly, being larger than the others and having the appearance of denticles. |7 is displaced to the inferior border of the mandible, and its roots are curved distally and not yet completely formed. A radiolucent follicular space surrounded by a thin, radiopaque lamina is still visible around its crown mesially and occlusally. |8 is absent, and the unopposed |7 has over-erupted. Note the image of the hyoid bone superimposed upon the roots |7. OLM

The Facial Bones 139

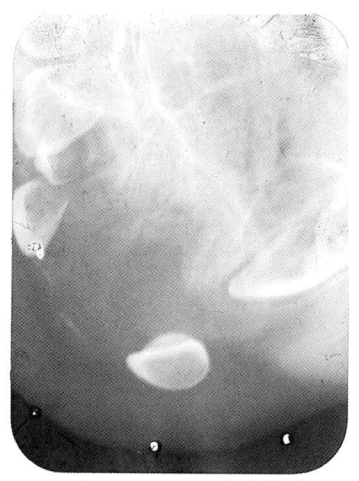

Neuroectodermal tumour of infancy
7.54 This lesion arises in the anterior part of the maxilla of young infants, causing an expansile, soft tissue mass. In this two-month-old infant, an approximately circular radiolucent mass occupies the incisor region causing displacement of A labially and B distally. The labial alveolus is expanded and eroded, only a small, thin remnant of radiopaque cortical lamina remaining. The deep margin of the tumour can just be determined. The soft tissue outline of the lip is displaced anteriorly by the mass. P

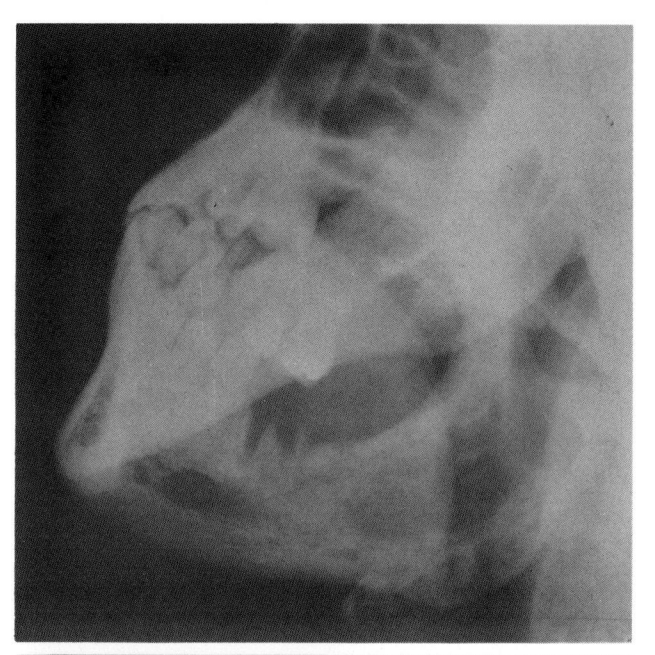

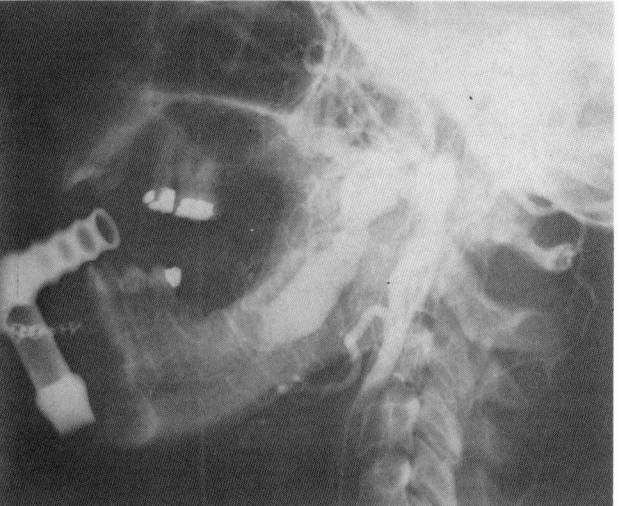

Haemangioma
7.55 (top) and 7.56 (bottom) Most haemangiomas are hamartomas and are usually poorly demarcated from the tissue in which they arise. In this central cavernous haemangioma of the mandible, although there are several obvious radiolucent defects, noticeably in the regions of the third molar/ramus and mental foramen, most of the bone shows abnormal structure. The trabecular pattern generally has a fuzzy appearance and randomly arranged throughout all the bone are pinhead sized radiolucencies, probably arising from vessels running through the bone in the direction of the X-ray beam. There are also several irregular, longitudinally running, radiolucent channels between the two main parts of the lesion. Note the recent extraction socket |6 from which there was profuse haemorrhage. The extent of the lesion is determined more clearly by carotid angiography (Fig. 7.56). The radiopaque contrast medium defines the lesion in the molar/ramus region, although its more anterior part had not yet been filled when this angiogram was taken. OLM & L

140 *A Radiological Atlas of Diseases of the Teeth and Jaws*

Fibrous dysplasia
7.57 (top), 7.58 (middle) and 7.59 (bottom) In its early stages, this hamartomatous lesion is composed of fibrous tissue and poorly mineralised bone trabeculae, and is therefore radiolucent. As it enlarges, the amount of mineralised tissue increases, but to a markedly variable degree in different lesions, so that it can present a variety of radiological appearances. In this monostotic lesion of the mandible of an 18-year-old, it is variably radiolucent and radiopaque, the radiopacities being randomly scattered throughout and irregularly shaped. The mass had been present for at least eight years and prevented the eruption of 5̄4̄| which are displaced, their crowns being surrounded by normal radiolucent follicular spaces. The overlying alveolar ridge is expanded and its radiopaque cortex intact. The inferior part of the lesion is more radiolucent with an irregularly loculated appearance and the inferior border of the mandible is slightly enlarged (Fig. 7.58). There is expansion of the buccal cortical plate (Fig. 7.59) which remains intact. The margins of the lesion are poorly defined, irregularly shaped, and blend imperceptibly with the adjacent normal bone. Note the retained roots 6̄|, beneath the mesial one of which there is a small, peripheral radiolucency. P, OLM & LTO

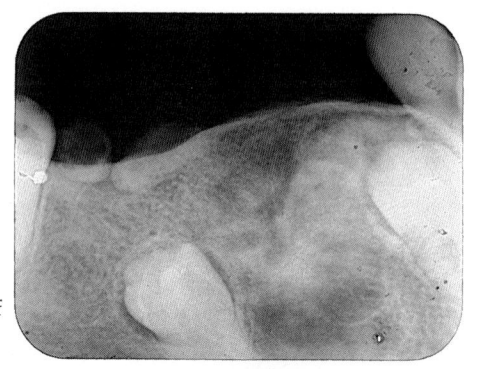

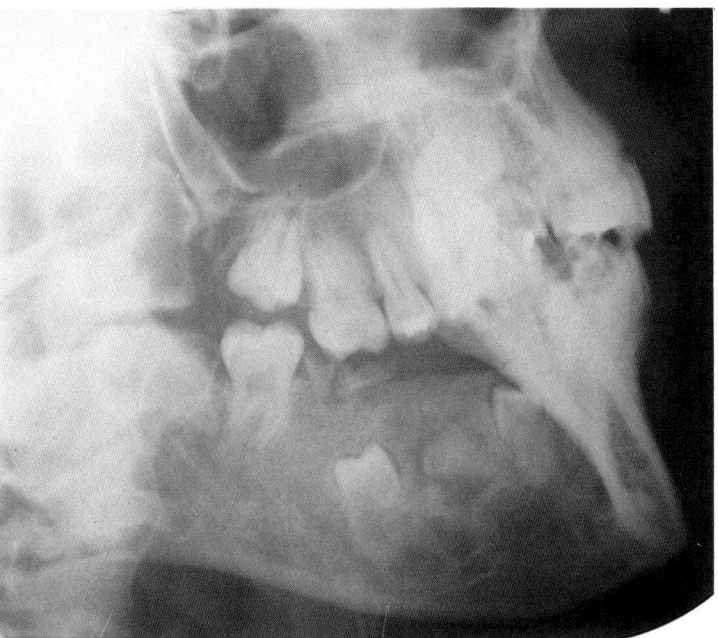

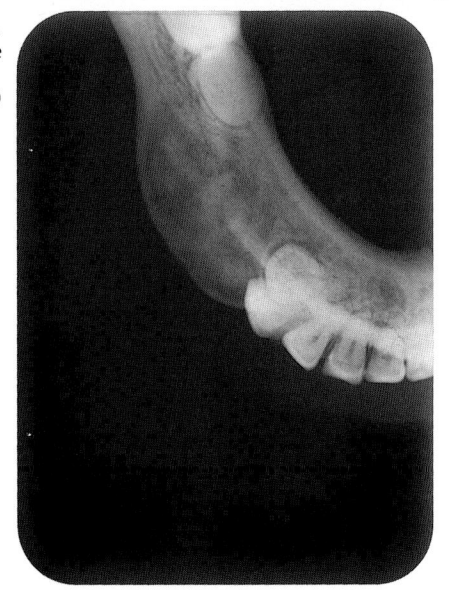

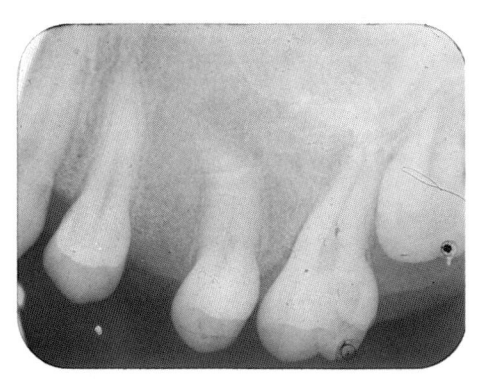

7.60 In this more mature lesion in the maxilla of a 19-year-old, the normal trabecular pattern of the alveolar bone has been replaced by a diffuse radiopacity of uniformly stippled appearance. The alveolar bone is expanded and ⌊5 displaced distally. The normal anatomical features of the region have been obscured by the lesion, and both the lamina dura around the roots ⌊45 7 and the boundaries of the maxillary antrum are indistinct. Note that ⌊6 is absent and ⌊8 is developing normally. P

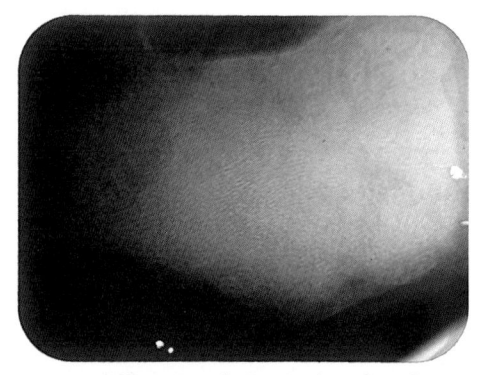

7.61 A fully mature lesion in the edentulous maxilla of an adult, which is uniformly radiopaque throughout and displays the typical 'orange peel' appearance. It has caused marked expansion of the alveolar ridge as demonstrated by the increased distance between the floor of the antrum and the bone surface. P

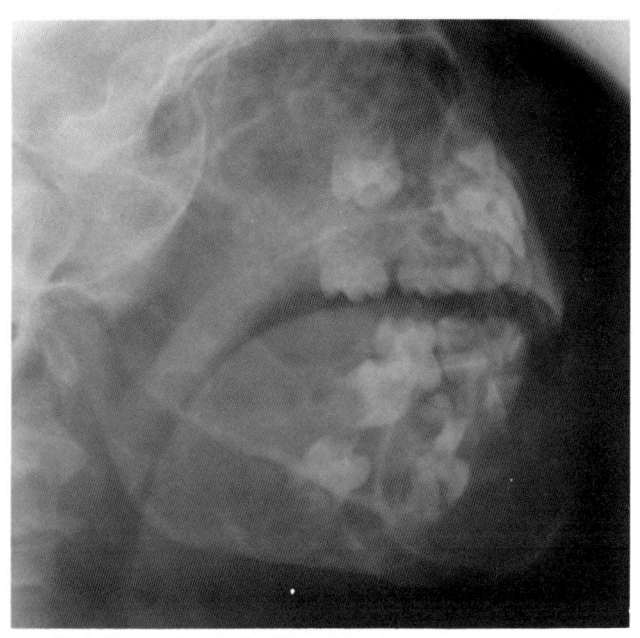

Familial fibrous dysplasia (Cherubism)

7.62 This condition affects the jaws in early childhood and results in their expansion by a mass of fibro-cellular tissue in which relatively little bone formation occurs. The condition classically involves all four quadrants, and they exhibit a multi-cystic pattern of radiolucency with varying numbers of radiopaque septa running between the locules. Although this view alone is not ideal, involvement of the entire jaws can be determined, together with expansion and thinning of the cortical bone, particularly in the anterior, inferior and coronoid regions of the mandible. OLM

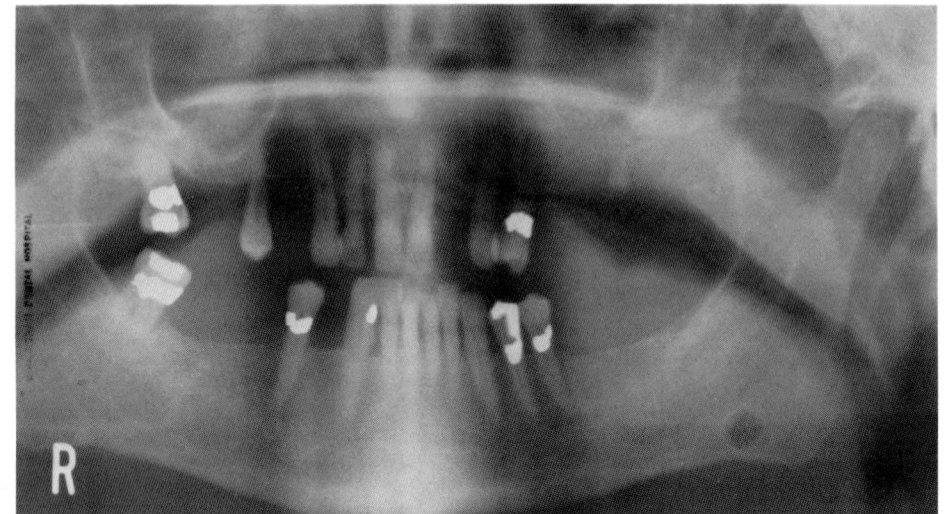

142 *A Radiological Atlas of Diseases of the Teeth and Jaws*

Stafne's bone cavity
7.63 This developmental defect of the mandible, which arises from the inclusion of aberrant submandibular salivary gland tissue, typically occurs beneath the inferior alveolar canal at the base of the ramus. It forms a well defined, mostly circular radiolucency surrounded by a thin, radiopaque lamina of cortical bone. Submandibular sialography may be of help in confirming the diagnosis. Note the generalised bone loss of chronic periodontitis and a retained root in the |6 region. PR

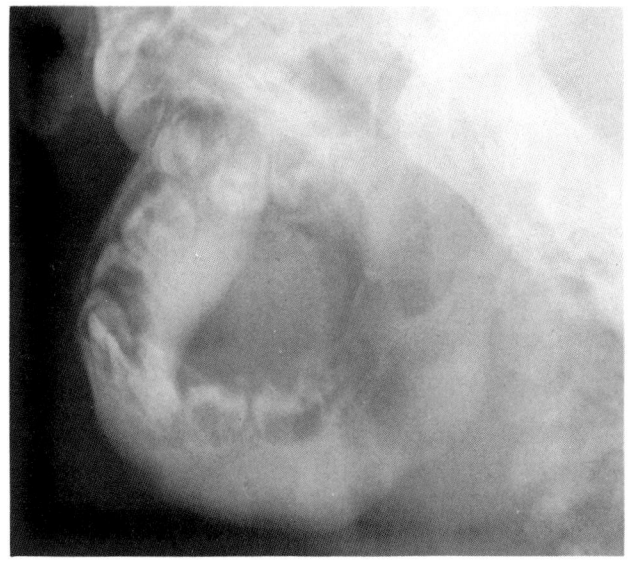

Infantile cortical hyperostosis (Caffey–Silverman syndrome)
7.64 Symmetrical, bilateral involvement of the mandible is a usual feature of this disorder. The condition usually arises during the first three months of life, as in this two-month-old child in whom there has been formation of much periosteal bone, particularly along the inferior border, resulting in enlargement and deformation of the jaw. A faint 'onion skin' layering of the bone can be discerned, presumably a consequence of succesive increments of bone deposition. As the child develops, the excess bone usually undergoes resolution. Note that the development of the primary molars and first permanent molar are unaffected. OLM

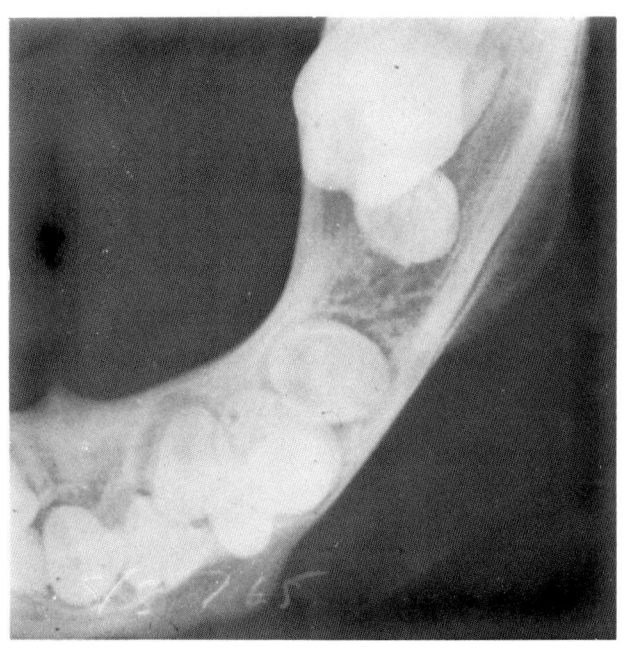

Periostitis
7.65 In young patients, localised infections within the mandible may be accompanied by reactive changes in the overlying periosteum. These are often best displayed on occlusal films, as in this example, where a localised deposition of reactive bone is present buccally in the premolar/molar region. Several lamellae of new bone have been formed giving an 'onion skin' appearance. LTO

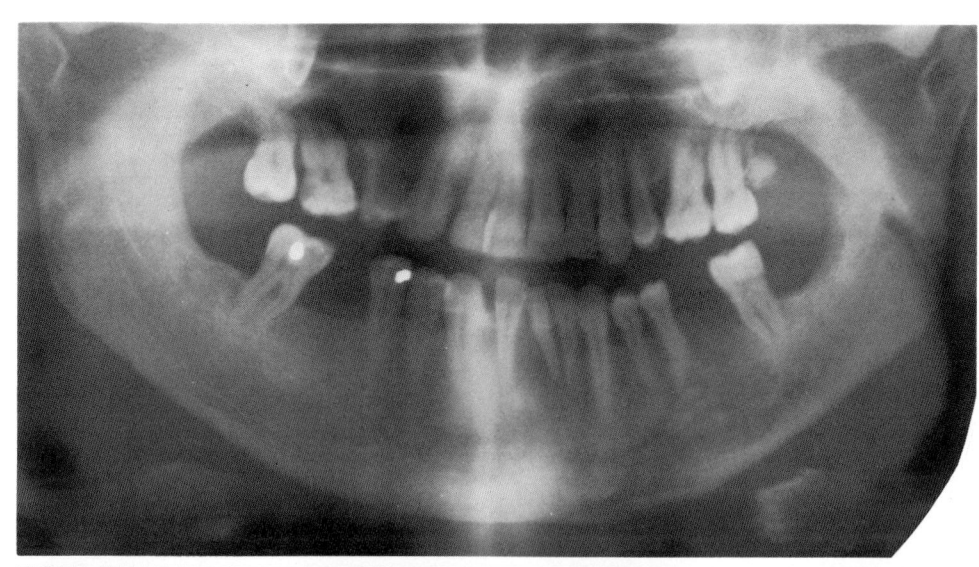

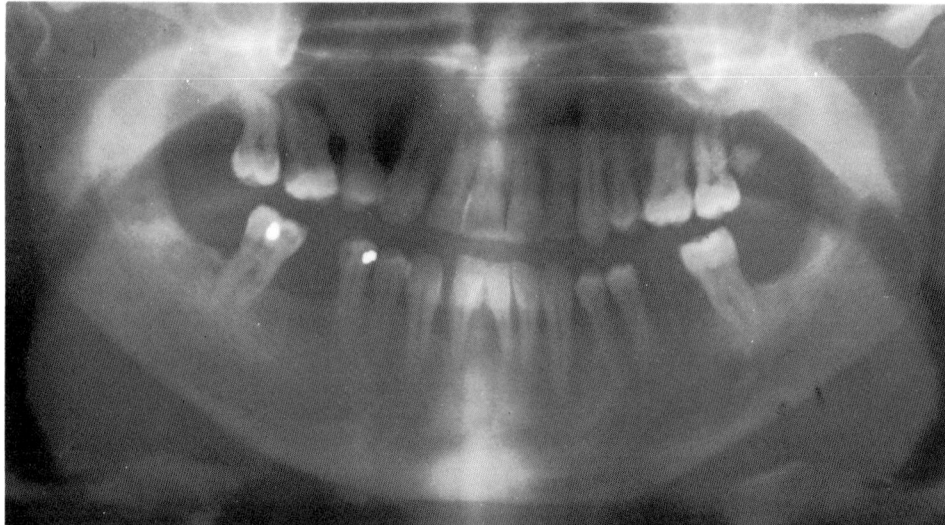

Chronic osteomyelitis 7.66 (left) and 7.67 (bottom left) As with all inflammatory lesions arising *de novo* within bone, radiological changes are uncommon before ten days, and they have therefore usually entered the chronic phase before such changes are apparent. In this lesion of the left mandible twelve days after the extraction ̅6, there is a poorly defined, indistinct, radiolucent defect with irregular outline in the ̅2–8 region, within which the margins of the inferior alveolar canal are indistinct. As such lesions progress, localised areas of dead bone (sequestra) are formed, which produce irregular radiopacities. Several such areas, together with a clearly defined, elongated sequestrum at the inferior border of the mandible in the ̅345 region, are present. The radiolucent image of the ̅6 socket is already indistinct, suggesting a more rapid process of bone resorption than would normally be expected. After four weeks of antibiotic therapy (Fig. 7.67), the lesion is resolving and the trabecular pattern has become more distinct, but several clearly defined radiolucent defects are still present in the body of the mandible in the ̅456 and ̅7 regions. Distinct radiopaque sequestra are present in the former area and disto-apically ̅5. The sequestrum previously identified at the inferior border has undergone rarefaction and there is evidence of periosteal new bone formation. Note also the periapical radiolucency 6̅ which has a large distal carious lesion, the generalised chronic periodontitis and the tooth remnant ̅8. PR

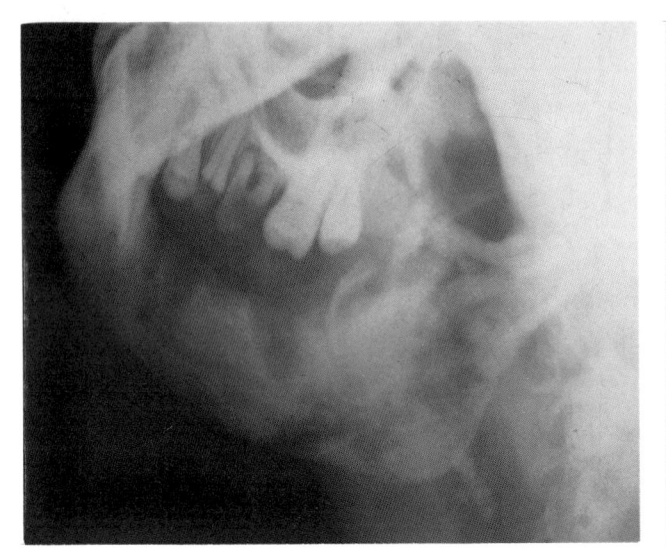

7.68 An extensive lesion affecting the body, ramus and angle of the mandible. There is a poorly defined radiolucency of irregular outline involving most of the ramus and within which are scattered irregular radiopacities, some of which are sequestered remnants of dead bone. There are numerous radiolucent perforations of the cortical bone, representing the cloacae and sinuses, which may be seen clinically. The extraction sockets |45 78 formed the portal of entry for the causative micro-organisms. Note the hyoid bone superimposed upon the |8 socket and the mineralised epiglottis lying obliquely over the angle of the mandible. OLM

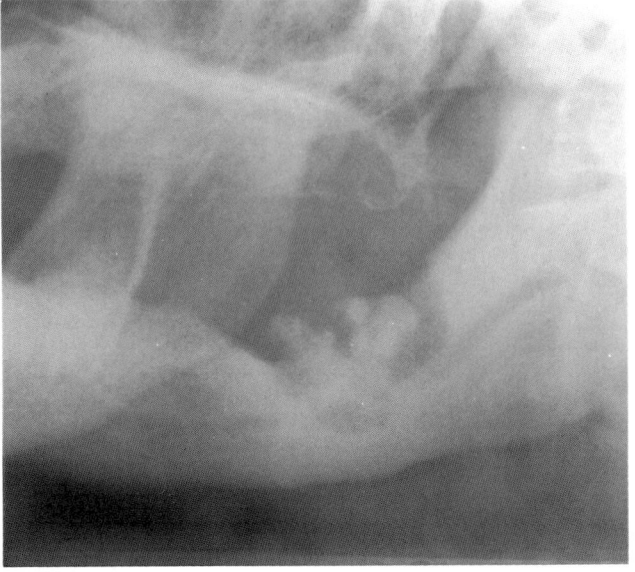

7.70 A long-standing lesion in an edentulous mandible with extensive sequestrum formation. There is a clearly defined, scalloped, radiolucent defect in the molar region, within which lie several irregularly shaped radiopaque sequestra. The slightly increased radiopacity of the surrounding bone indicates the presence of reactive osteosclerotic bone formation. Although the lesion is superimposed upon the inferior alveolar canal, there was no disturbance of neural function. OLM

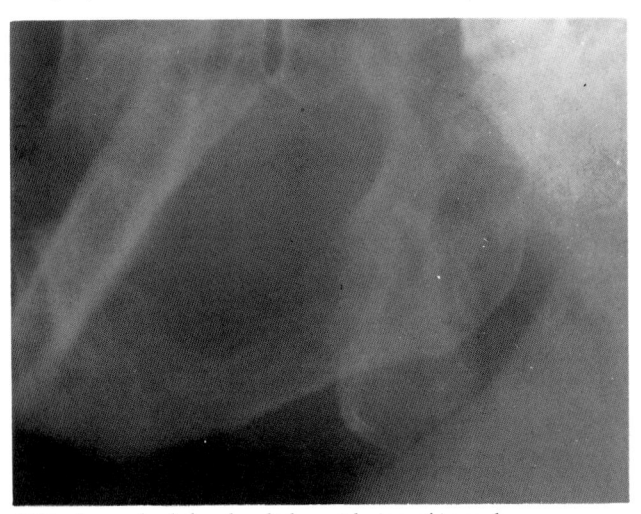

7.69 A poorly defined radiolucent lesion of irregular outline predominantly in the alveolar part of the |4–8 region of an edentulous mandible. Scattered, irregularly shaped radiopacities are present mainly within its anterior part, indicating the presence of sequestra. OLM

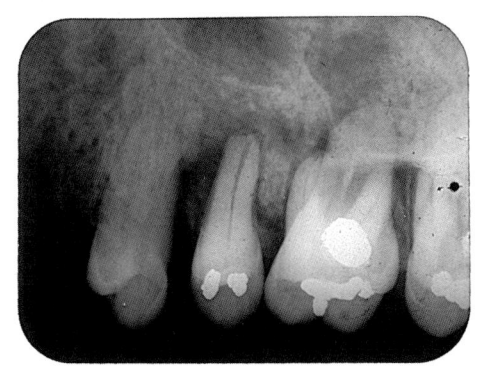

7.71 Osteomyelitis is less common in the maxilla, but may occasionally occur. In this small lesion localised to the alveolar part of the |56 region, a diffuse, poorly defined area of radiolucency is present around the apices of these teeth and involving the interdental septa. There is loss of the lamina dura, and small radiopaque sequestra are present interdentally |45 and in the main part of the lesion. Note the loss of bone mesially in the trifurcation |6, and that the thin, radiopaque lamina which outlines the floor of the antrum and dips down posteriorly overlying the apical half of the roots |6, is less distinct than normal. The apical part |5 is irregular, indicating the presence of resorption. P

The Facial Bones 145

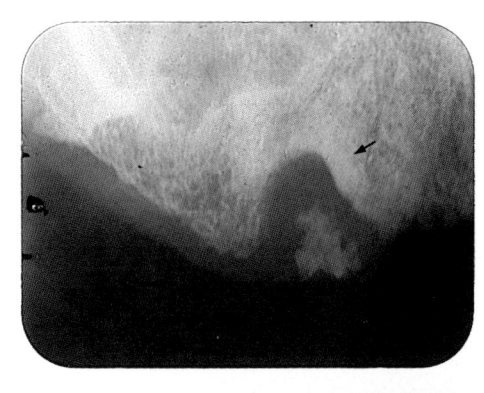

7.72 A long-standing lesion in the premolar region of an edentulous maxilla which has progressed to the formation of a sequestrum which is clearly separated from the residual bone. The sequestrum, which lies in a deep radiolucent defect in the alveolus, has the trabecular pattern of bone. Adjacent to the sequestrum, the bone is slightly more radiopaque due to reactive osteosclerosis, and there is a small tooth fragment antero-superiorly (arrow). Note the overlying soft issue outline. P

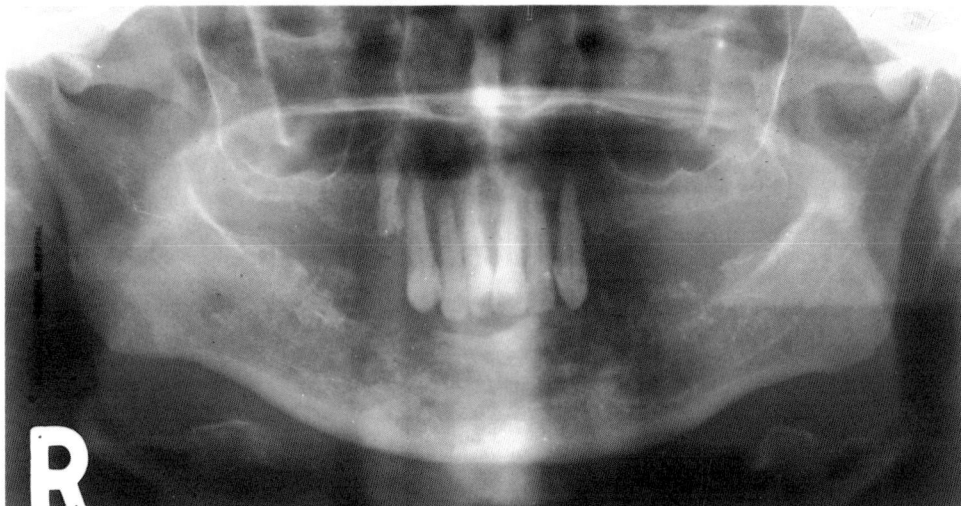

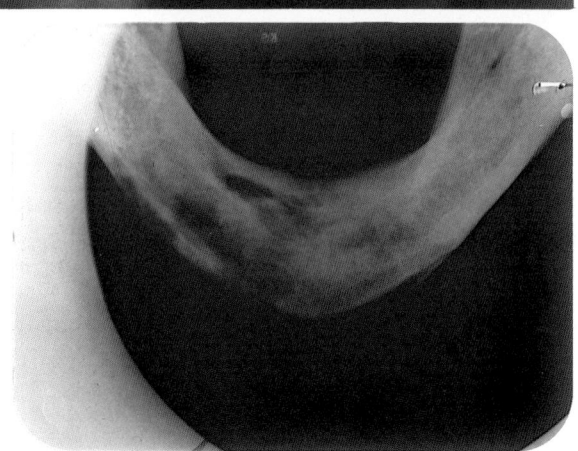

Osteoradionecrosis
7.73 (left) and 7.74 (bottom left) A long-standing lesion of an edentulous mandible of at least ten years duration in a patient who had received X-irradiation some years ago for a squamous cell carcinoma of the floor of the mouth. There is an ill defined, irregular radiolucency of the body of the mandible extending from 6| to |6, and in several places reaching down to its inferior border. Within the affected area, the normal trabecular pattern of bone is absent and has a coarsely mottled structure, among which are some clearly defined areas of radiolucency. A large radiopaque sequestrum is present in the alveolar part of the incisor region. Note the retained 4| root. PR & LTO

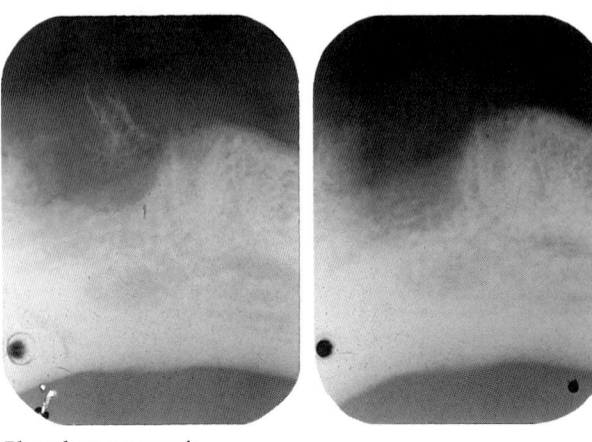

Phosphorus necrosis
7.75 (left) and 7.76 (right) Exposure to phosphorus may result in necrosis of the jaws, a condition which can be persistent and progressive. In this example in the alveolar part of the mandibular incisor region, a radiolucent area is present which contains a clearly demarcated radiopaque sequestrum of bone. The sequestrum was removed, but some six months later (Fig. 7.76) the lesion was still present with evidence of further sequestration as demonstrated by its more indistinct border and numerous small radiopacities within it. P

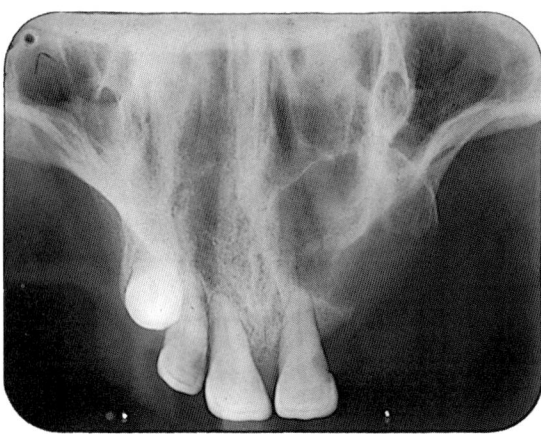

7.78 This lesion in the left maxilla forms a circular radiolucency, mostly surrounded by a distinct, thin, radiopaque lamina. The buccal outline of the maxilla is expanded where there is an area of darker radiolucency together with an absence of cortical outline, indicating perforation of the buccal bone. This cyst has expanded to encroach upon the apex of $\underline{1}$, although its position clearly indicates that it has not arisen from this tooth. Further radiographs confirmed that the lamina dura $\underline{1}$ was intact. Note the oval image of the nasolacrima canal posteriorly and the outline of the antrum postero-laterally to the cyst. USO

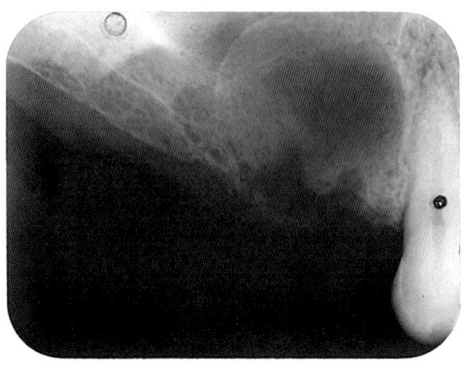

Dental cyst (residual cyst)
7.77 A small, circular, clearly defined, radiolucent lesion in the $\underline{54}$ region which is surrounded by a thin, radiopaque lamina. The remnants of the $\underline{54}$ sockets are present, and the alveolus is expanded and markedly thinned. The appearance of a circular, radiolucent area surrounded by a thin, radiopaque lamina of bone is characteristic of this type of benign expansile lesion. P

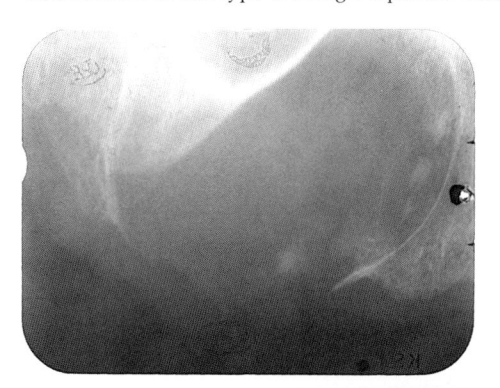

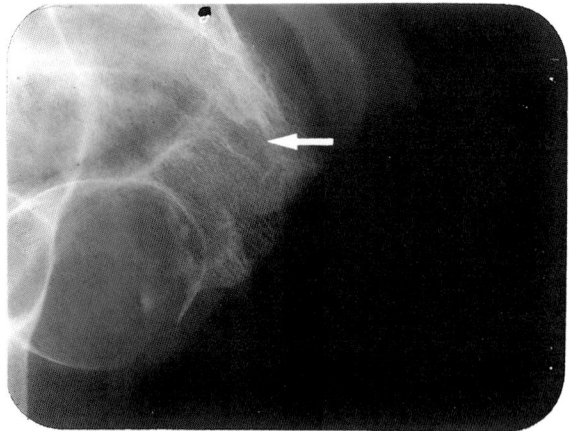

7.79 (upper) 7.80 (lower) This cyst in the right side of an edentulous maxilla forms a clearly defined, circular radiolucency which is surrounded, except on the alveolar surface, by a thin, radiopaque lamina. There are several, small, irregular, radiopaque areas in the mesio-alveolar aspect of the lesion, indicating deposits of dystrophic mineralisation. The image of the root of the zygomatic arch is superimposed upon the cyst in both films. Note the incisive fossa (arrow). P & UOO

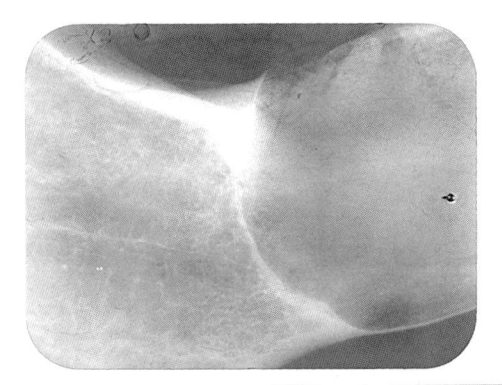

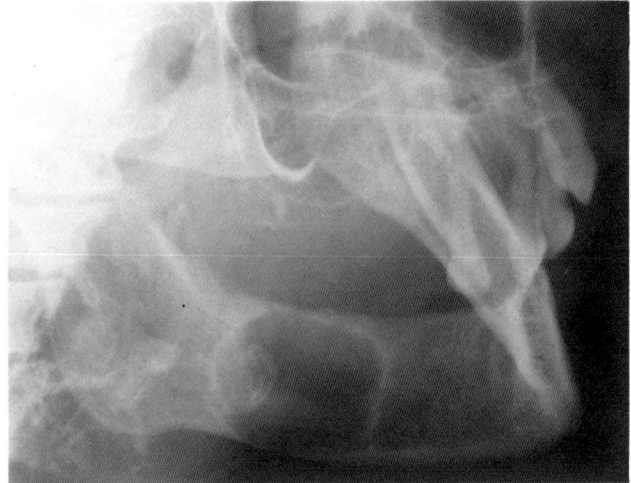

7.81 (top) and 7.82 (bottom) A cyst in the $\overline{8-6|}$ region of an edentulous mandible with thinning of the cortical bone at the inferior border. The approximately circular radiolucency is surrounded by a thin, clearly defined, radiopaque lamina and contains an ovoid, more radiolucent area centrally, indicating thinning of the lingual or buccal cortical plates. Note the image of the hyoid bone overlying the lesion, the mental foramen anterior to it, and the retained root in the $\underline{8|}$ region (Fig. 7.82). P & OLM

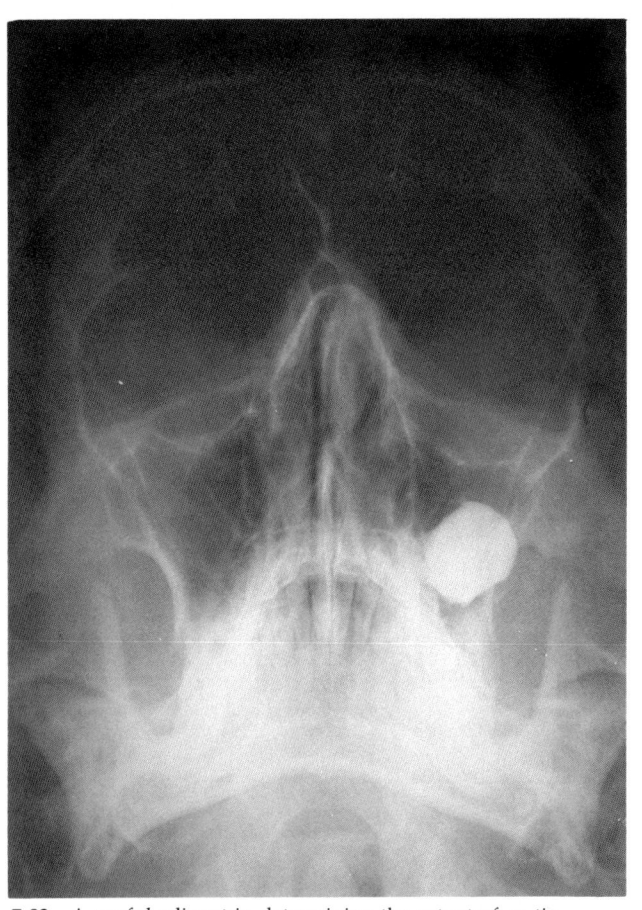

7.83 A useful adjunct in determining the extent of cystic lesions in the maxilla, or when there is difficulty in deciding whether a radiolucent area is cystic or merely part of the antrum, is to inject radiopaque contrast medium into the area. If it is cystic, the cavity of the lesion becomes filled with radiopaque medium forming a circular mass of smooth outline typical of an expansile cyst. OM

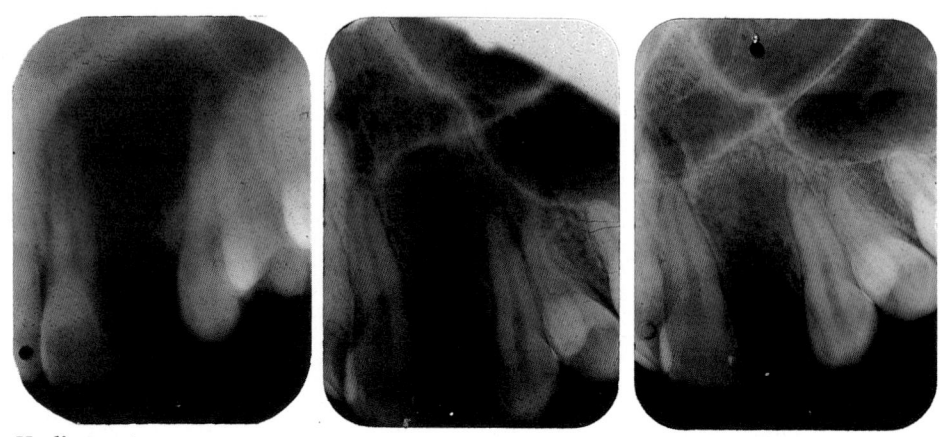

Healing cyst

7.84 (left), 7.85 (middle) 7.86 (right) Healing of a bony cavity after enucleation of a residual dental cyst |2 region and primary closure of the wound. Although the lamina dura (Fig. 7.84) around the roots of |1 3 is indistinct apically, the teeth were vital. Four months post-operatively (Fig. 7.85), the lamina dura and periodontal ligament space |1 3 are present, and much of the cavity has been filled in from its periphery by fine trabeculations arranged radially, particularly at the nasal aspect of the defect. By 12 months (Fig. 7.86), the defect is filled in completely, although there is still some radial arrangement of the trabeculae. Note the incisive foramen superimposed |1 apically, the lateral border of the floor of the nose, and the floor of the antrum. P

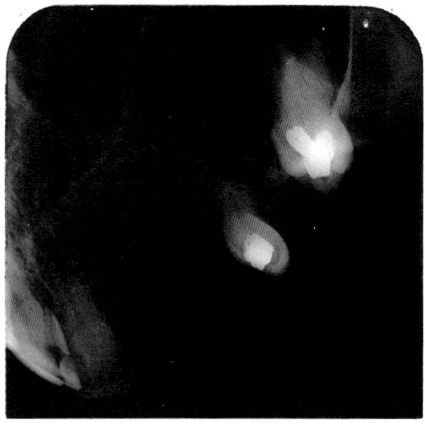

7.87 Three months after enucleation of a residual dental cyst |234 region and primary closure of the wound, the circumferential radial arrangement of new bony trabeculae in the defect is apparent. Its central part is still radiolucent, indicating that bony repair has not yet reached this far. Note the thin cortical laminae demarcating the lateral border of the floor of the nose and the floor of the antrum. UOO

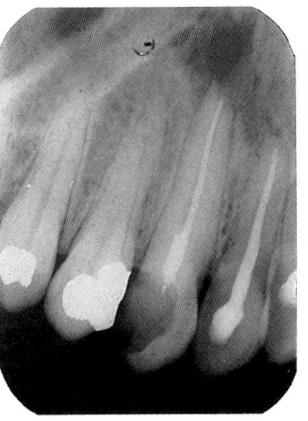

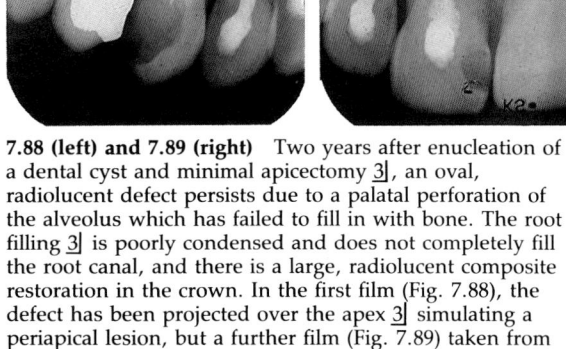

7.88 (left) and 7.89 (right) Two years after enucleation of a dental cyst and minimal apicectomy 3|, an oval, radiolucent defect persists due to a palatal perforation of the alveolus which has failed to fill in with bone. The root filling 3| is poorly condensed and does not completely fill the root canal, and there is a large, radiolucent composite restoration in the crown. In the first film (Fig. 7.88), the defect has been projected over the apex 3| simulating a periapical lesion, but a further film (Fig. 7.89) taken from another direction indicates its true position (parallax). The radiopaque lamina of the lateral border of the floor of the nose is superimposed upon the defect. P

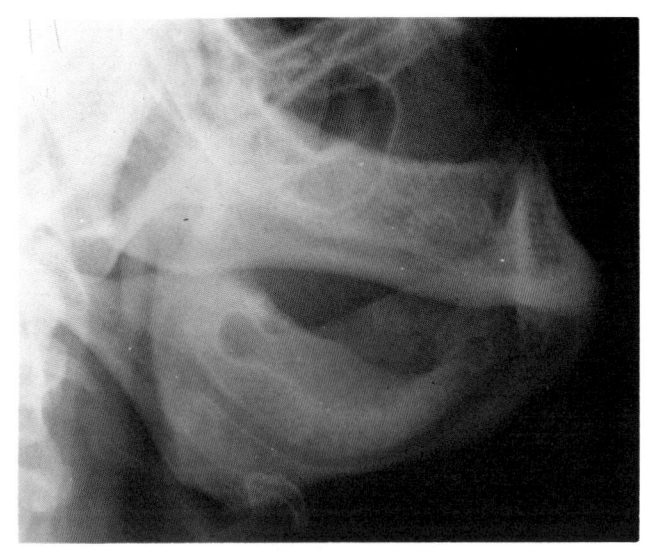

The Facial Bones 149

7.90 Six months after the treatment of a large cyst of the right body and ramus of the mandible by enucleation and primary closure, there are radially arranged trabeculae of reparative bone around the periphery of the bony defect which can still be determined. A key-hole shaped area of radiolucency remains where bony repair has not occurred. At this stage of healing, substantially more trabeculae than are necessary for normal function have been deposited, so the tissue is relatively radiopaque. Note the displaced inferior alveolar canal. OLM

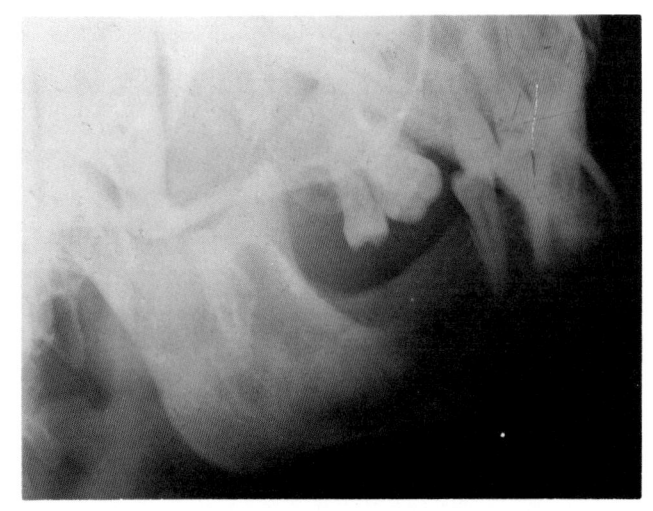

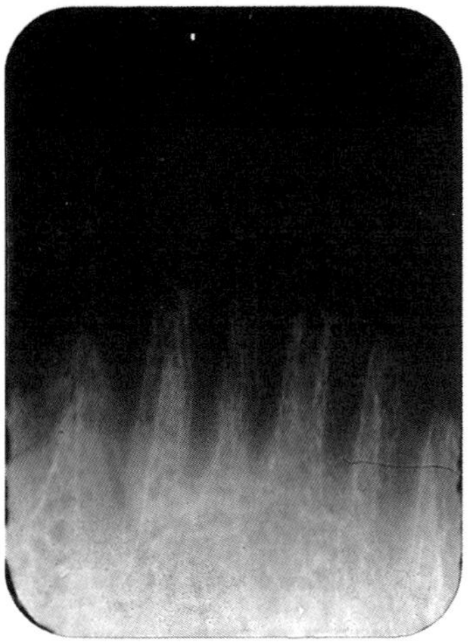

Extraction socket
7.92 Sockets of the mandibular incisors and canines following recent extraction of the teeth. The lamina dura is still intact around the margins of the sockets and there is no evidence of bony repair. The crest of the interdental septum $\overline{21}$ has been fractured and is displaced slightly medially. P

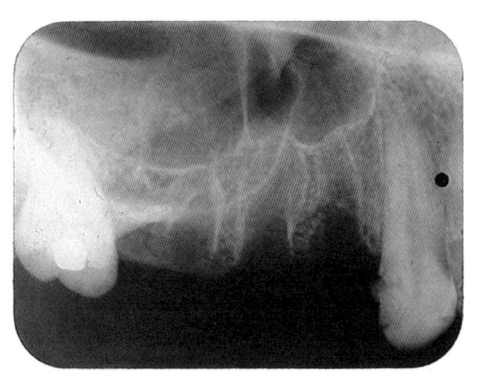

7.93 Maxillary premolar sockets, several weeks after extraction of the teeth. The interdental septa and the lamina dura around the sockets are still clearly visible, and there is early infilling of their apical parts with bone. Note the radiopaque lamina of the antral floor with a thin septum running vertically above $\underline{5|}$ socket, and the root of the zygomatic process overlying $\underline{65|}$ sockets. P

7.91 A residual cyst in the right body and ramus of the mandible 12 months after treatment by enucleation and primary closure. The outline of the original bony defect is indistinct, especially anteriorly. The defect is now fully filled in with bone which, at its centre in the more recently healed part of the lesion, is more radiopaque with a radial arrangement of the trabeculae. Peripherally, the process of bone remodelling is further advanced, and a more normal trabecular pattern is present. The inferior alveolar canal has been displaced inferiorly by the original lesion. Note the prominent mental foramen. OLM

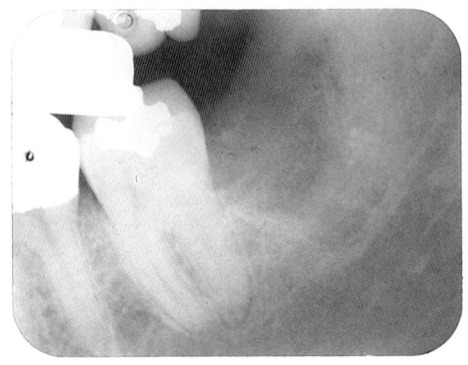

7.94 The rate of bone repair of a tooth socket is very variable and can be influenced by many factors. In this |8 socket, approximately six weeks after the tooth extraction, the lamina dura outlining the original margin is still discernible, although not clearly defined, indicating that remodelling is in progress. The socket is largely filled in with poorly mineralised reparative bone, and thus is still relatively radiolucent. P

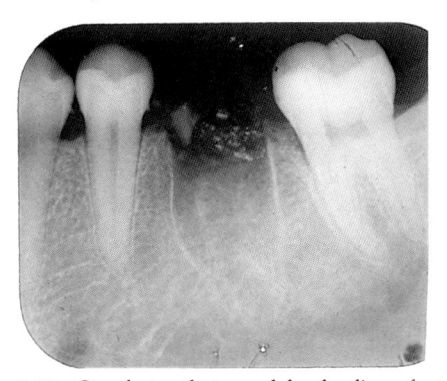

7.95 One factor that can delay healing of a tooth socket is the presence of foreign material. In this |6 socket, approximately six weeks after tooth extraction, the apical parts are healing normally and are infilled with reparative bone, although the lamina dura is still just discernible. The coronal part contains several radiopaque bodies and there is no evidence of bony repair. The larger mesial body is a root fragment, while the numerous, fine, more dense particles are remnants of filling material. P

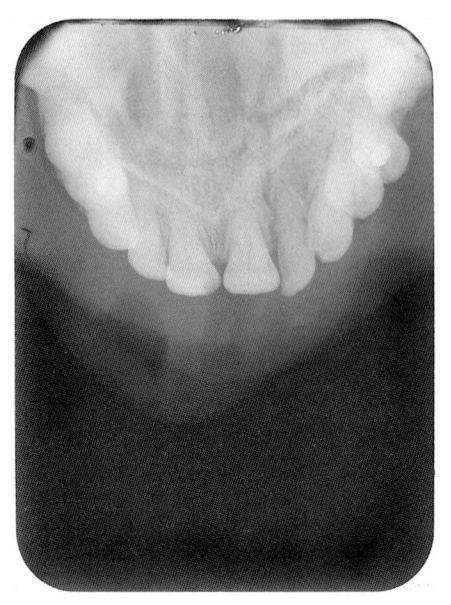

Fracture of the alveolus
7.96 The radiolucent fracture line in the upper left quadrant of this alveolus extends from the |2 socket across the hard palate to the |6 region. The fragment bearing |2345 is displaced, resulting in widening of the fracture line and incisal displacement of |2 relative to |1. Note the outline of the labial and nasal soft tissues. USO

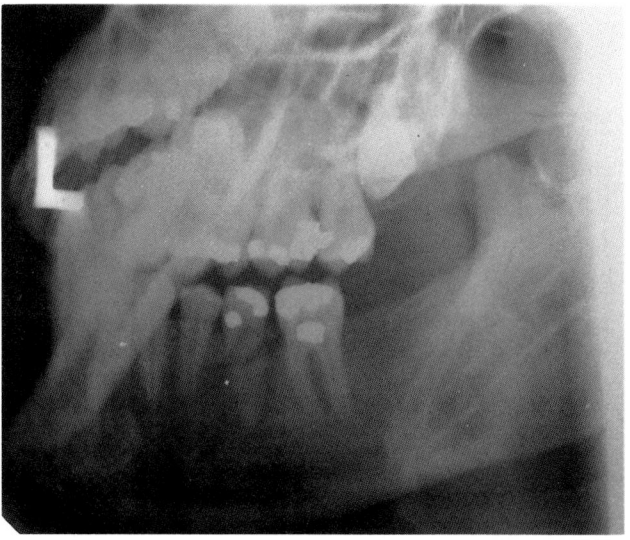

7.97 A comminuted dento-alveolar fracture of the left mandibular premolar and canine region. One radiolucent fracture line extends antero-inferiorly from the crest of the alveolus mesially |6 across the middle part of the roots |45. A second line runs more steeply in a similar direction from the alveolar crest overlying |5 crossing the apical parts of the roots |34. The root of |5 is fractured with occlusal displacement of its crown and there is widening of the periodontal ligament space apically |34. The tooth bearing fragment of the alveolus is minimally displaced. OLM

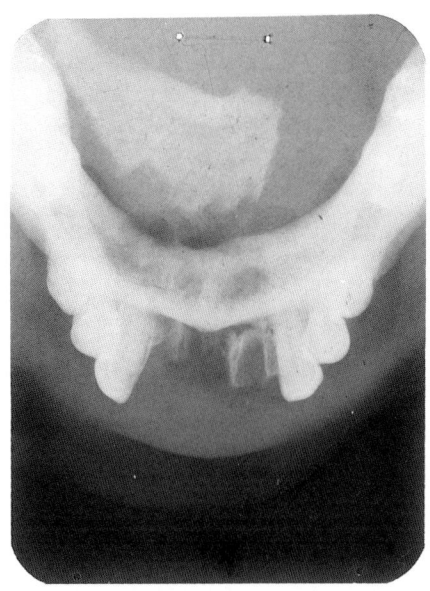

The Facial Bones 151

7.98 An unusual fracture in which the lingual bony plate anteriorly has been separated from the mandible and displaced posteriorly by contraction of its attached muscles. $\overline{21|12}$ have been avulsed and the trabeculations of the cancellous bone in the edentulous mandible are clearly visible due to loss of the lingual cortical plate. The scalloped outline of the alveolar crests is displayed on the displaced fragment together with the genial tubercles on its upper margin. LTO

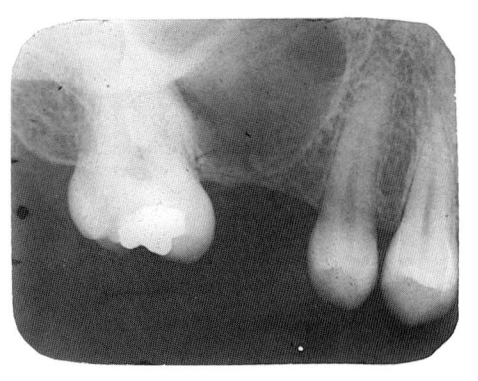

Fracture of the maxillary tuberosity
7.100 Fracture of the tuberosity is likely to occur following attempted extraction of maxillary molar teeth when the alveolus is weakened, either by the presence of unsuspected unerupted teeth, particularly if they have undergone fusion (concrescence) with the roots of the tooth to be extracted, or by the encroachment of the antrum into the alveolus as in this example. A radiolucent fracture line runs antero-inferiorly from the mesial aspect of the apical part $\underline{7|}$, through the bone forming the wall of the antrum, to the crest of the edentulous ridge. The more posterior part of the fracture line is obscured by the root of the zygoma. The course of the fracture line into the bone beyond the limits of the antrum distinguishes it from a vascular channel lying in the bony wall of the antrum (Fig. 3.12). P

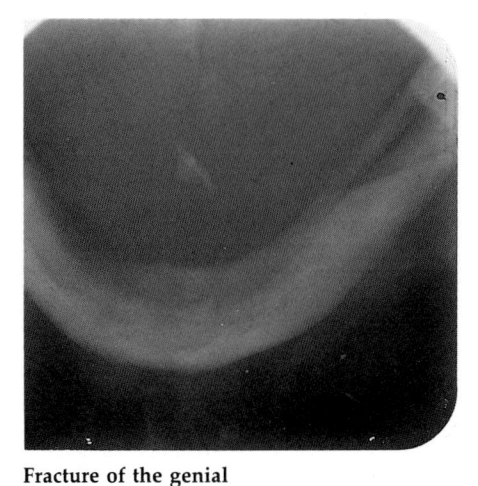

Fracture of the genial tubercles
7.99 Spontaneous fracture of the genial tubercles from an edentulous mandible with displacement of the fragment posteriorly due to muscle contraction. LTO

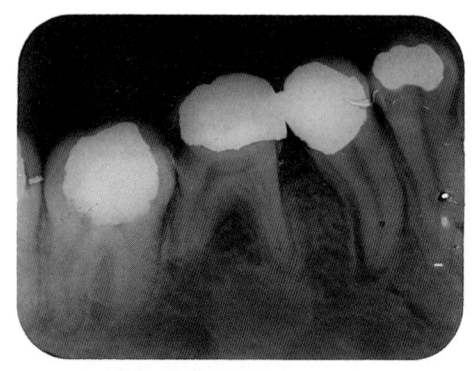

Fracture of the mandible
7.101 A fracture in the premolar region which is only partly displayed on this film, and for which further films would be required to determine its full extent. The radiolucent fracture line extends inferiorly from the base $\overline{5|}$ socket and the tooth has been displaced occlusally with widening of the periodontal ligament space all round. Note the area of radiopacity associated with the apical part of the mesial root $\overline{6|}$, being an area of osteosclerosis. This tooth has been extensively restored coronally, and there is blunting and shortening of the apices of both roots, indicating the presence of resorption. P

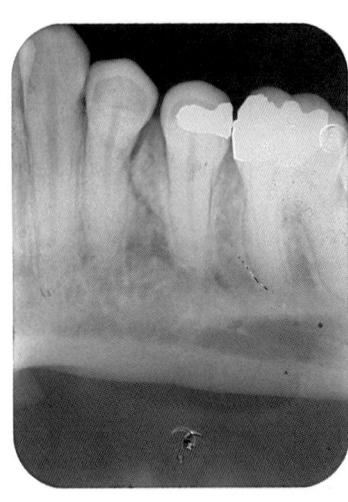

152   *A Radiological Atlas of Diseases of the Teeth and Jaws*

7.102 (left) and 7.103 (below)   A crack fracture of the left body of the mandible between $\overline{45}$ with no displacement of the bone ends. The fracture line runs from the distal aspect of $\overline{4}$ obliquely backwards to the inferior border of the mandible. The correct perspective of the fracture line is shown better on the panoramic radiograph (Fig. 7.103) than on the intra-oral film on which the image is foreshortend. Note the presence of amalgam fragments distal to $\overline{7}$. P & PR

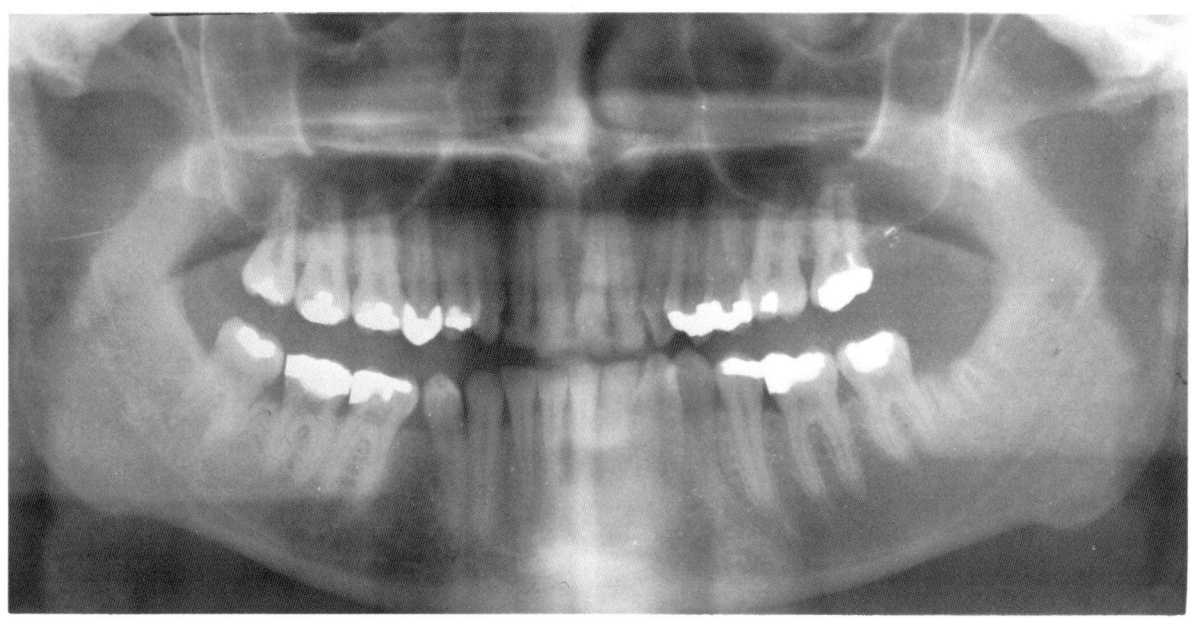

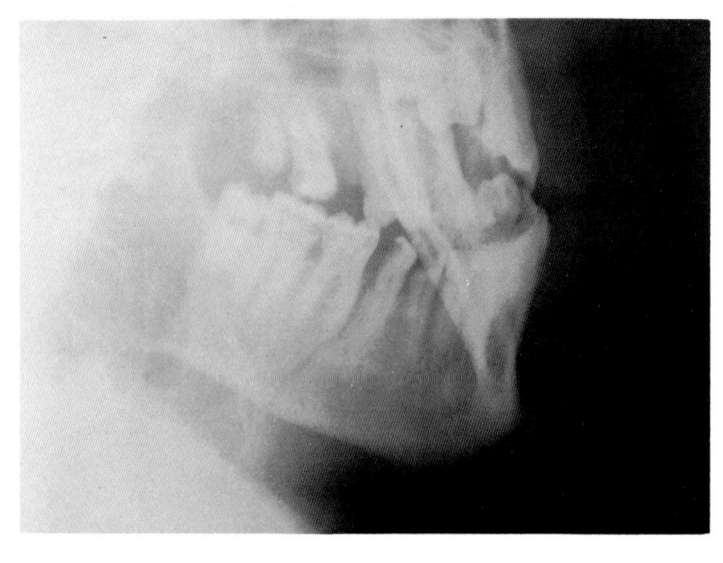

7.104   Fracture of the right body of the mandible extending through the mesial aspect of the socket of the mesial root of $\overline{6}$ obliquely to the inferior border, with only slight displacement of the fragments. Note the many carious lesions. OLM

The Facial Bones 153

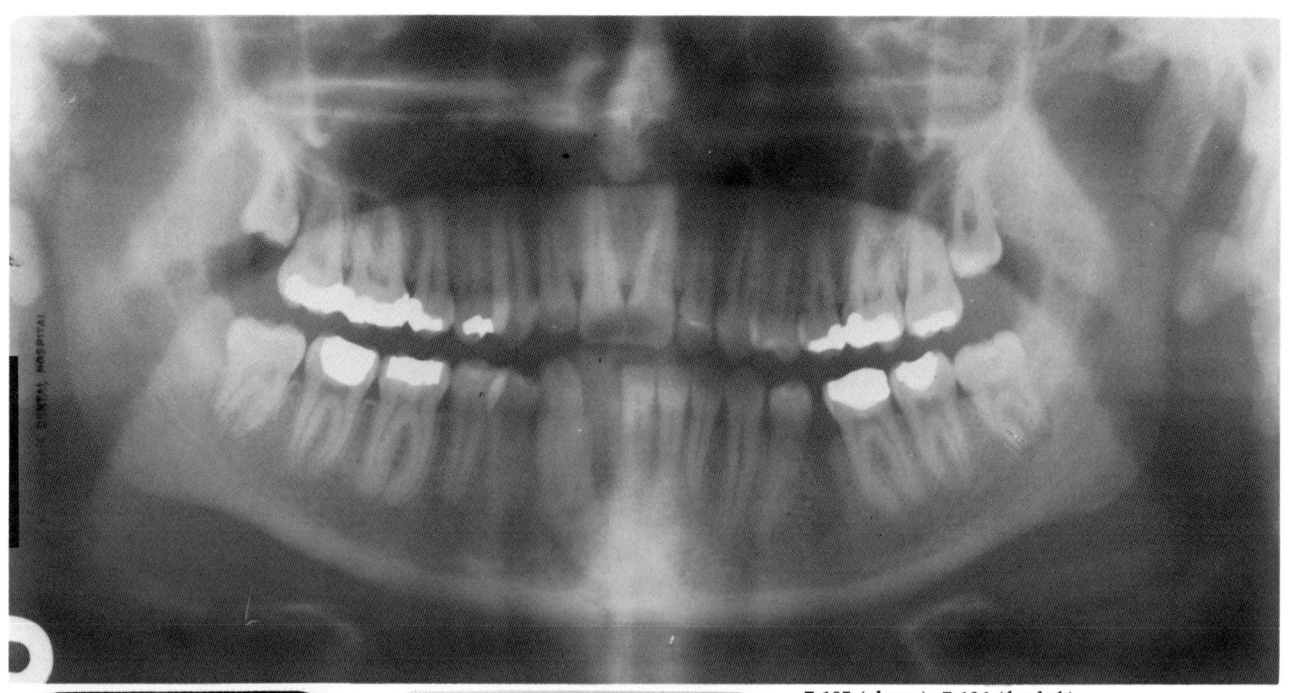

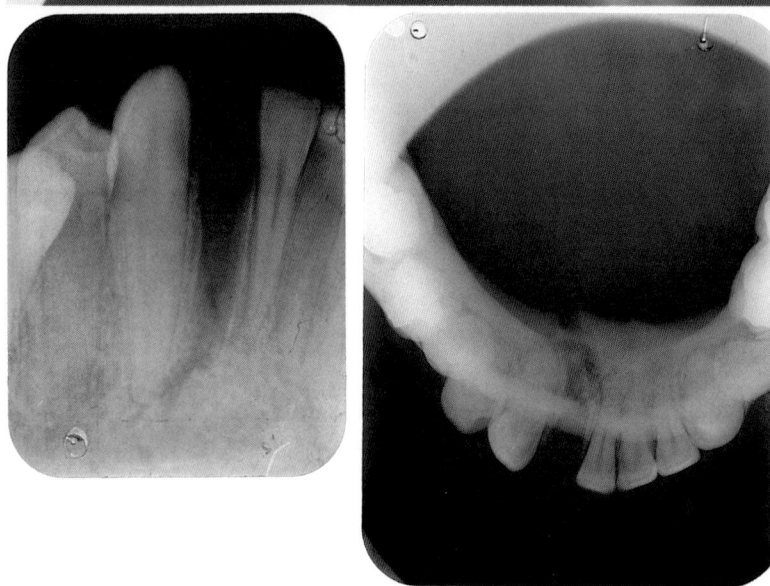

7.105 (above), 7.106 (far left) and 7.107 (left) Fractures of the mandible in the $\overline{32|}$ region and bilaterally of the condyles following direct trauma to the point of the chin (Fig. 7.105). $\overline{2|}$ was avulsed and the fracture line runs through the wall of the socket to its base (Fig. 7.106) and obliquely in a V-shape to the inferior border of the mandible, the apex of the V pointing distally. There is separation of the ends of the bone fragments, which is particularly well shown on the occlusal film (Fig. 7.107). Both condyles have been fractured through their necks by transmission of the force of impact through the mandible, but there is minimal displacement of the condylar heads (Fig. 7.105). Note the healing socket $|\overline{5}$. PR, P & LTO

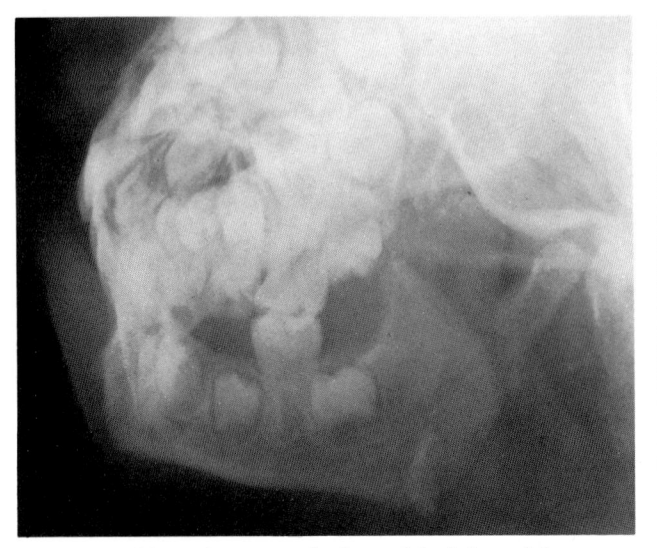

154 *A Radiological Atlas of Diseases of the Teeth and Jaws*

7.108 An oblique fracture at the base of the left condylar neck in a seven-year-old child. The fracture extends into the coronoid process anteriorly, with obvious displacement, but its full extent cannot be fully determined from this one radiograph. Interpretation of fracture lines in this site may be complicated by superimposition of the radiolucent shadow of the pharyngeal air space upon the ramus as in this example. OLM

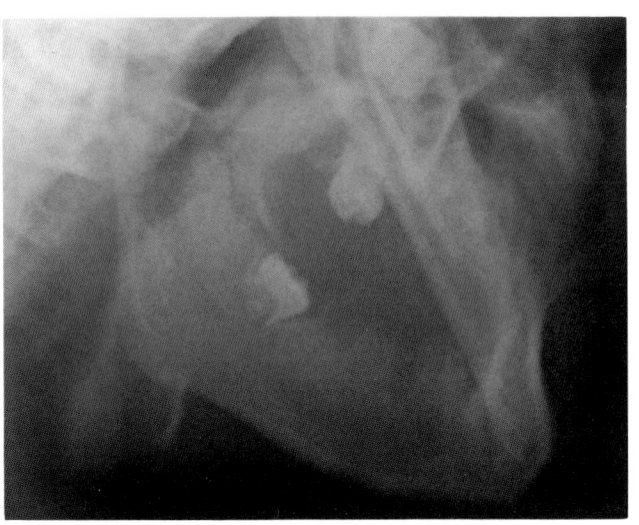

7.110 A fracture of the base of the coronoid process of the right ramus in a 16-year-old. The fracture line extends postero-superiorly from the distal aspect 8⌋, which is incompletely formed, to the anterior part of the sigmoid notch. Although there is a suspicion of a fractured condyle also, the degree of superimposition of other structures in this view of the condylar region makes interpretation difficult, and other views would be necessary to confirm the diagnosis. Note the many recent extraction sockets. OLM

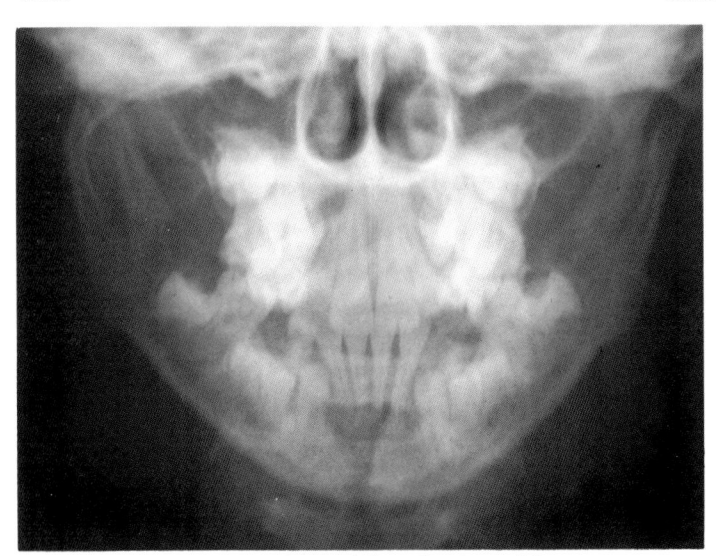

7.109 Fractures, resulting from a fall on the chin, of the anterior part of the mandible and neck of the right condyle in a nine-year-old child. The anterior fracture runs approximately vertically, passing between ⌊12. The condylar fracture has arisen indirectly from transmitted force and the condylar head is displaced medially by the pull of the lateral pterygoid muscle. PA

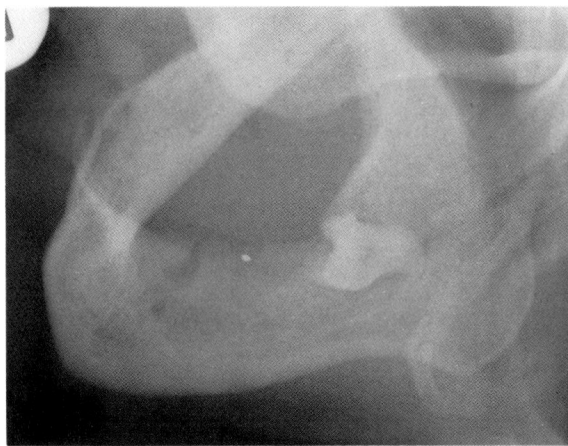

7.111 An oblique fracture running from the apex of the tooth socket to the posterior border of the left, ascending ramus of the mandible, which occurred during attempted removal of the unerupted, horizontally impacted ⌊8. Note that there has been little surgical removal of bone prior to attempted elevation of the tooth, and that its root is hooked apically. There is also a ⌊5 root fragment with a periapical radiolucency. The image of the hyoid bone overlies the angle of the mandible. OLM

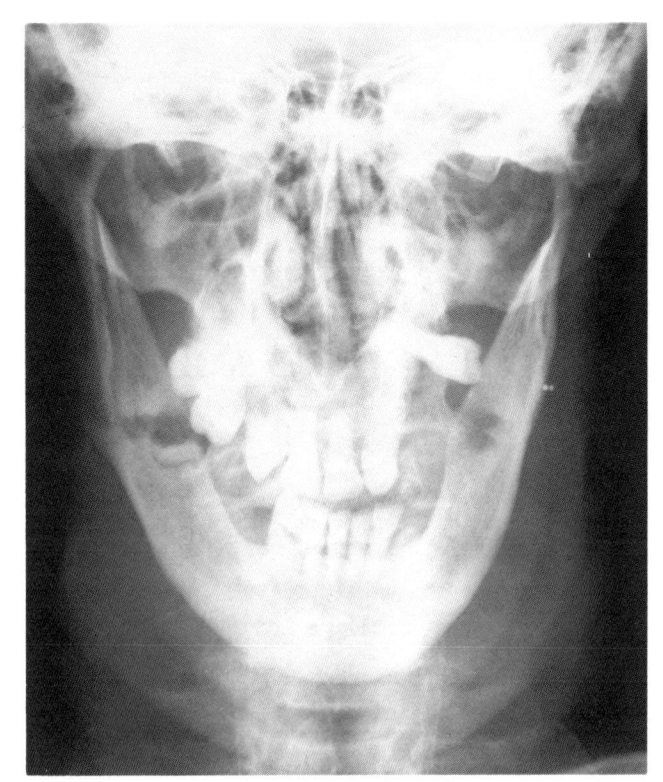

7.112 An iatrogenic fracture of the mandible, which occurred during the attempted removal of 8̅|, runs from the tooth socket obliquely backwards to the angle. The mesial root of the tooth is retained. Note the medial displacement of the ascending ramus from the pull of its attached muscles, the |8̅ socket and the transversely positioned |8. PA

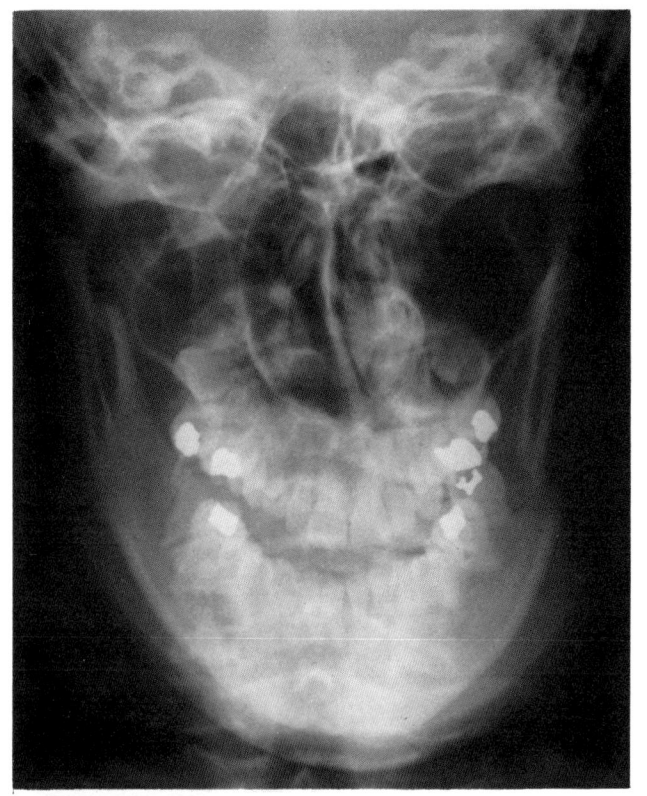

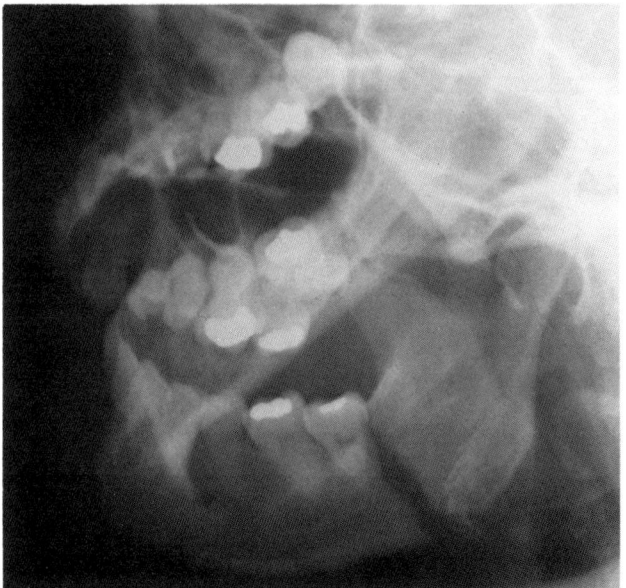

7.113 (top) and 7.114 (bottom) A unilateral oblique fracture of the left body of the mandible running through the distal aspect of the |8̅ socket to the inferior border close to the angle. The posterior fragment has been displaced inwards (Fig. 7.113) and upwards (Fig. 7.114) by contraction of the attached muscles as a consequence of the unfavourable plane of the fracture. The extent of the displacement can be assessed from the disparity in the levels of the inferior border and inferior alveolar canal in the two fragments (Fig. 7.114). PA & OLM

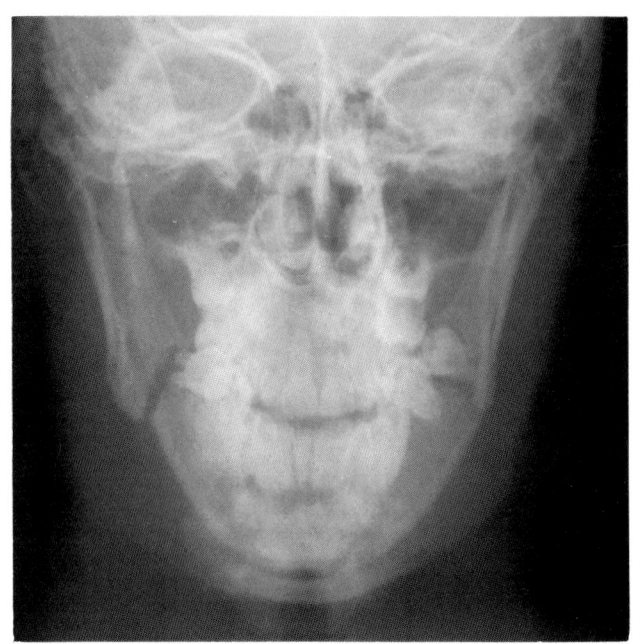

156 *A Radiological Atlas of Diseases of the Teeth and Jaws*

7.115 Bilateral fractures of the mandible through the sockets of two mesially impacted wisdom teeth, with marked separation of the bone ends at both sites. Unerupted teeth constitute an area of weakness in the jaws, and when present the fracture line often passes through their sockets. PA

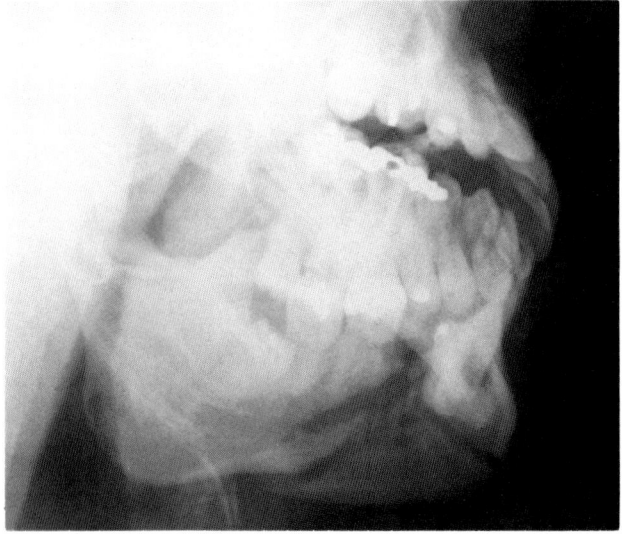

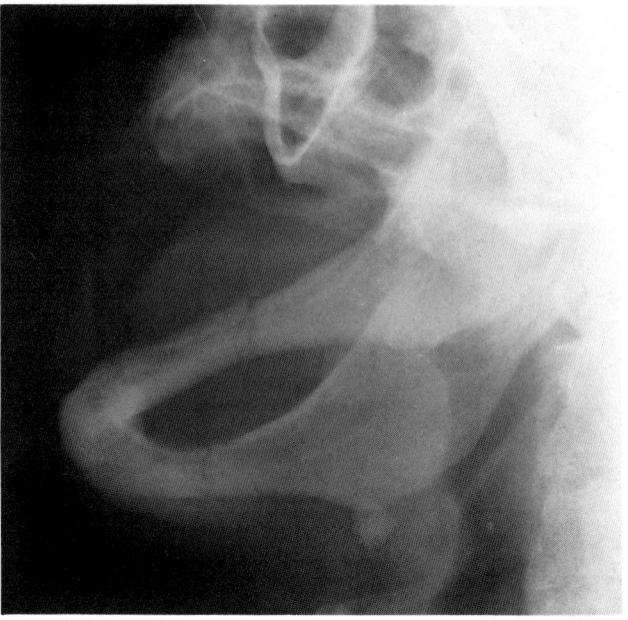

7.117 Bilateral fractures of the body of an edentulous mandible with only slight displacement of the anterior fragment. Due to the obliquity of the fracture on both sides, the radiolucent fracture lines of the inner and outer cortical plates appear separate, but converge at the upper and lower borders of the mandible, thus confirming that there is only a single fracture on each side. Note the calcified lymph node beneath, and the calcified stylo-hyoid ligament, posterior to the angle of the mandible. OLM

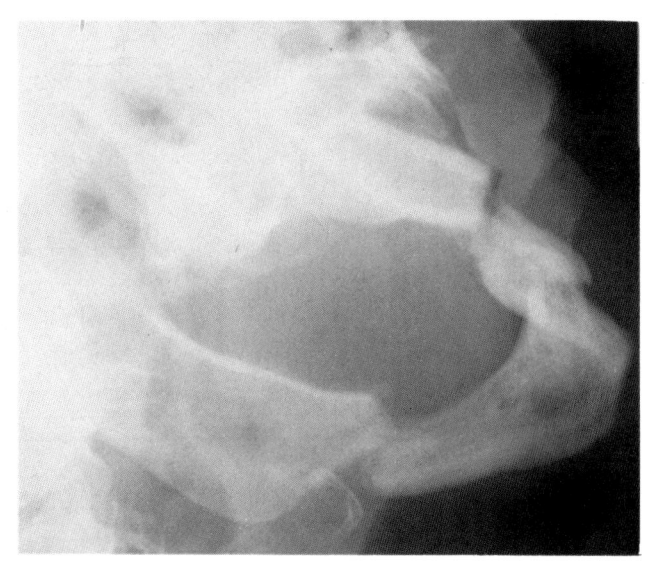

7.116 A comminuted fracture of the right body of the mandible resulting from direct violence. The posterior fragment has been displaced upwards resulting in a step deformity of the inferior border. Oblique fractures running through the inner and outer cortical plates often cause the appearance of a double fracture. Such an appearance is clearly shown posteriorly in this example, together with duplication of the image of the mental foramen. OLM

7.118 Bilateral fractures of the body of an edentulous mandible with gross displacement of the fragments causing a 'bucket handle' deformity. This disruption has resulted from a combination of severe trauma and downwards muscle pull on the anterior, and upward pull on the posterior fragments. OLM

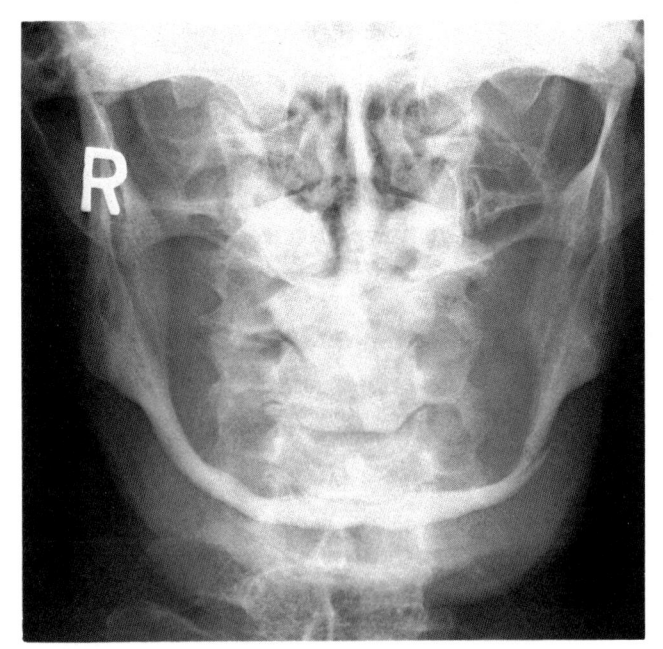

7.119 A crack fracture of the left body of an atrophic mandible in an elderly patient with minimal displacement of the bony fragments. There is swelling of the soft tissue outline of the face overlying the fracture. Note that the atrophic changes are confined to the tooth bearing part of the mandible. PA

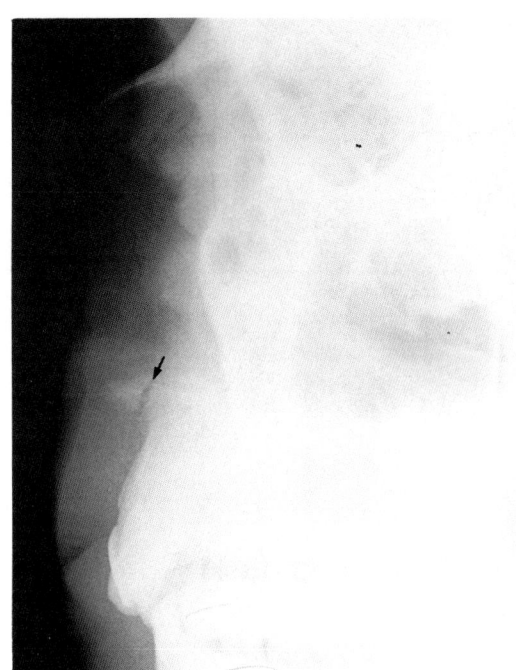

Fracture of the anterior nasal spine
7.122 A soft tissue exposure to demonstrate a fracture of the anterior nasal spine (arrow) with minimal displacement of the bone fragments. L

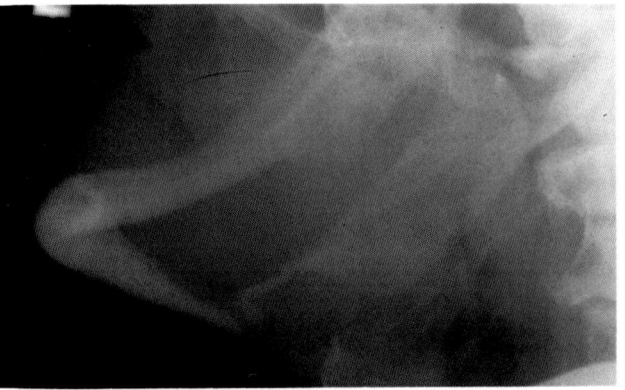

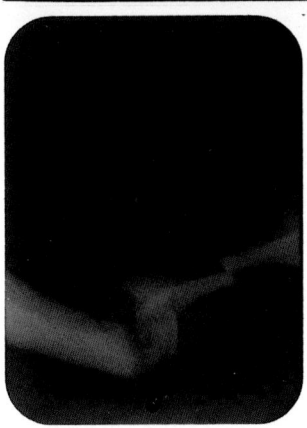

7.120 (above) and 7.121 (left) A comminuted fracture in the body of a markedly atrophic mandible in an elderly patient. There are at least two small fragments, both of which are displaced, and the posterior part of the mandible has been pulled upwards and forwards by its attached muscles. OLM & P

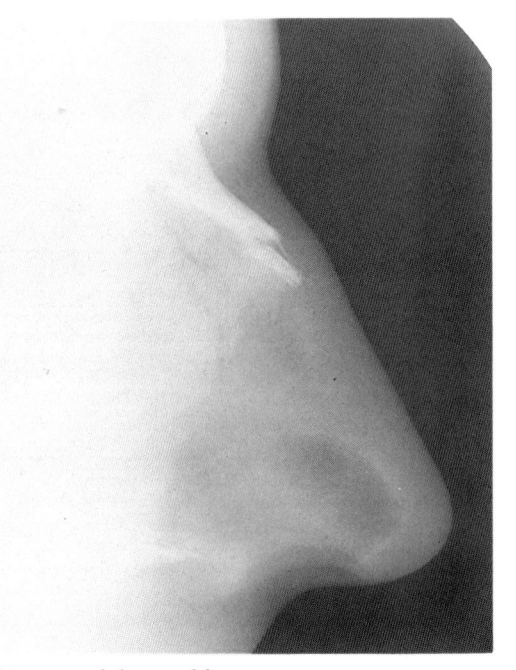

Fracture of the nasal bones
7.123 A soft tissue exposure to demonstrate a fracture of the nasal bones with downward displacement of the anterior fragments. L

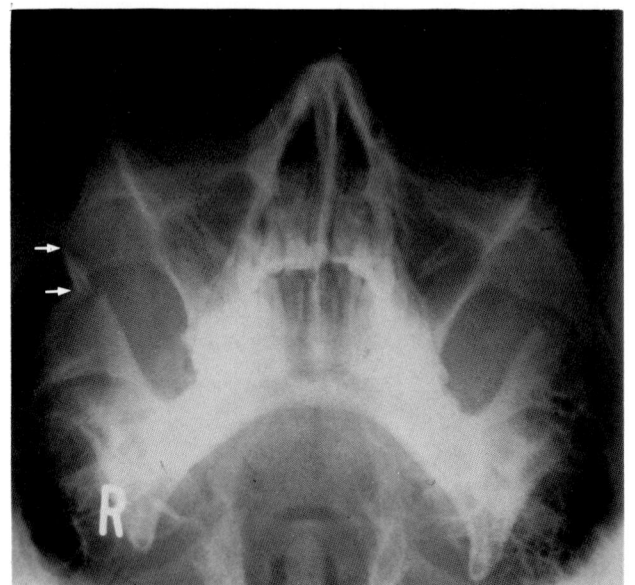

Fracture of the zygomatic complex

7.124 Three fractures (arrows) of the right zygomatic arch resulting in the formation of two separate fragments, both of which have been displaced inwards towards the coronoid process of the mandible, thus causing limitation of its movement. Note that the remainder of the zygomatic complex is intact. OM

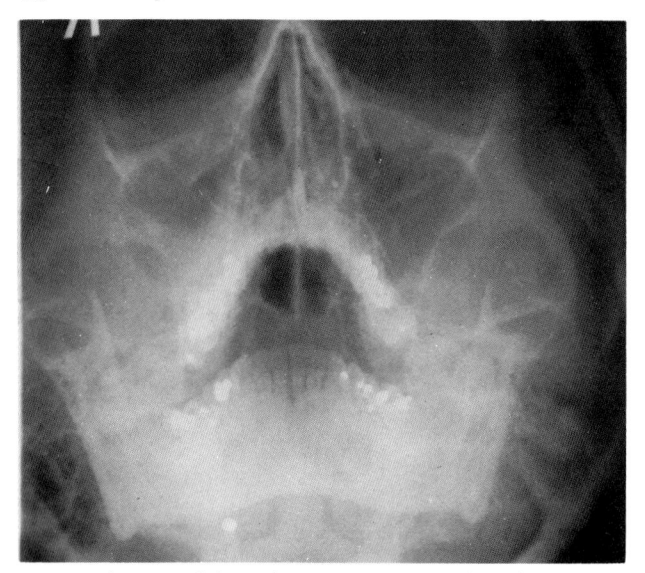

7.125 A fracture of the right zygoma crossing the inferior orbital margin medial to the infraorbital foramen superiorly, and passing through the lateral wall of the antrum and the inferior margin of the root of the zygoma inferiorly. At both margins, there is discontinuity and a step deformity across the fracture line, and the malar bone is slightly displaced. The outline of the antrum is only slightly distorted and there is some antral cloudiness due to haemorrhage into the cavity. Note the raised radiopaque shadow of the overlying soft tissues running obliquely across the inferior part of the orbit indicating that they are swollen. OM

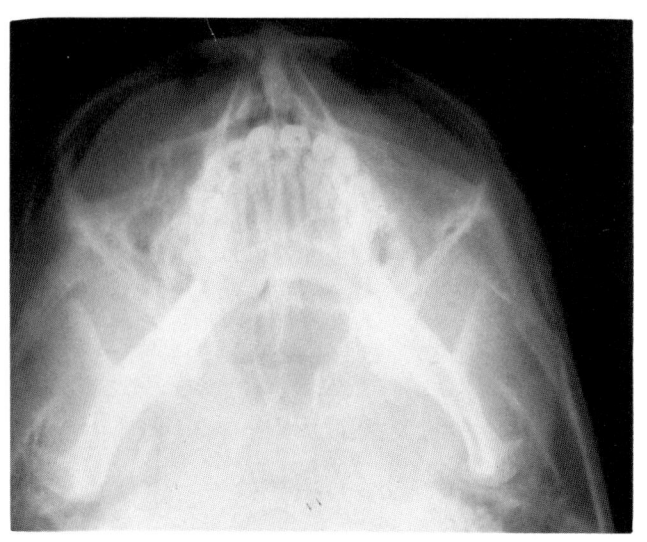

7.126 A fracture of the right zygoma viewed to display its marked inward displacement, as demonstrated by its close proximity to the coronoid process of the mandible. There is discontinuity of the inferior orbital margin, with a pronounced step deformity and at least one separate bone fragment (comminution) lying vertically in the fracture line. The outline of the antral cavity is markedly distorted and there is separation of the zygomatico-temporal suture. Again, the swelling of the overlying soft tissues is apparent from the raised radiopaque shadow occupying most of the orbital cavity. OM 30

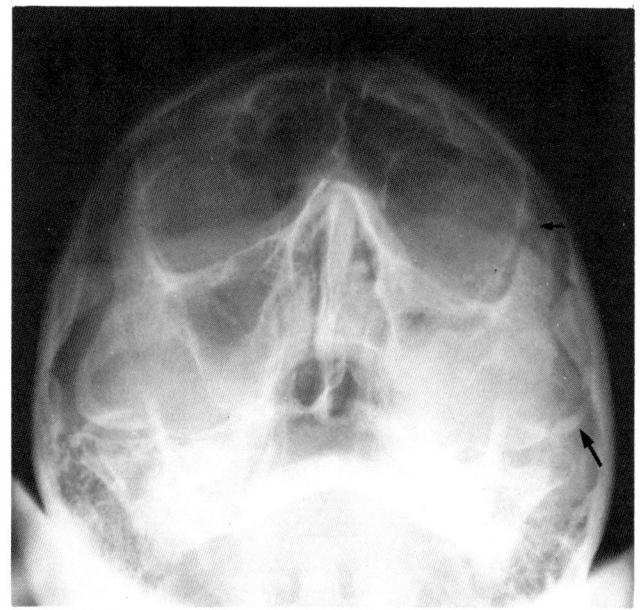

7.127 A fracture displacement of the left zygomatic complex. The inferior orbital margin appears intact, although it is lying inferiorly compared with the opposite side. There is a comminuted fracture of the zygomatic arch with at least one separate fragment (large arrow) and the fronto-zygomatic suture is widely separated (small arrow). Haemorrhage into the antral cavity has caused cloudiness (radiopacity) of the antrum and obscured its bony outline infero-laterally. OM

The Facial Bones

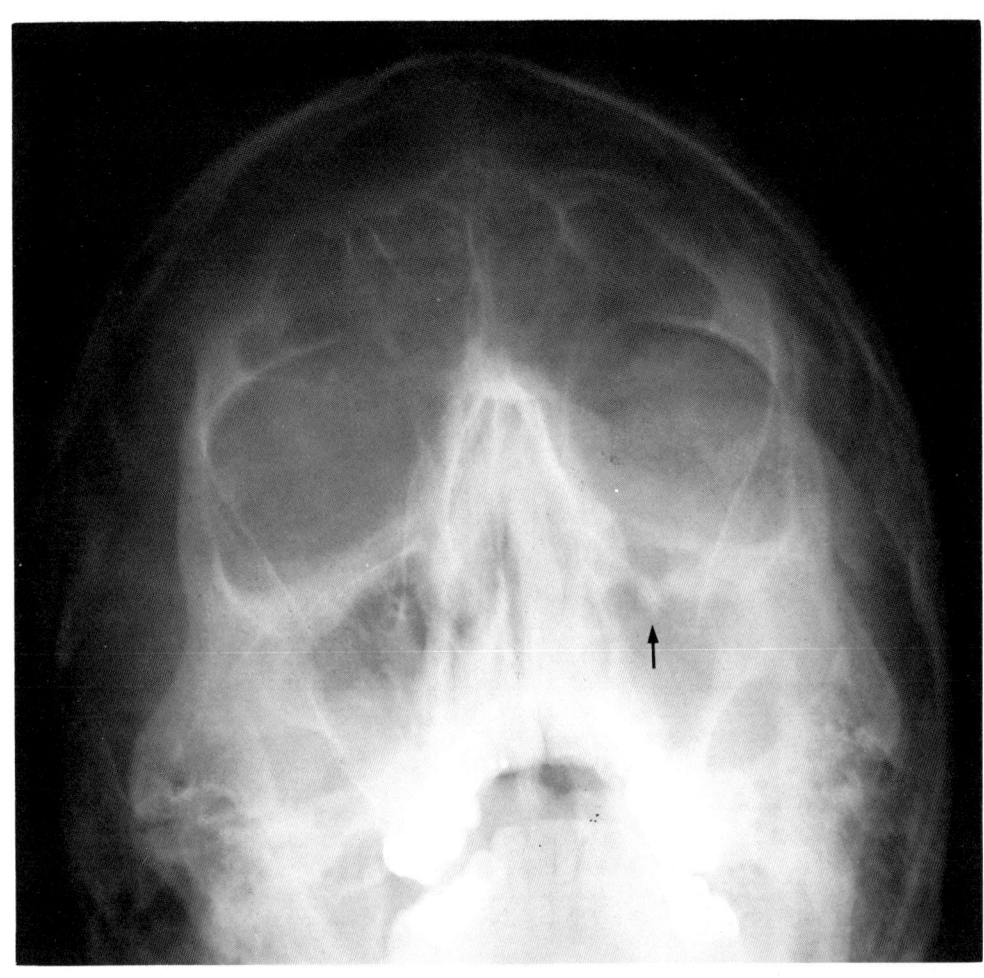

Fracture of the orbital floor
7.128 A 'blow out' fracture of the floor of the left orbit resulting from compression trauma to the globe of the eye. The inferior orbital margin remains intact, but there is downward displacement of the fragments from the thin part of the floor of the orbit, forming a 'trapdoor' appearance (arrow). The antral cavity is radiopaque due to haemorrhage into it. Note the dome-shaped, radiopaque outline superimposed over the inferior two-thirds of the orbital cavity due to infra-orbital oedema. OM

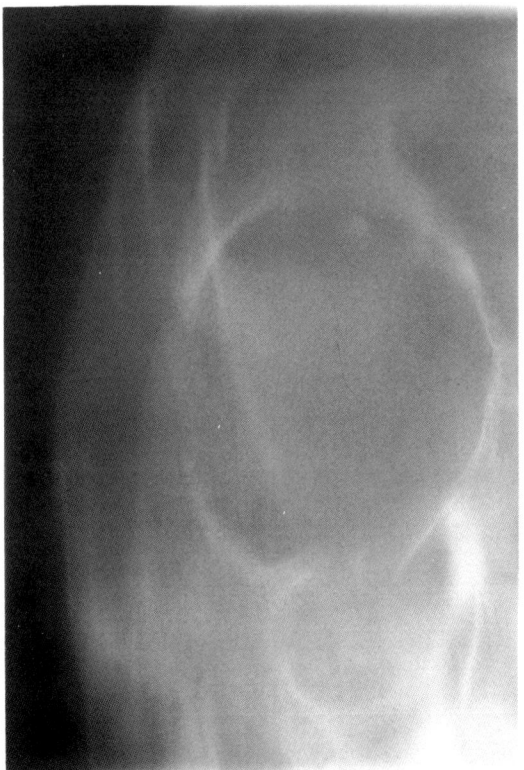

7.129 Tomograms are very helpful in determining the position of such lesions. In this example, the defect in the continuity of the radiopaque, bony lamina of the orbital floor, and the contents of the orbit herniated into the upper part of the maxillary antrum forming a 'hanging drop' appearance, are both clearly displayed. TG

160 *A Radiological Atlas of Diseases of the Teeth and Jaws*

Fracture of the maxilla 7.130 (top) and 7.131 (bottom) Bilateral fractures of the maxilla passing through the lateral wall of both antra (Fig. 7.130) and involving the floor of the nose (le Fort type II). There are step deformities in the lateral wall of both antra (arrows). Both antra are radiopaque, the right one diffusely so, and the left one exhibiting a distinct horizontal upper border to the opacity, indicating a fluid level. In the lateral view (Fig. 7.131), the radiolucent fracture line is more clearly displayed passing obliquely upwards and backwards through the lateral wall of the antrum from just superior to the anterior nasal spine anteriorly. Note the vertically running radiopacity superimposed over the midline of the vault of the skull, due to dystrophic mineralisation in the falx cerebri of this middle aged patient (Fig. 7.130). OM & L

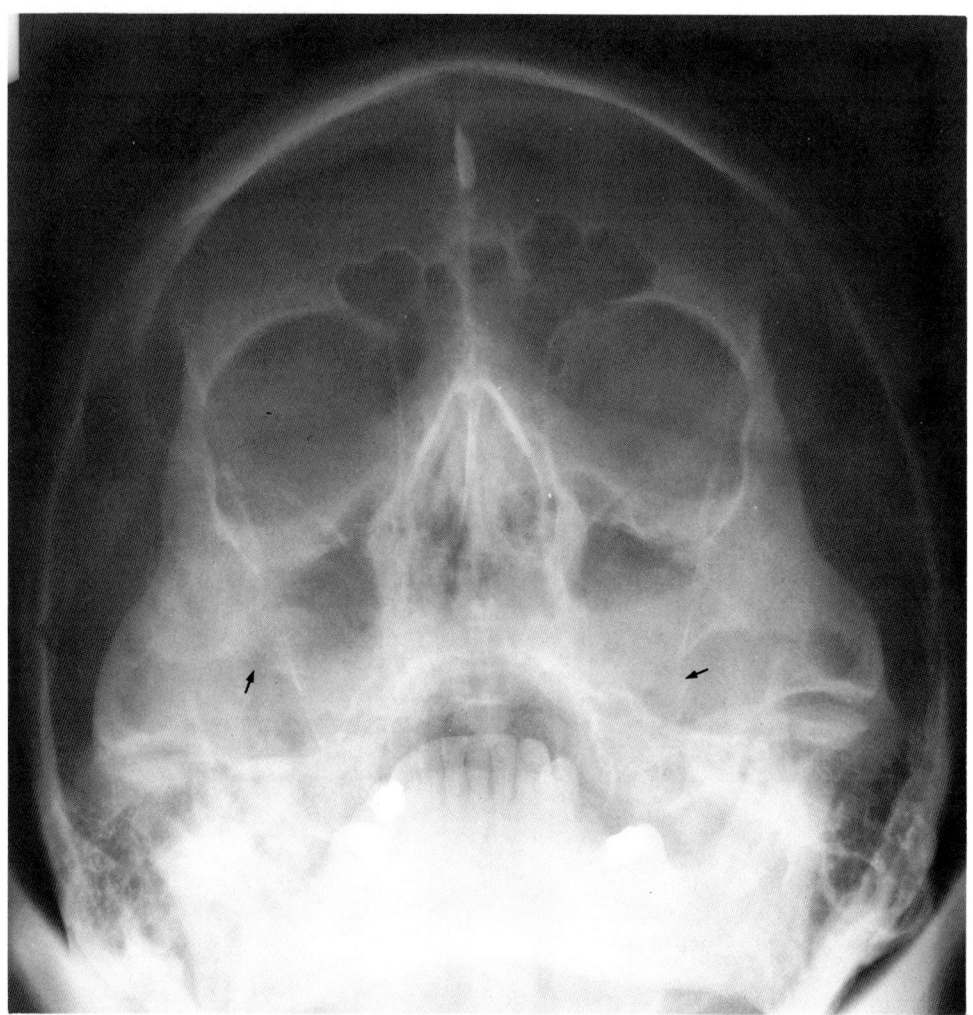

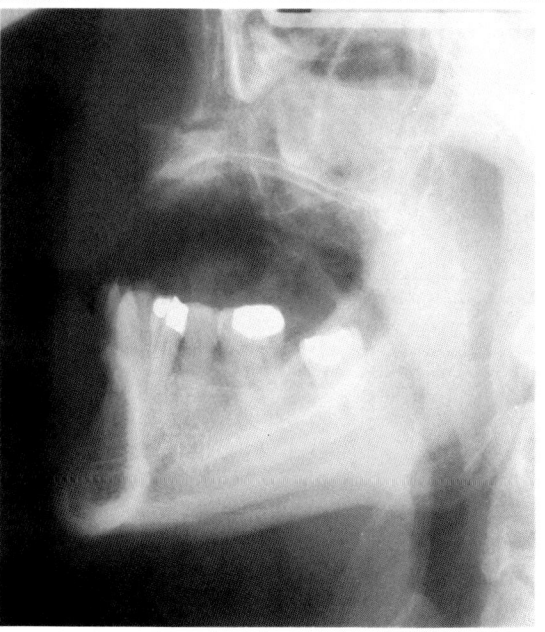

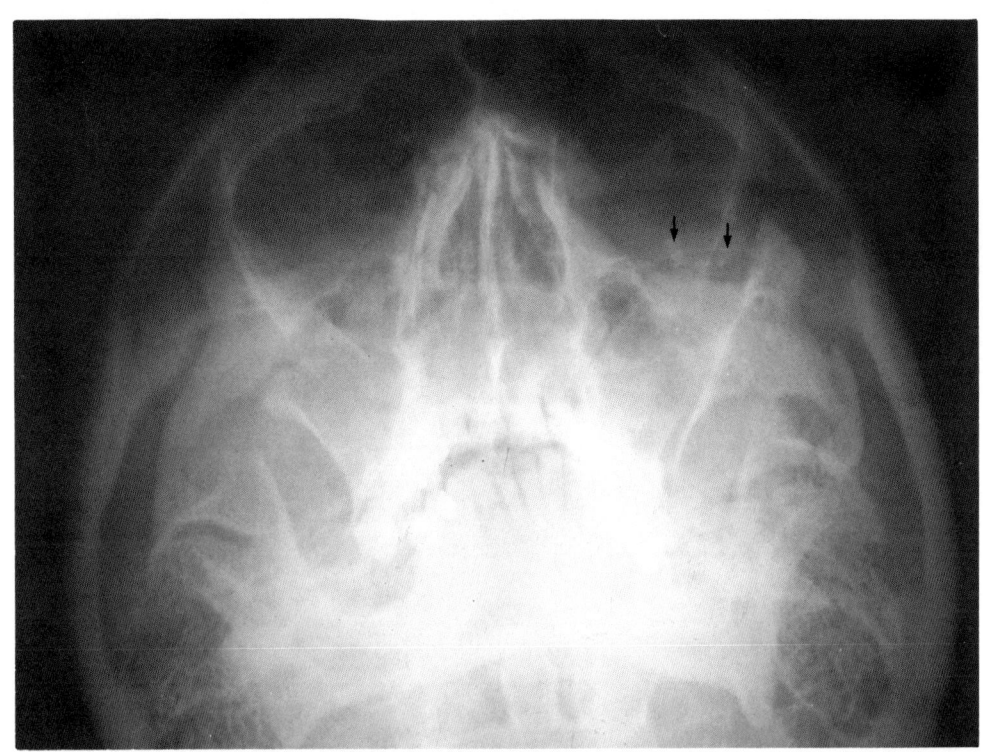

7.132 Multiple fractures of the mid-facial skeleton (le Fort type III), including the bodies of both maxillae running down from the orbital floors, and the left zygomatic arch with wide separation of the fronto-zygomatic suture. Note the bony fragments in the area of the left orbit (arrows) and the bilateral radiopacity of the maxillary antra. OM

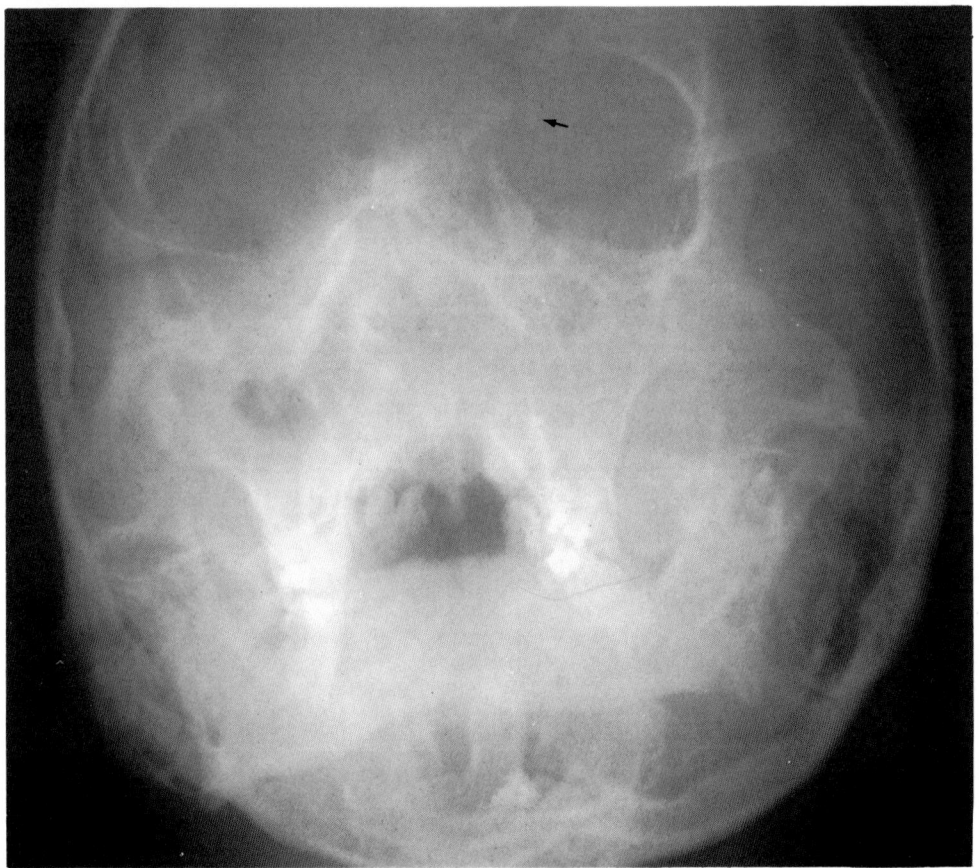

Fracture of the fronto-naso-ethmoid complex
7.133 Severe comminuted and depressed fractures of the fronto-naso-ethmoid complex with loss of the right supra-orbital margin resulting in gross distortion of the normal radiographic anatomy. A bone fragment has been displaced from the supero-medial margin of the left orbit and is lying infero-medially (arrow) within the orbital cavity. There are other fractures of the facial skeleton, particularly of the right maxilla, which are poorly demonstrated in this radiograph. OM

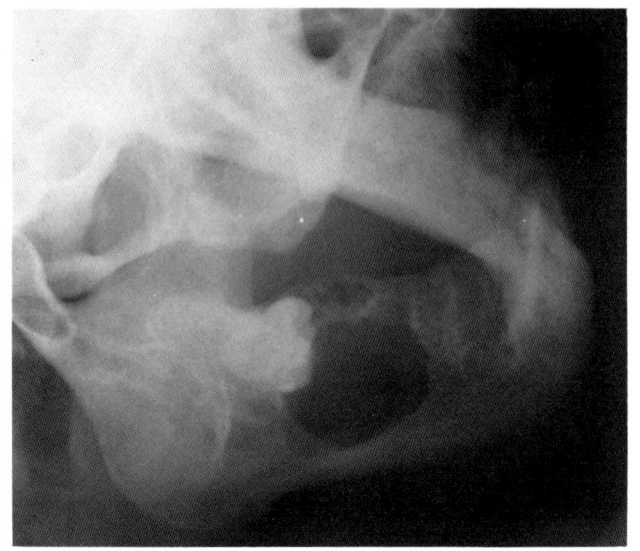

162   *A Radiological Atlas of Diseases of the Teeth and Jaws*

Ameloblastoma
7.134   This lesion has a variable radiographic appearance and may be confused with a number of other conditions, notably dentigerous cysts and odontogenic keratocysts. This example is associated with the crown of a horizontally placed, unerupted third molar in the right body of an otherwise edentulous mandible. It consists of an approximately circular, radiolucent area in the lower part of the mandible, with a smaller, more oval loculated area superiorly in the expanded edentulous ridge. The main locule is clearly defined and contains a more radiolucent area centrally, indicating extreme thinning or perforation of a cortical plate. OLM

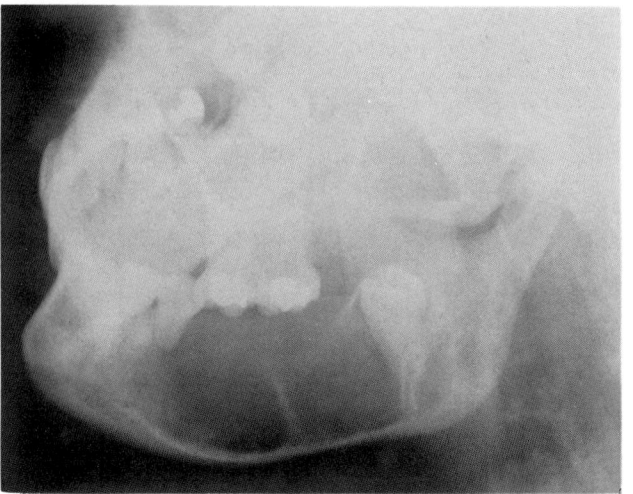

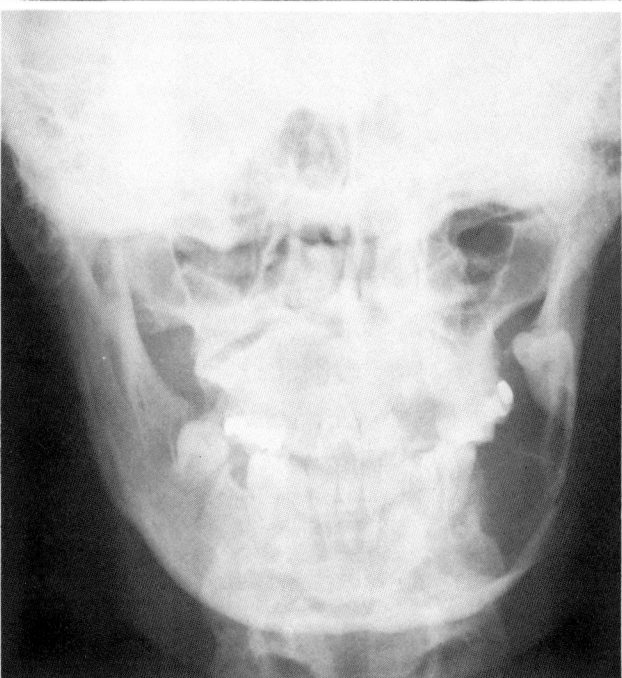

7.135 (top) and 7.136 (bottom)   A lesion of the left body of the mandible, associated with a vertically placed, unerupted third molar. The radiolucent area extends from the canine region anteriorly to the mid-portion of the ascending ramus posteriorly (Fig. 7.135). It is a basically unilocular, well defined lesion, which is less clearly outlined anteriorly, with an incomplete, vertical septum arising from its midpoint inferiorly. There is thinning of the cortical bone at the inferior border of the mandible, and thinning and expansion of the alveolar ridge and buccal bone (Fig. 7.136). The inferior alveolar canal has been displaced posteriorly and inferiorly, and there is apical resorption |5. Note that the image of the hyoid bone is superimposed over the apical part of |8. OLM & PA

The Facial Bones 163

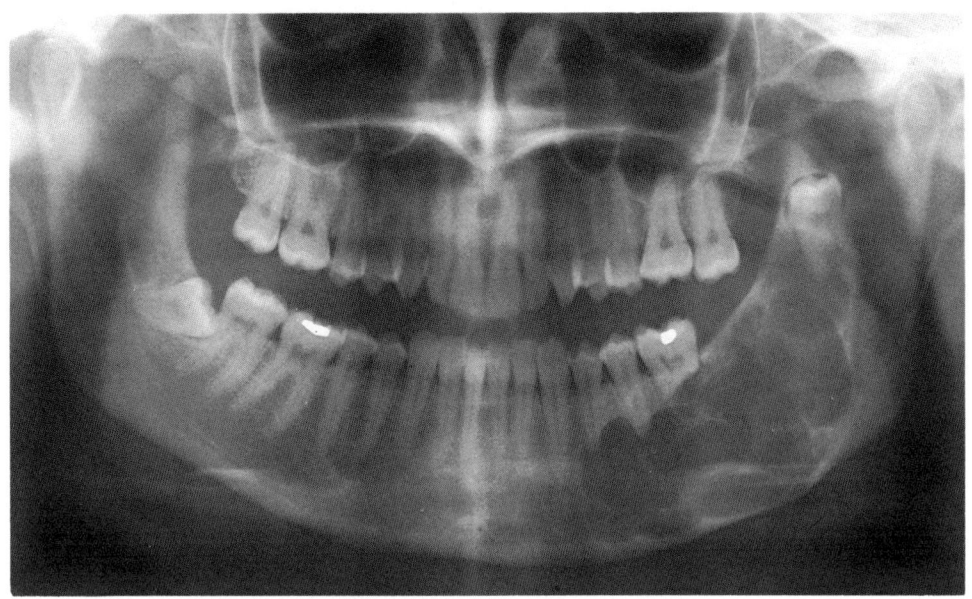

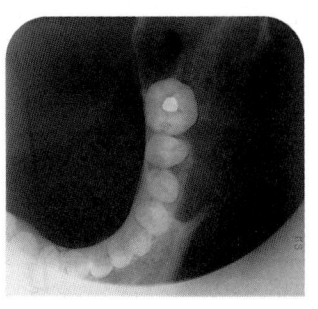

7.137 (left) and 7.138 (right) Since ameloblastomas spread predominantly through the marrow spaces, they more typically have a multilocular appearance. This lesion of the left mandible extends from |3 anteriorly and involves the majority of the ascending ramus (Fig. 7.137). It has a well defined, scalloped margin and the cortical bone at the inferior border of the mandible is thinned, but remains intact. There is resorption of the roots of |456 and also of the unerupted |7 which has been displaced to the base of the coronoid process. There is expansion and thinning of the cortical bone lingually (Fig. 7.138) and buccally where the outline is discontinuous due to its perforation. PR & LTO

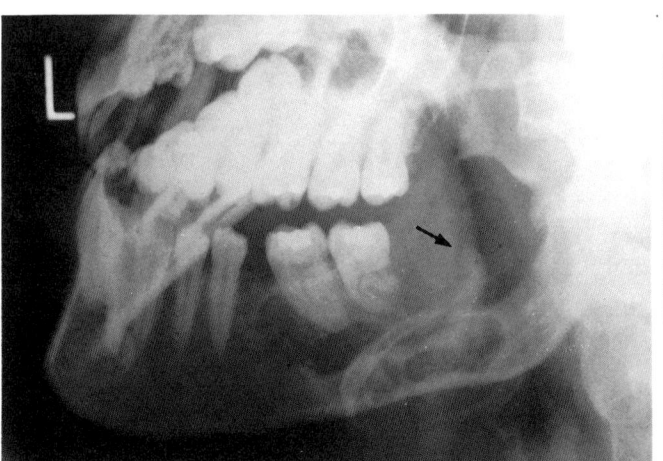

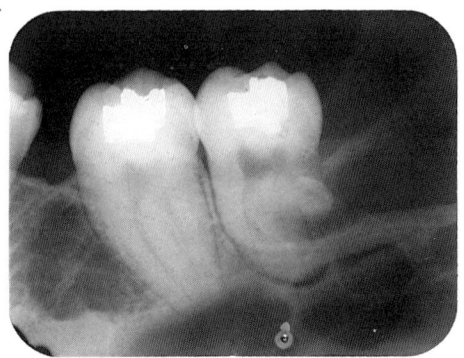

7.139 (left) and 7.140 (right) Another multilocular lesion of the left mandible extending from the first molar region anteriorly to half-way up the anterior part of the ramus posteriorly (Fig. 7.139). The radiolucent tumour has a scalloped, well defined margin and contains several radiopaque bony septa. The inferior border of the mandible is thinned but continuous, and the alveolar margin in the retromolar area is indistinct and has a soft tissue swelling overlying it. Note the images of the hyoid bone and the epiglottis (arrow) superimposed upon the lesion, the latter of which is apparent due to the extensive bone destruction. The distal root |8 is foreshortened and of greater radiopacity than the mesial root (Fig. 7.140) due either to its displacement buccally by the tumour during development or to resorption. OLM & P

164 *A Radiological Atlas of Diseases of the Teeth and Jaws*

7.141 (top), 7.142 (middle) and 7.143 (bottom) A large, predominantly unilocular, radiolucent lesion of the left mandible occupying the ramus, and which has produced thinning and expansion of the cortical bone inferiorly, anteriorly and posteriorly (Fig. 7.141). Nearly the entire ramus is radiolucent and only a small amount of radiopaque bone remains in the region of the angle, where a bony septum curves into the tumour mass. There is expansion of the coronoid process and flattening of the sigmoid notch. |8 is displaced antero-inferiorly to the lower border of the mandible, and its crown appears to be projecting into the radiolucent defect, thus simulating a dentigerous cyst. Note the images of the hyoid bone and epiglottis again superimposed upon the lesion. On the intra-oral radiograph (Fig. 7.142), a dentigerous relationship of the crown of |8 to the lesion is again suggested and the thin, radiopaque lamina on the outer aspect of the expanded ramus indicates that the cortical bone is still intact. In addition, there is expansion of the buccal and lingual (arrows) aspects of the ramus (Fig. 7.143), the buccal cortical outline being indistinct. OLM, P & PA

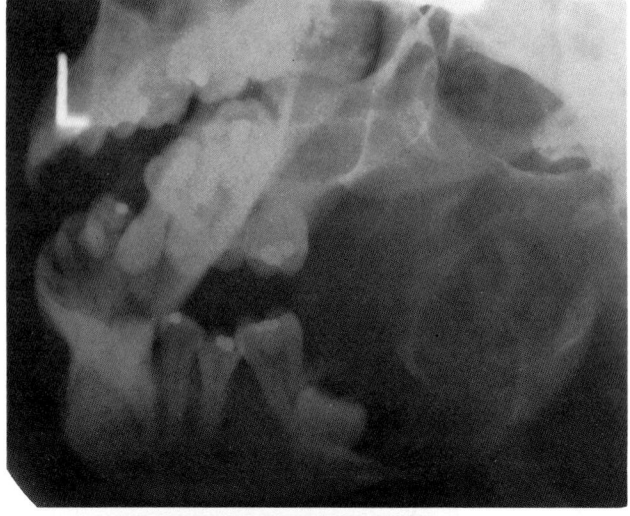

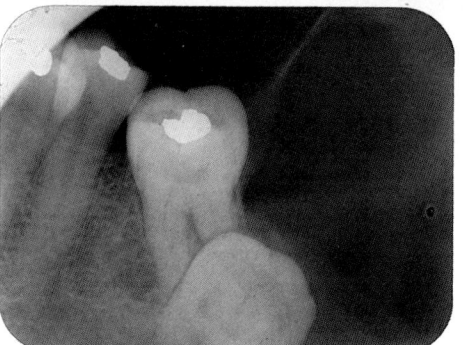

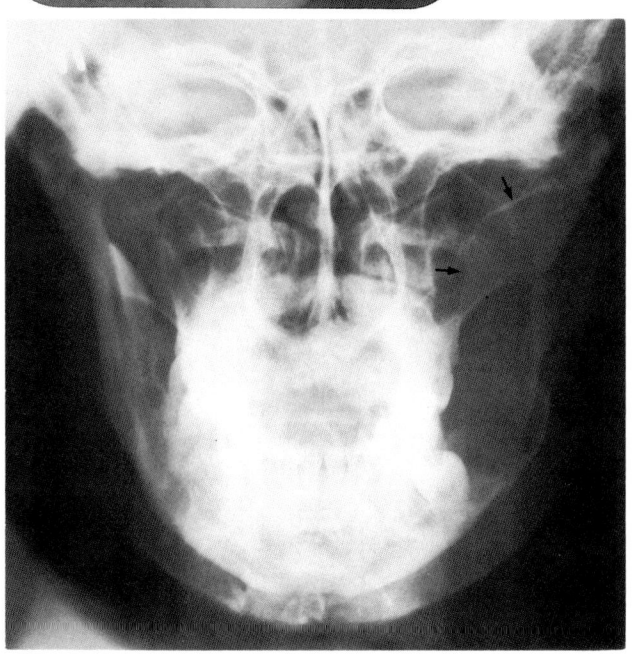

7.144 (top), 7.145 (middle) and 7.146 (bottom) A large unilocular type of ameloblastoma in a 14-year-old, in which the tumour growth occurs essentially into a cyst cavity (ameloblastomatoid cyst). The radiolucent defect extends from the first molar region anteriorly and occupies the entire ramus, apart from the condyloid process, posteriorly (Fig. 7.144). There is thinning of the cortical bone inferiorly, anteriorly and posteriorly, and expansion anteriorly, inferiorly and in the region of the sigmoid notch, which is flattened. 8̅| is partially formed and displaced into the coronoid process. 7̅| is displaced antero-inferiorly. The radiolucent defect is superimposed upon 7̅|, causing an appearance similar to that of a dentigerous cyst. Note the outline of the incompletely calcified hyoid bone superimposed on the lesion. The more occlusal position of 7̅| on the intra-oral film (Fig. 7.145) relative to that in the previous illustration is consequent upon the upward projection of the image of the tooth, which lies buccally to 6̅|, due to the greater upward angulation of the X-ray tube. The buccal position of 7̅| is confirmed in the postero-anterior view (Fig. 7.146), which also illustrates buccal and lingual expansion of the ramus. OLM, P & PA

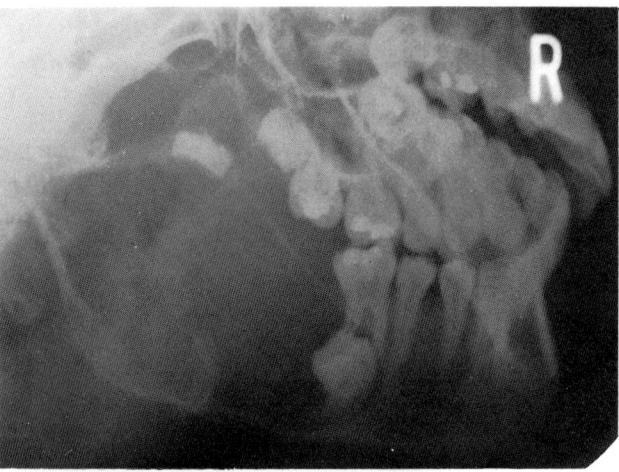

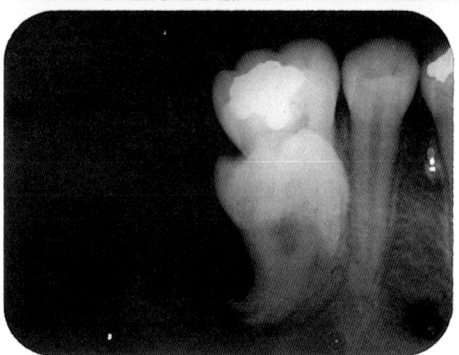

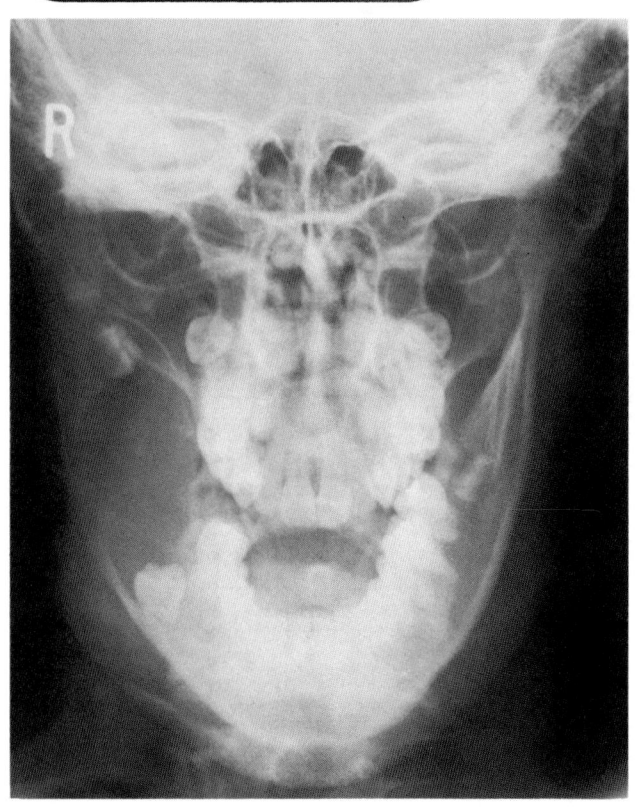

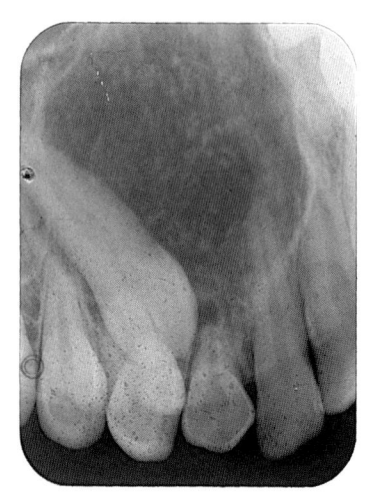

Adenomatoid odontogenic tumour
7.147 This benign expansile tumour arises characteristically in the anterior part of the jaws and is often associated with the crown of an unerupted tooth, thus simulating a dentigerous cyst. In this example in an 18-year-old, the clearly defined, radiolucent lesion is associated with the mesial aspect of the unerupted 3| where the lamina dura and follicular space are absent. It is partly surrounded by a thin, radiopaque lamina. Not infrequently, such lesions contain a number of radiopaque foci of dystrophic mineralisation, which are present in this tumour. C| is retained, although there has been some apical resorption. P

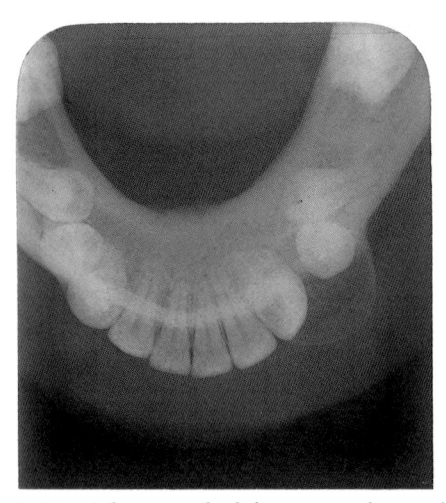

7.148 A lesion in the left canine and premolar region of the mandible not associated with an unerupted tooth. It has produced a circular, radiolucent defect with marked buccal expansion of the bone around which the thinned cortical lamina remains intact. The radiopaque lamina demarcating the medial wall of the lesion is superimposed upon the images of the canine and first premolar teeth, between which there is a diastema. Again, a number of radiopaque foci of mineralisation are present and in this view are shown characteristically towards the centre of the mass rather than at its periphery. Note the lingual inclination of the crowns 5|5, both of which are instanding. LTO

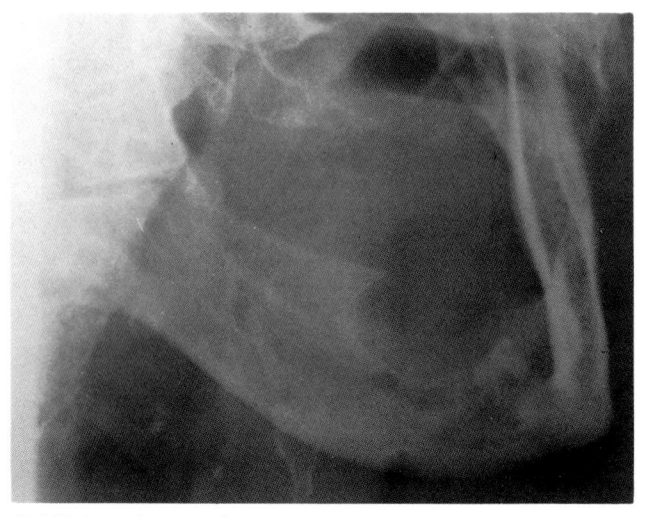

Calcifying odontogenic cyst
7.149 This lesion is essentially an expansile cystic tumour, which in some instances contains areas of dystrophic mineralisation and is occasionally associated with an odontome. It has, therefore, a variable radiographic appearance. In this example, there is an ovoid, clearly defined, radiolucent lesion in the right premolar region of an edentulous mandible. It is bounded by a thin, radiopaque lamina of cortical bone except superiorly, where the alveolar bone has been eroded. Two areas of darker radiolucency within the lesion indicate that one of the cortical plates has been thinned. Note the mental foramen lying just beneath the cyst. OLM

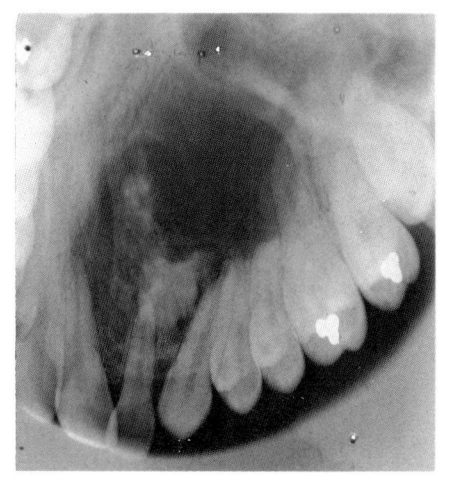

7.150 Another lesion in the left maxilla containing areas of dystrophic mineralisation. There is a clearly defined, round radiolucent area extending from |1 to |6. Numerous irregularly shaped masses of variable size and of uniformly dense radiopacity are present in the anterior part of the lesion. The lamina dura is absent around the apices of |345 which are blunted, indicating the presence of resorption, and their roots have been displaced by the tumour together with |1. UOO

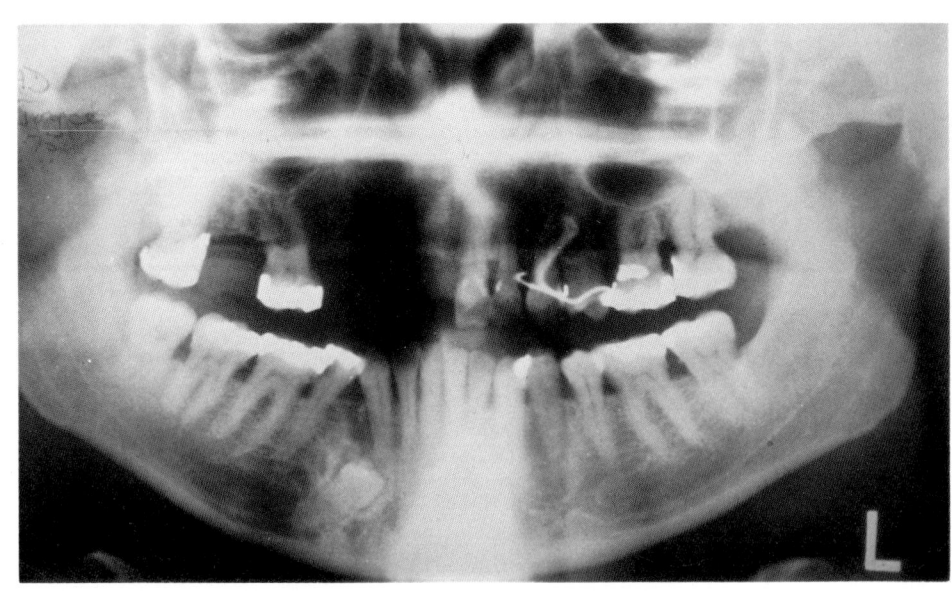

Calcifying epithelial odontogenic tumour (Pindborg tumour)

7.151 This tumour is sometimes associated with an unerupted tooth, as in this example involving $\overline{4|}$. There is a loculated radiolucent lesion lying between $\overline{5|}$ and $\overline{3|}$, the roots of which are displaced away from it. $\overline{4|}$ is displaced inferiorly and its crown is surrounded by a normal follicular space and cortical lamina, except superiorly where the lesion is present. Note the patient is wearing an upper partial denture with wire clasps. PR

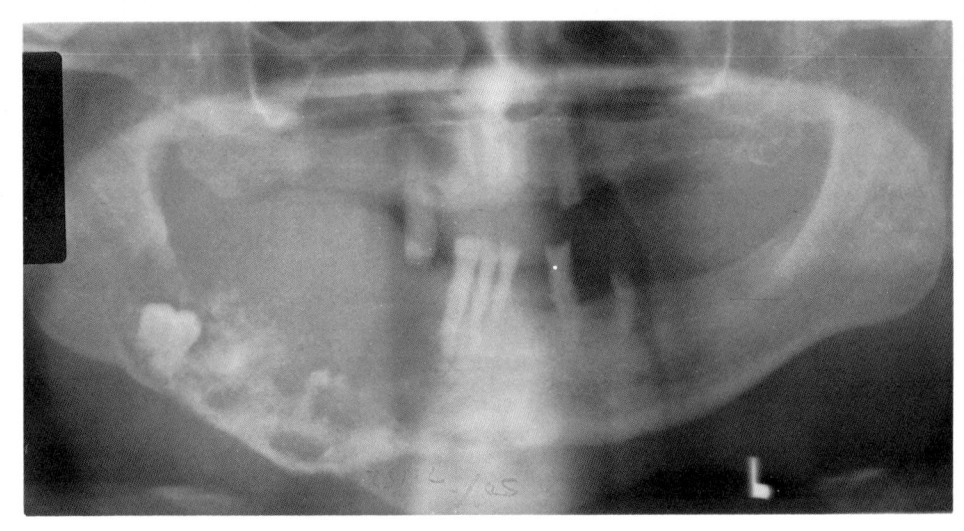

7.152 A very large tumour of long standing in the right mandible of an elderly patient. It is basically a radiolucent lesion with a clearly defined margin posteriorly, and is poorly defined anteriorly where it has crossed the midline. Superiorly, there is complete destruction of the alveolar bone and a large soft tissue swelling, whereas the cortical bone of the inferior border of the mandible has been expanded, and in places markedly thinned. A malformed, unerupted $\overline{8|}$ is present in the posterior part of the lesion, which contains numerous, irregular, radiopaque structures some of which are residual bone trabeculae, and other areas of dystrophic mineralisation within the mass. The cortical margins of the inferior alveolar canal, although clearly present in the ramus, are absent within the tumour. Note the heavy deposits of calculus on the remaining erupted teeth, which show advanced loss of alveolar bone. PR

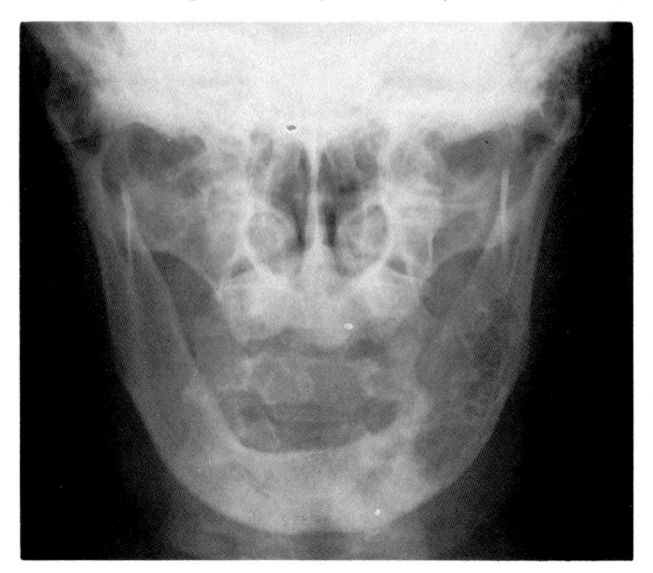

168 *A Radiological Atlas of Diseases of the Teeth and Jaws*

Odontogenic myxoma

7.153 A large lesion of the left body and ramus of an edentulous mandible, which forms a clearly defined, radiolucent defect with scalloped outline. Within the area, randomly arranged radiopaque bony septa are present in a reticular pattern, forming the 'honeycomb' appearance characteristic of this lesion. The cortical plate is expanded lingually and thinned on all surfaces. PA

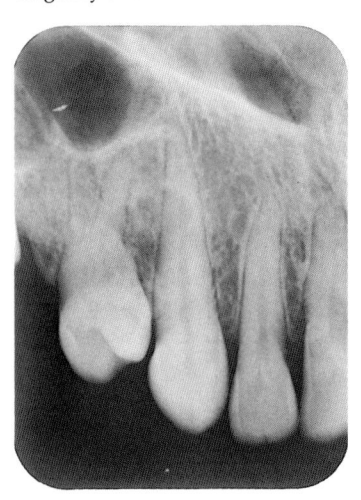

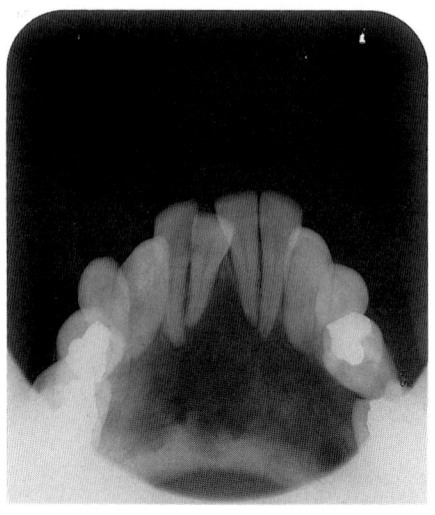

7.155 A much larger lesion in the anterior part of the mandible, occupying almost the entire height of the bone. The radiolucent lesion has a loculated, clearly defined margin and contains several thin, radiopaque septa. There is displacement of the roots 1|1 distally and loss of the lamina dura around the apical halves of all four incisors. Occasionally such an aggressive lesion is associated with pregnancy, as in this example. LAO

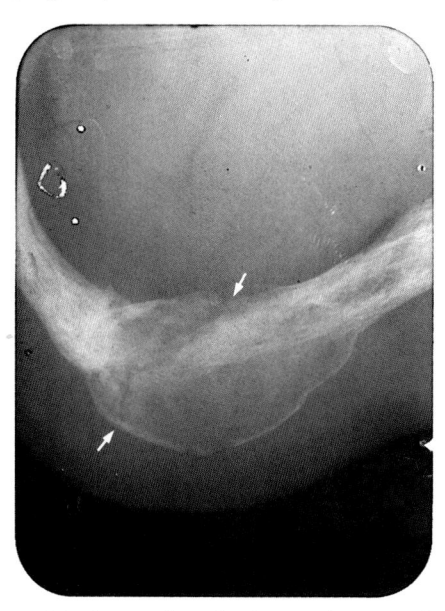

Central giant cell tumour

7.154 Most central giant cell tumours are granulomas and are confined to the tooth bearing parts of the jaws. This small, radiolucent granuloma has a clearly defined, loculated outline overlying the roots 43|. It is only partly surrounded by a thin, radiopaque lamina and several trabeculations run across it. The periodontal ligament space and lamina dura around the adjacent teeth remain intact. P

7.156 A granuloma in the anterior part of an edentulous mandible in an elderly patient. There is pronounced expansion and thinning of the labial cortical bone producing a 'soap bubble' appearance typical of this lesion. In addition, there is slight lingual expansion. The extent of the lateral margins is unclear, and there is a pathological fracture (arrows) running obliquely across the lesion from the midline lingually to the 2| region labially. LTO

The Facial Bones 169

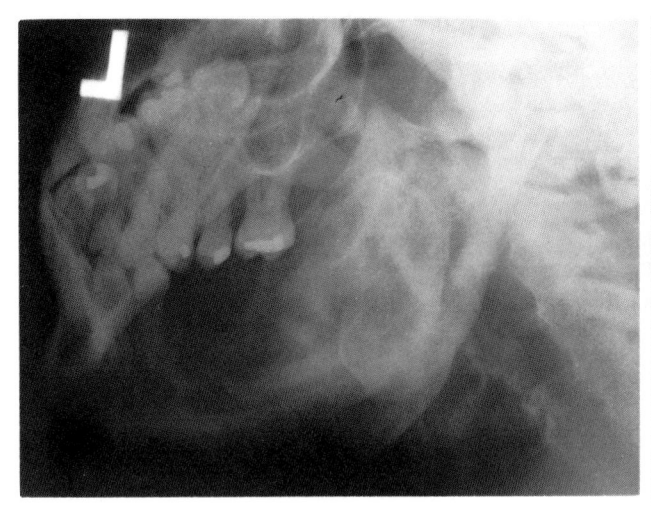

7.157 (above) and 7.158 (right) Sometimes aggressive giant cell tumours are classified as osteoclastomas. This large tumour occupies the ramus and body of the left mandible as far forward as $\overline{|3}$ (Fig. 7.157). In the ramus, it extends into the coronoid process and has caused expansion of the anterior border and flattening of the sigmoid notch. This expansile benign tumour has a clearly defined margin apart from the $\overline{|34}$ region and is essentially radiolucent, although there are numerous, coarse, radiopaque trabeculations running through it. The image of the hyoid bone is projected across the middle of the lower part of the ramus. In addition, there is marked lingual and buccal expansion, the former projecting beyond the inferior border in the oblique lateral mandibular view. Note that the inferior alveolar canal is demonstrated in both films. OLM & PA

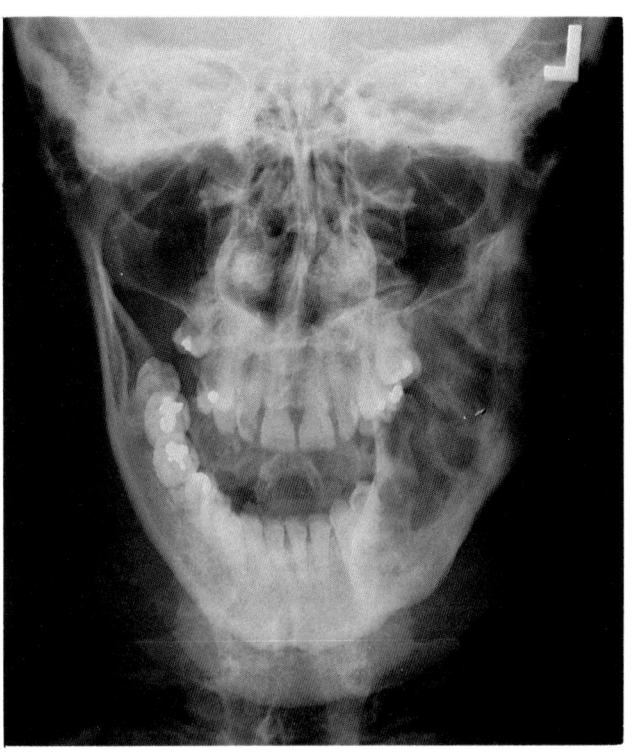

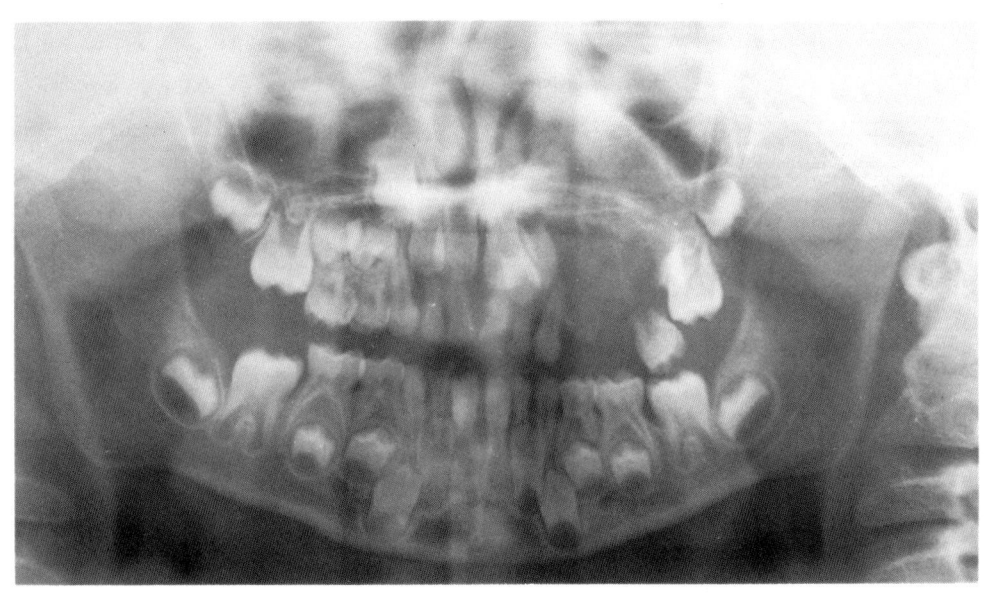

Ossifying fibroma
7.159 This expansile, approximately circular mass in the left maxilla of a six-year-old has displayed the antral floor superiorly, and has expanded the alveolus inferiorly. $|\underline{E}$ has been displaced occlusally and distally, and much of the roots is missing. $|\underline{45}$ are absent. The unerupted $|\underline{3}$ has been displaced mesially and overlies the unerupted $|\underline{12}$. The mass is variably radiopaque and radiolucent since it is composed of a mixture of fibrous tissue within which centres of ossification and mineralisation are randomly arranged. PR

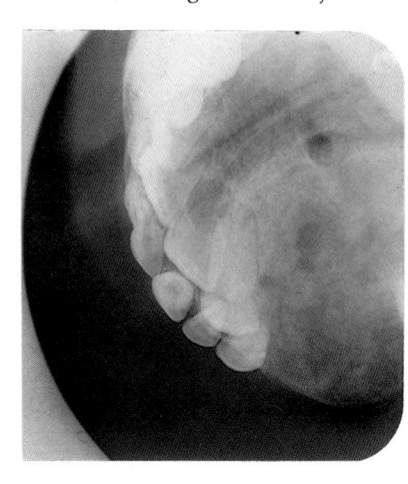

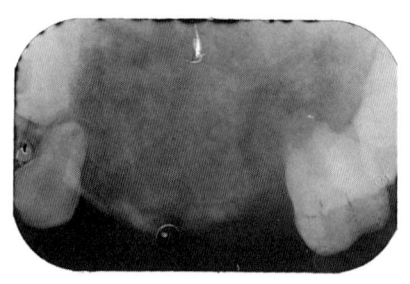

170 A Radiological Atlas of Diseases of the Teeth and Jaws

7.160 (left) and 7.161 (above) On the intra-oral films of the same patient as in Fig. 7.159, its internal structure is more clearly demonstrated as randomly arranged granular radiopacities in a radiolucent background. Somewhat atypically, the lesion blends with the adjacent bone and is not demarcated with a clear margin. UOO & P

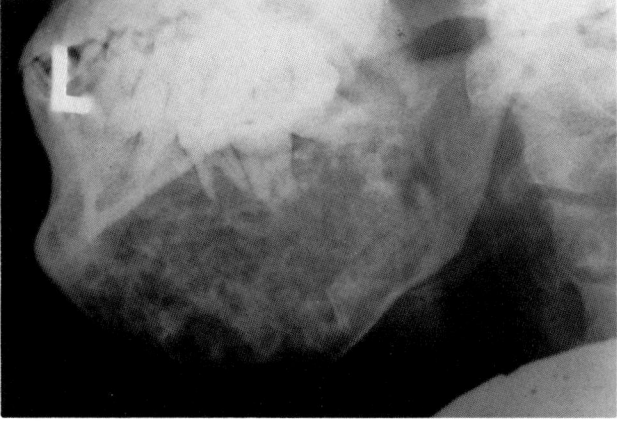

7.162 (above) and 7.163 (right) An extensive lesion in an adult, which has caused expansion of the mandible buccally, lingually and inferiorly. The lesion extends from the midline anteriorly to the base of the coronoid process posteriorly, and its posterior margin is clearly defined. A thin cortical lamina persists inferiorly, but buccally and lingually is indistinct, and the buccal outline is undulated. The lesion is composed of randomly arranged, relatively coarse radiopacities of varying density in a radiolucent background. As such lesions develop, the radiopacities tend to become increasingly coarse and numerous as more mineral is deposited within it. The premolar and molar teeth have been displaced by the tumour. OLM & LTO

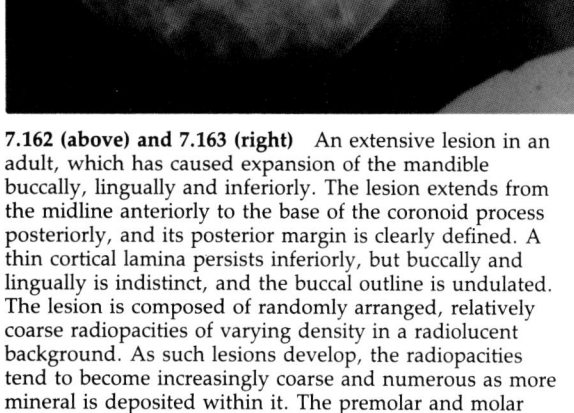

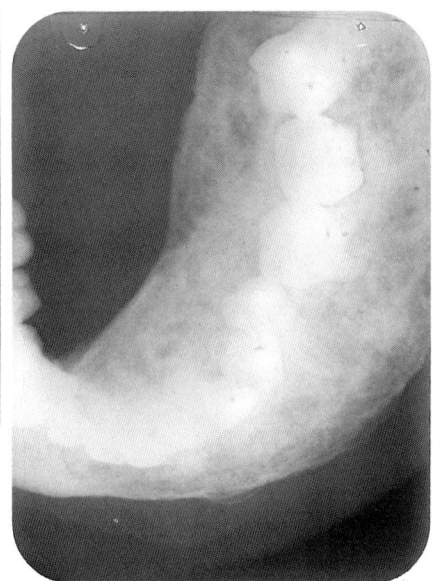

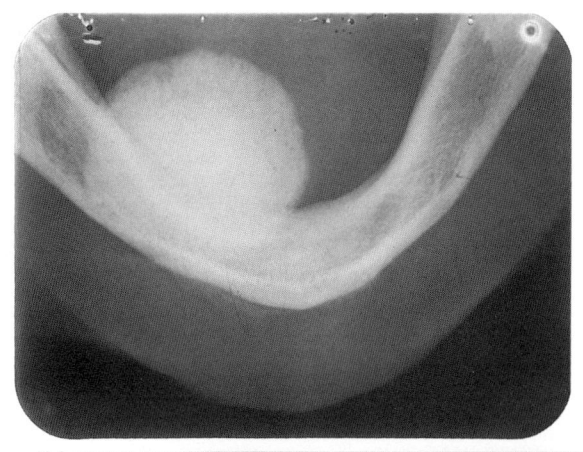

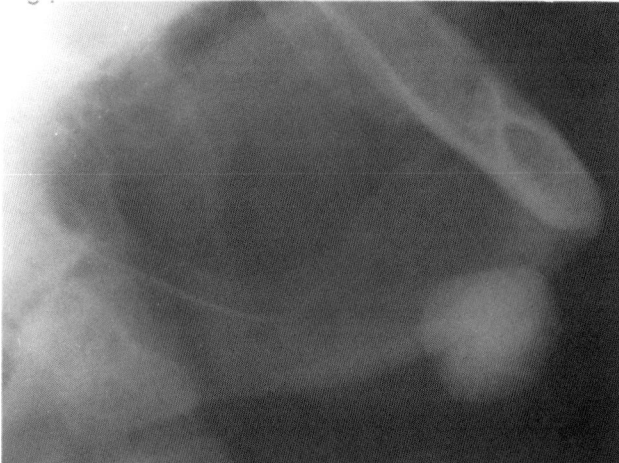

The Facial Bones 171

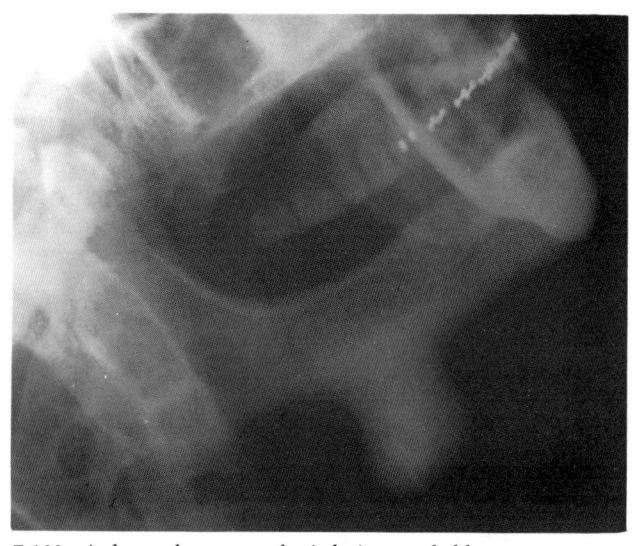

7.166 A dense, bony, exophytic lesion, probably a compact osteoma, projecting inferiorly from the lower border of an edentulous mandible. It is a uniformly radiopaque mass, the radiopacity extending into the inferior border of the mandible at the base of the lesion. The image of the body of the hyoid bone is superimposed upon the mass. Note the presence of the upper denture with porcelain teeth, the anterior ones being pin-retained. OLM

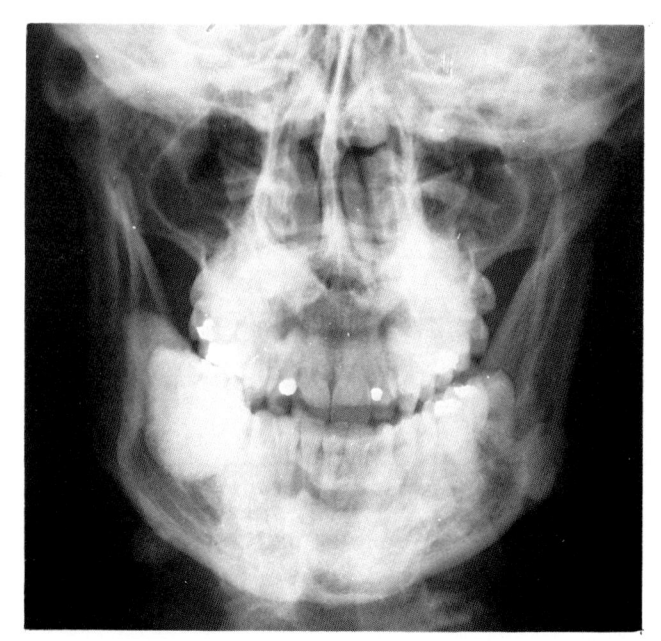

Osteoma
7.164 (top) and 7.165 (bottom) A compact (ivory) osteoma arising from the inferior border of an edentulous mandible. The approximately circular mass which projects lingually (Fig. 7.164) is densely radiopaque with a more granular pattern in its peripheral part. Being composed of dense compact bone, its radiopacity is similar to that of the cortical bone at the inferior border of the mandible. LTO & OLM

7.167 Multiple osteomas of the jaws may occur in Gardner's syndrome, as in this example in which a tumour is present in both sides of the mandible. The densely radiopaque mass in the right body is clearly defined and circumscribed by a radiolucent follicular space which is partly demarcated by a thin, radiopaque cortical lamina, particularly posteriorly and laterally. The lesion at the left angle is less densely radiopaque, although it also has a clearly defined margin, and is protruding laterally. A similar lesion protrudes from the inferior border of the right body. PA

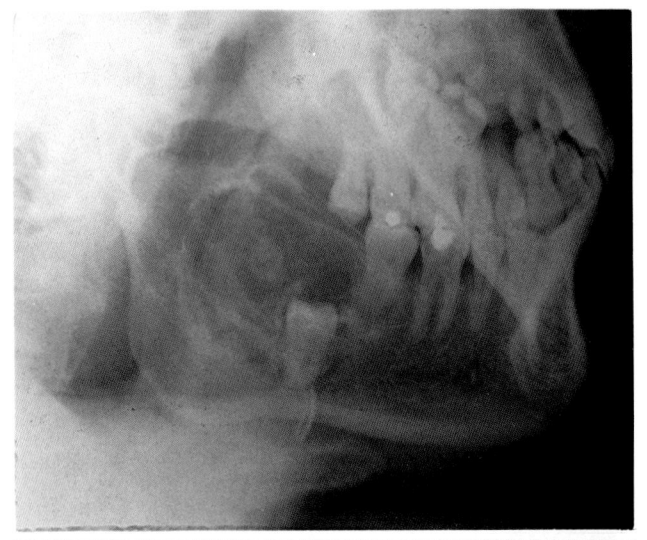

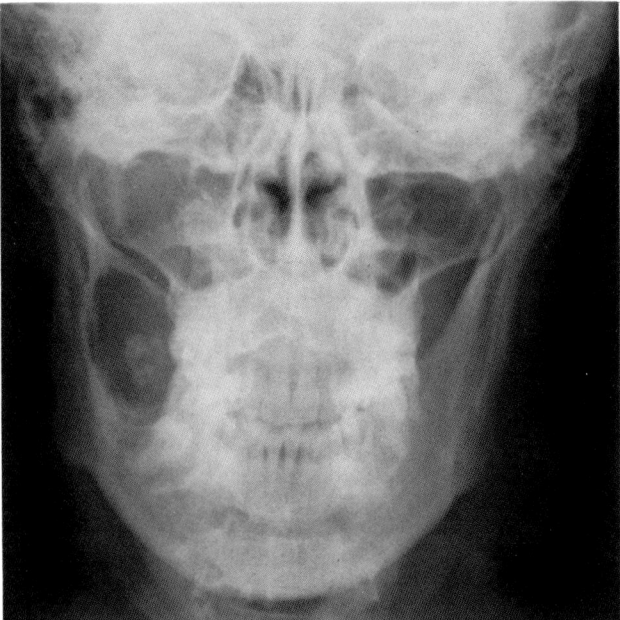

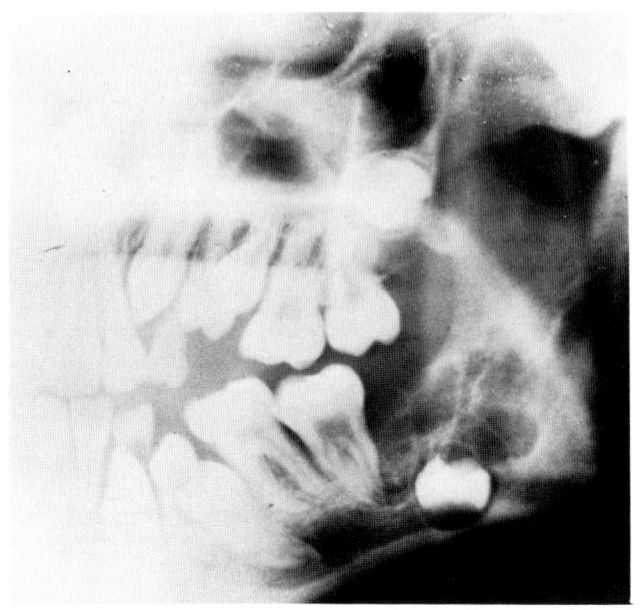

Chondromyxoid fibroma
7.170 This lesion, which rarely affects the jaws, forms a multiloculated, radiolucent defect which, in this example, is present in the third molar region of the mandible. The locules are clearly defined and contain numerous randomly arranged trabeculations within them. The third molar, which is incompletely formed, has been displaced to the lower border of the mandible. Note several permanent teeth are still unerupted and $\frac{D}{D}$ are retained. OLM

Central fibroma
7.168 (top) and 7.169 (bottom) A lesion of the right mandible, occupying the ascending ramus and molar region. It extends from the base of the coronoid process to the mesial aspect 7|, and has a clearly defined margin with a thin, radiopaque, cortical lamina. 8| has been displaced inferiorly by the lesion, which is radiolucent and contains several randomly arranged, delicate, radiopaque trabeculae and an area of more dense mineralisation towards its centre. There is marked lingual expansion of the mandible, which has resulted in the projection of two apparently separate margins to the lesion superiorly on the oblique lateral film. Note the image of the hyoid bone superimposed over the inferior part of the lesion and the 8| (Fig. 7.168). OLM & PA

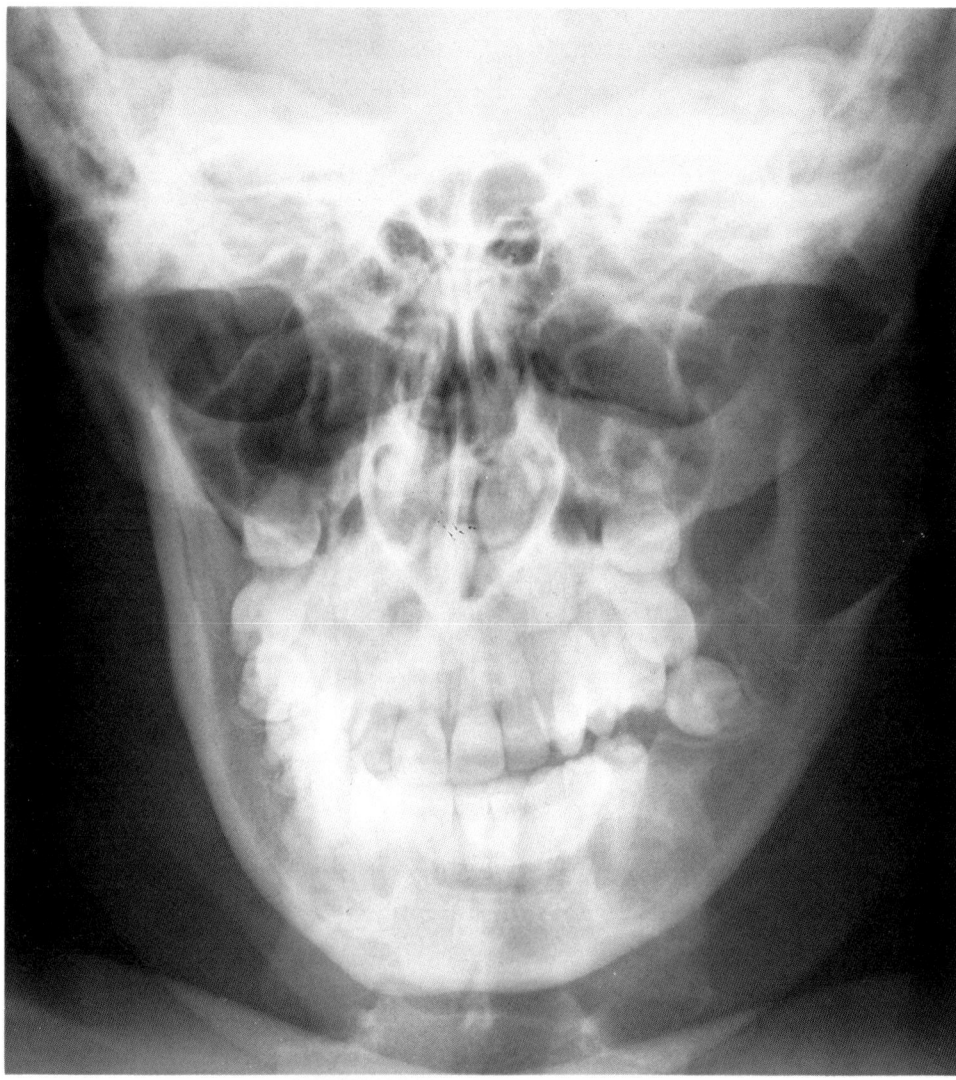

Central neurilemmoma 7.171 (top) and 7.172 (bottom) A large tumour in the left ramus of the mandible of a 20-year-old. It has a clearly defined outline, particularly at its inferior margin, which has a radiopaque lamina. This benign, expansile neoplasm has caused thinning of the cortical bone buccally, but posteriorly it has been mostly resorbed (Fig. 7.172). Such neural tumours usually form a defect which has obvious continuity with the unaffected part of the inferior alveolar canal, but because of the position of this tumour at the posterior end of the canal this relationship is not clearly displayed. Note that the image of the hyoid bone is superimposed over the lesion. PA & OLM

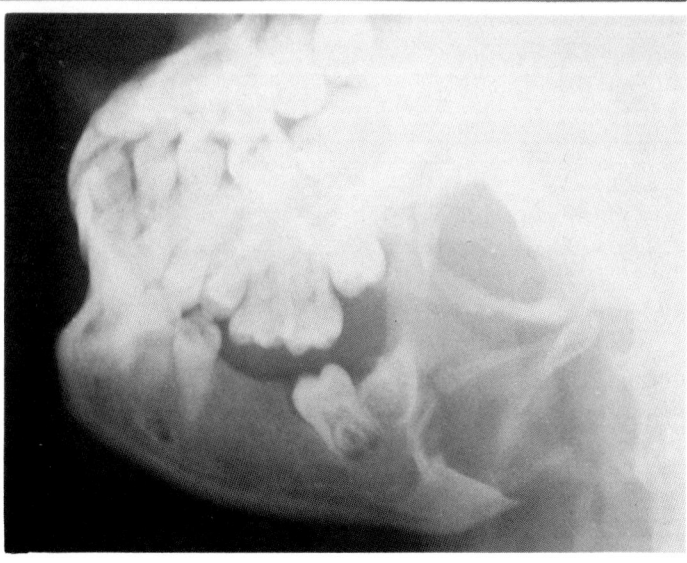

Aneurysmal bone cyst

7.173 An oval, radiolucent lesion with clearly defined outline surrounded by a thin, radiopaque, cortical lamina is present in the left body of the mandible. There are numerous, coarse trabeculae running through the lesion, and antero-inferiorly a lobulated area of radiolucency suggesting marked thinning or perforation of a cortical plate. The alveolar surface of the lesion is slightly expanded, but the cortex is still intact. PR

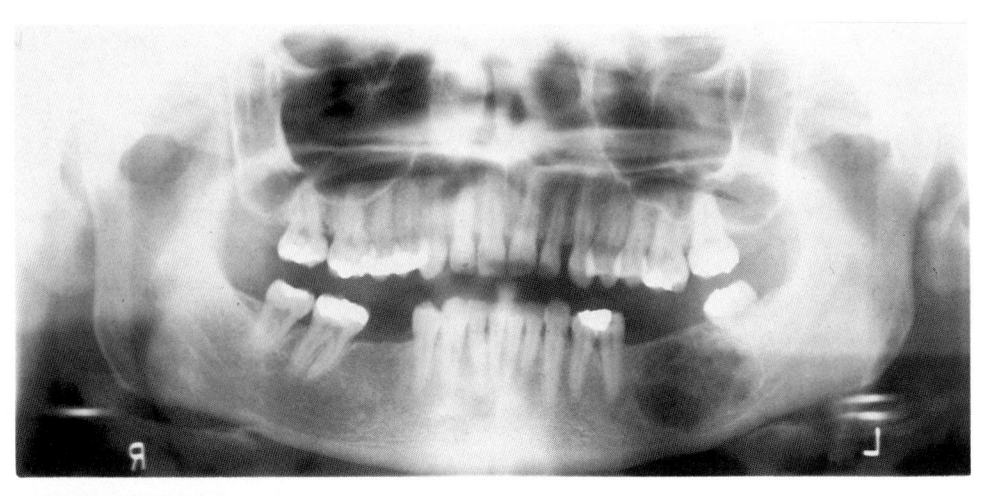

7.174 On some occasions, this cyst arises within a pre-existing lesion, as in this example in a 19-year-old, which probably developed within an ossifying fibroma. The lesion occupies the entire left body of the mandible and contains several variably shaped areas of radiolucency within a mass which is granularly radiopaque elsewhere. The inferior border of the mandible has been greatly expanded forming a typical 'soap bubble' abnormality, and there is also expansion of the alveolus crestally. The unerupted $\overline{8|}$ lies transversely in the posterior part of the lesion. OLM

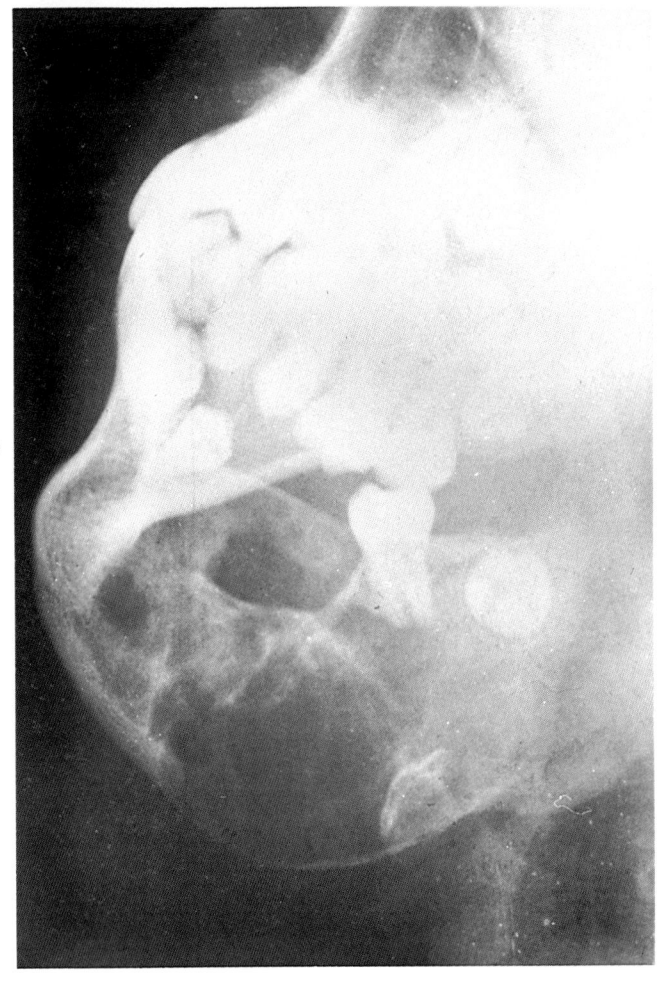

The Facial Bones

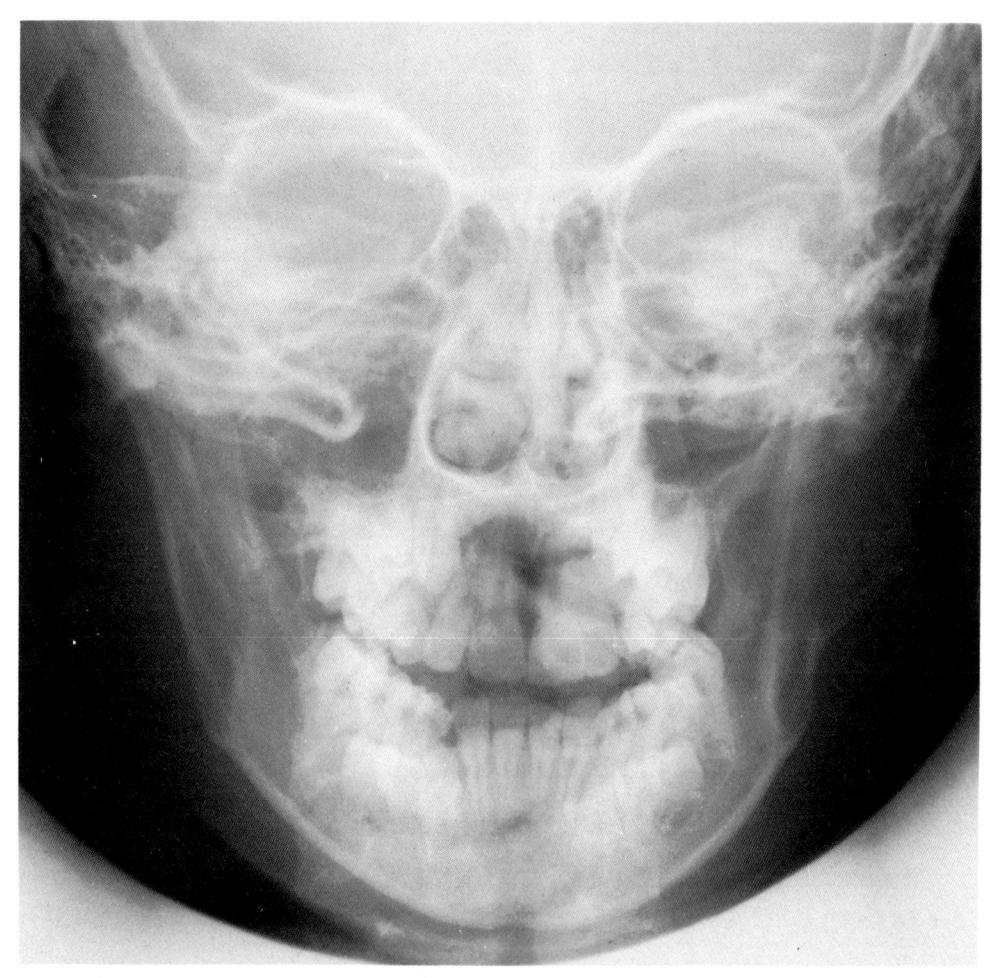

Solitary bone cyst (traumatic bone cyst, haemorrhagic bone cyst)
7.175 Most commonly, these lesions arise in adolescent males in the subapical part of the posterior region of the body of the mandible. In this site, expansion of the bone may be only slight and the lesion forms a characteristic scalloped pattern where it extends between the roots of the teeth. Occasional lesions may occur in the ramus, as in this example in a ten-year-old, in which site bone expansion may be more prominent. There is a large, clearly defined radiolucency in the left ramus which has caused marked buccal and lingual expansion of the cortical plates which remain intact. PA

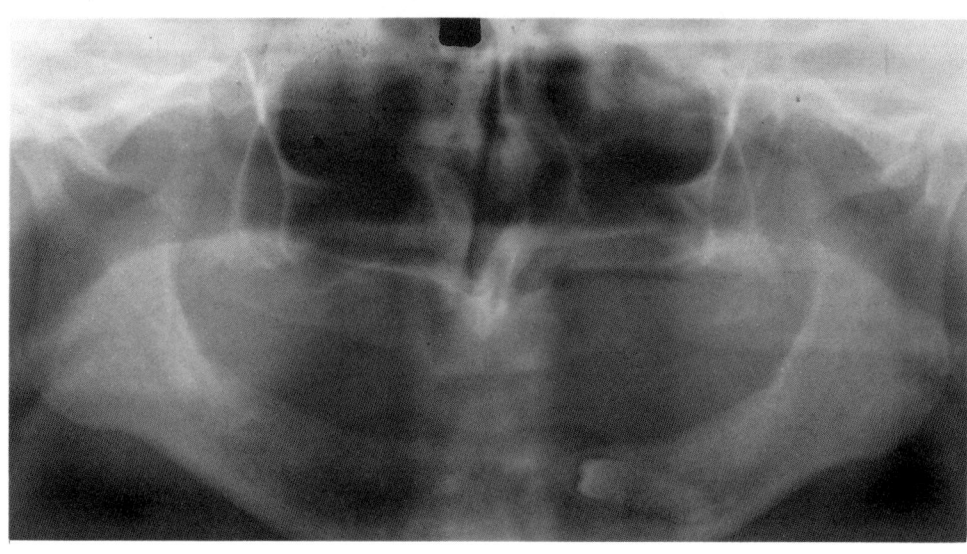

Pleomorphic adenoma
7.176 (left), 7.177 and 7.178 (overleaf) In the maxilla, this benign tumour, although arising in the mucosal salivary glands, may cause bone destruction. In this edentulous patient with a recurrent tumour in the left maxilla, there is a large, radiolucent defect with clearly defined ovoid outline. The alveolar ridge is expanded and the radiopaque lamina of the palatal shelf is absent on the affected side, the tumour occupying the lower part of the antral cavity.

176 *A Radiological Atlas of Diseases of the Teeth and Jaws*

7.176 (overleaf), 7.177 (left) and 7.178 (far left) (cntd)
Computerised tomography is very helpful in determining the extent of such lesions in the posterior part of the maxilla, and the axial (Fig. 7.177) and coronal (Fig. 7.178) views reveal the full extent of the tumour, and that it is a benign, expansile lesion rather than an invasive one. In the planes illustrated, the slightly radiopaque tumour (arrows) is shown expanding into the floor of the antrum and medially into the lateral wall of the nose. PR & CAT

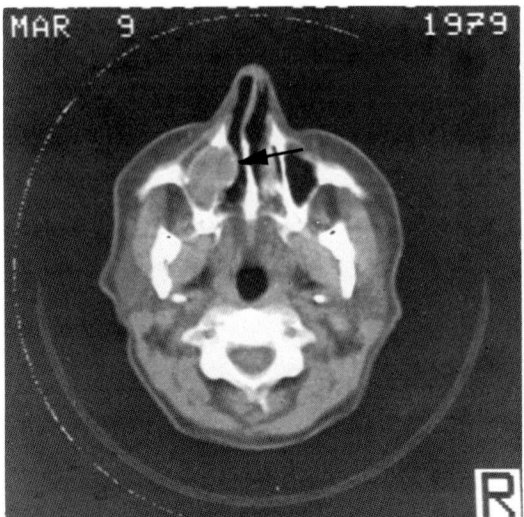

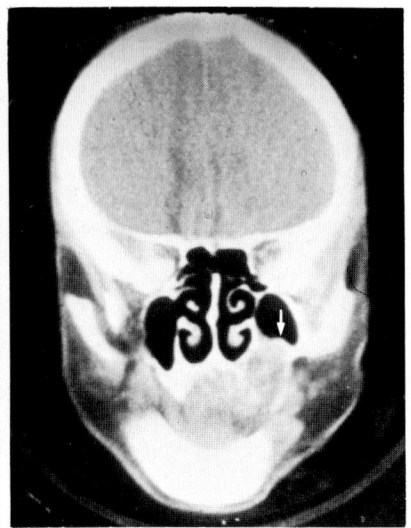

7.177

7.178

Histiocytosis X
7.179
In Hand–Schüller–Christian disease, classically there are multiple deposits of tumour leading to the triad of symptoms of exophthalmos, pituitary damage causing diabetes insipidus, and multiple bone lesions. The jaws are frequently involved, and if the lesions are extensive, extraction of the teeth may be necessary, as in this example, where there are two large deposits, one in the maxilla and one in the mandible. The lesions are radiolucent with clearly defined, rather lobulated margins, and contain occasional incomplete septa. The cortical bone in the alveolar part of both jaws is eroded. OLM

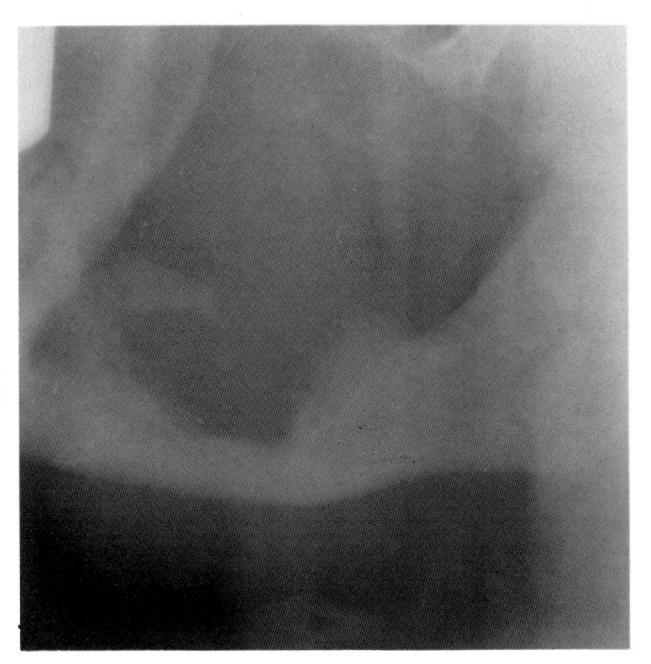

7.180 In this example, there is a radiolucent tumour deposit within the periapical and interdental tissues 1|123. The lesion has an irregular margin, although it is clearly defined, and there is loss of the lamina dura around the affected teeth. Such deposits may simulate periapical granulomas and present difficulty in diagnosis. USO

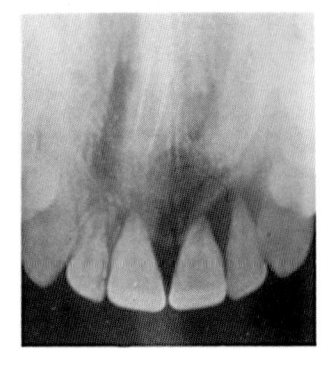

The Facial Bones 177

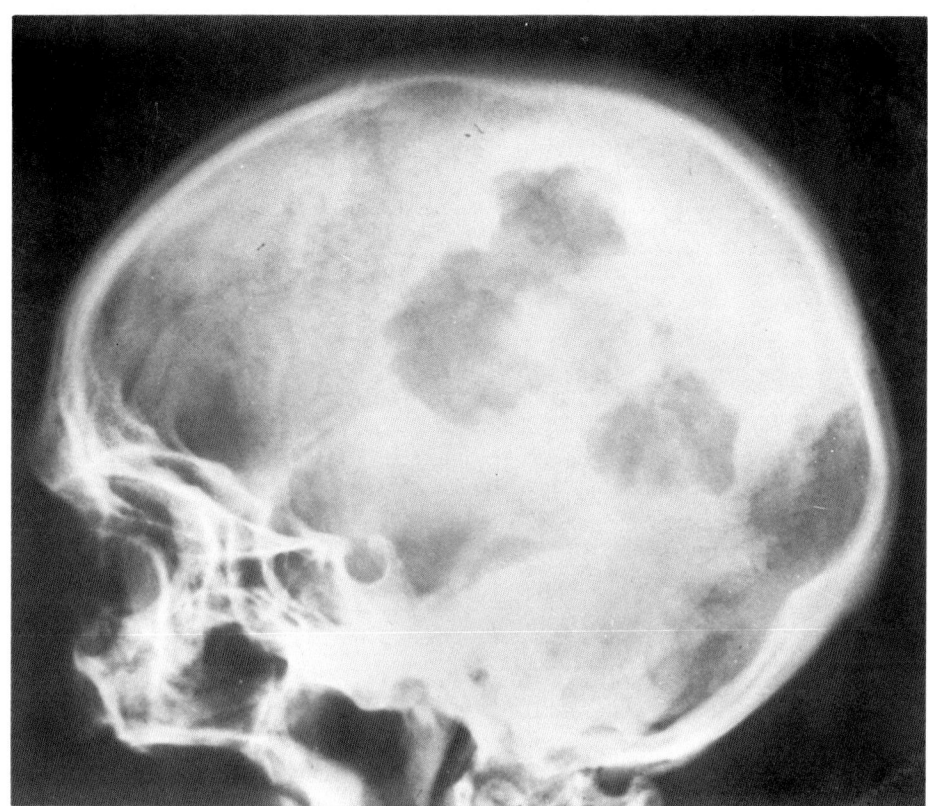

7.181
In Hand–Schüller–Christian disease and Letterer–Siwe disease, multiple deposits of tumour are often present in the skull. Several large, clearly defined radiolucent defects are present in the vault of the skull in this patient, although the sella turcica appears normal. Erosion of the latter may be a feature of Hand–Schüller–Christian disease due to infiltration of the posterior part of the pituitary gland, causing diabetes insipidus. L

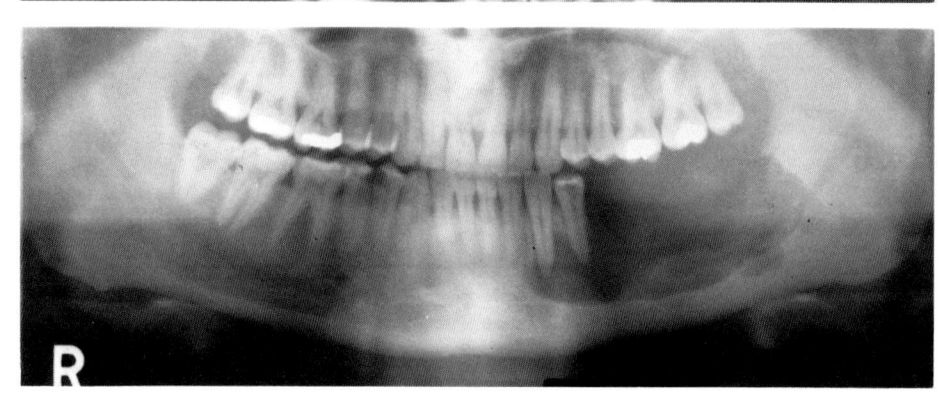

7.182 An extensive eosinophilic granuloma of the left mandible, extending from the lateral incisor region anteriorly to the base of the ascending ramus posteriorly. It is clearly defined with a scalloped outline, and variably radiolucent with darker areas suggesting there has been erosion of the cortical plates. There is destruction of the alveolar bone apically around |34 and widening of the periodontal ligament space mesially |3. PR

Squamous cell carcinoma
7.183 A tumour of the retromolar region of the oral mucosa, which has invaded the anterior aspect of the ramus of the left mandible. The infiltrative growth pattern of these tumours leads to the formation of poorly defined areas of radiolucency with irregular, ragged margins. Within the lesion are scattered, variously shaped radiopacities of different size, representing residual trabeculae of bone which have not yet been completely resorbed by the tumour. In this example, the lesion has spread anteriorly to |7, around which most of the alveolar bone has been destroyed and the cortical outlines of the internal and external oblique ridges of the anterior surface of the ramus are almost completely eroded, typical of a lesion that has grown into the mandible from the overlying tissues. A residual portion of the external oblique ridge can be seen within the lesion (arrow). Note the stud-shaped image of the transverse process of the atlas vertebra projecting laterally beyond the maxillary molars. PA

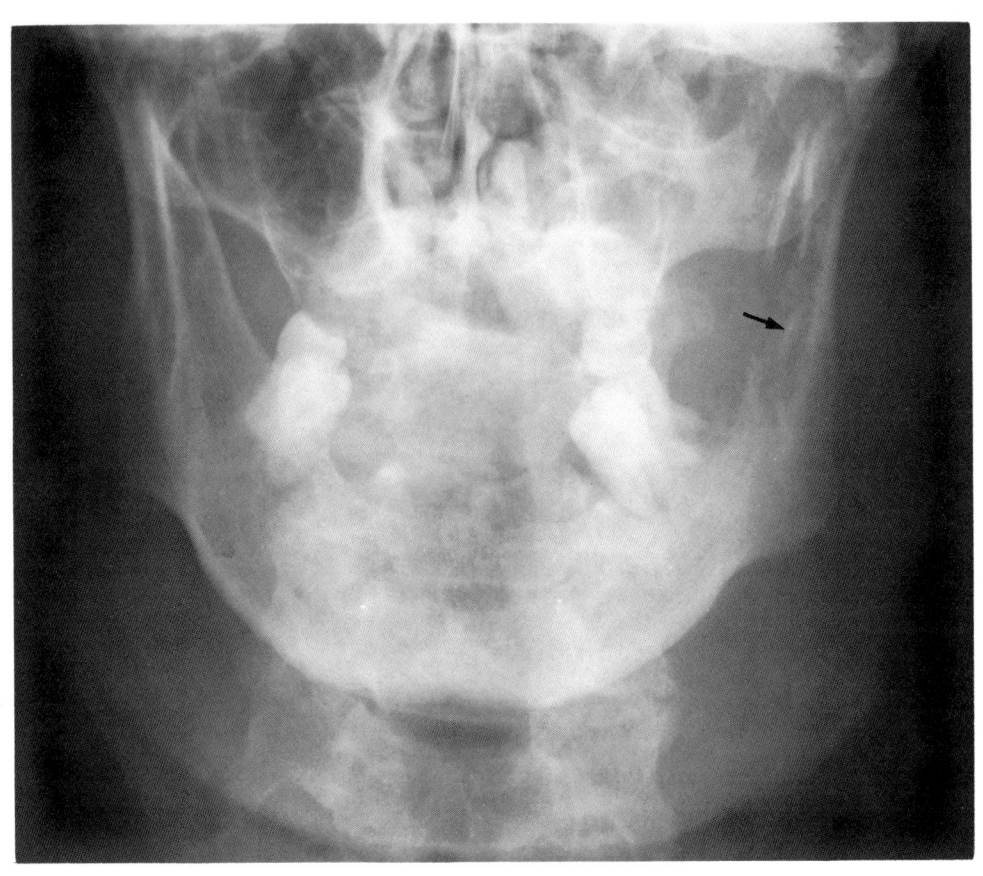

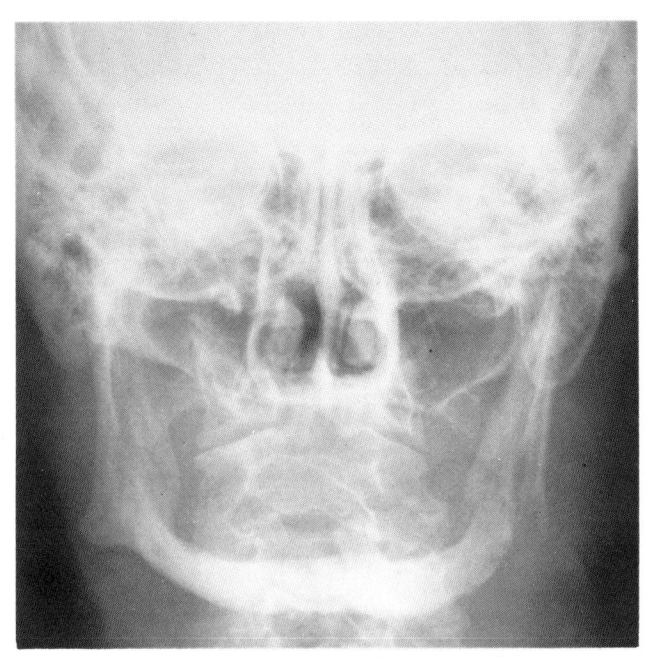

7.184 A tumour arising on the buccal mucosa with invasion of the left body and angle of an atrophic, edentulous mandible. There is an extensive, poorly defined, variably radiolucent defect with a ragged, 'moth eaten' appearance typical of an invasive tumour. The step-like irregularity of the inferior border, together with the loss of a distinct cortical outline, is indicative of a pathological fracture. The soft tissues lying infero-laterally to the mandible are swollen. PA

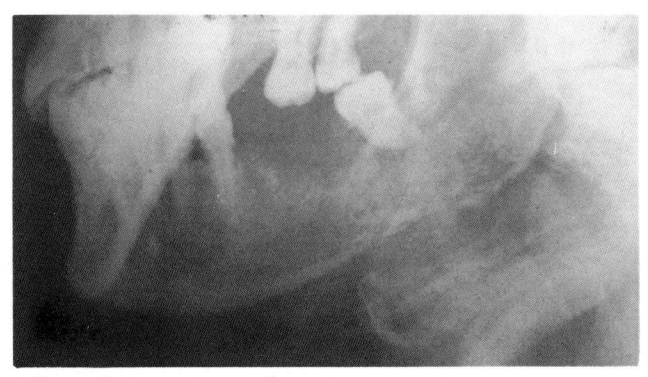

Primary intra-osseous carcinoma
7.185 Rarely, a carcinoma can arise from epithelial residues in the jaw bones, and thus the tumour grows from within, outwards. In this lesion of the body of the left mandible, there is an extensive, 'moth eaten' area of radiolucency which is poorly defined and extends from the |5 region to the posterior border of the ramus. Throughout the lesion, there are scattered, pin-head sized foci of radiolucency where the infiltrative pattern of bone destruction is more advanced. In the molar region at the inferior border of the mandible, the cortical bone has been eroded and there is a more confluent radiolucent defect in the alveolar process. Much of the alveolar bone around |8 has been destroyed. The diffuse loss of bone has resulted in difficulty in visualising the inferior alveolar canal over much of its course, although it can still be identified in the ramus and |8 region. OLM

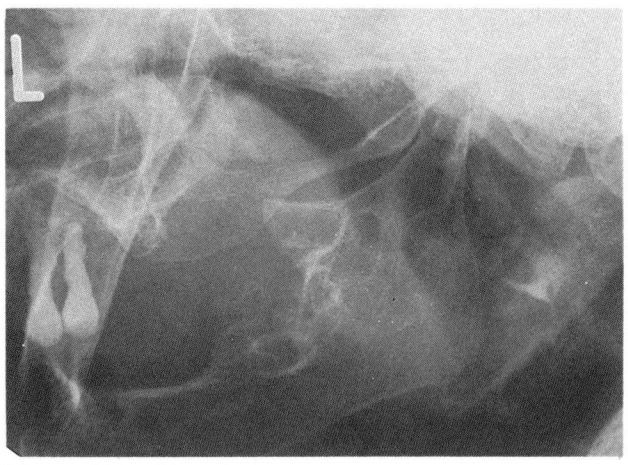

Muco-epidermoid carcinoma
7.186 This lesion, although invasive, is very variable in its rate of growth, and can therefore form a variety of radiographical appearances. In this example, a relatively slow growing tumour has arisen from the salivary glands in the mucosa covering the left retromolar region of the mandible and invaded the anterior part of the ramus which appears enlarged. There is an irregularly loculated, radiolucent defect, many of the locules being surrounded by radiopaque laminae. Partly because of its slow growth, reactive bone formation may occur and there are numerous, irregular, radiopaque trabeculae within it. OLM

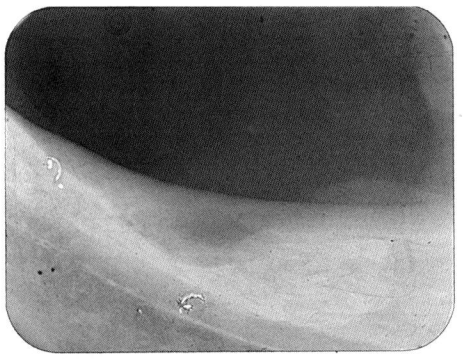

Basal cell carcinoma
7.187 These lesions typically arise on the skin of the face, but exceptionally may occur in other sites, including the oral mucosa, as in this example in the right retromolar region which has invaded the underlying mandible. There is a quite well defined, radiolucent defect with scalloped outline in the retromolar fossa, and loss of the radiopaque cortical margin of the internal oblique ridge. P

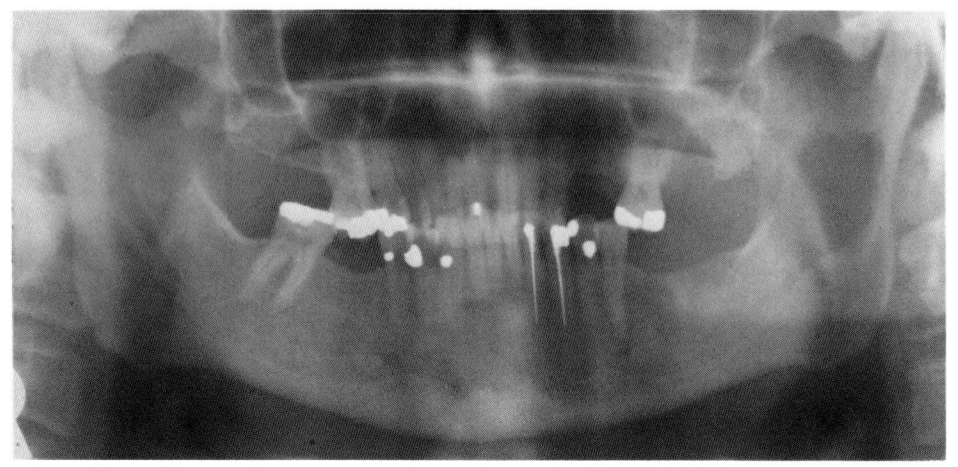

180 *A Radiological Atlas of Diseases of the Teeth and Jaws*

Metastatic carcinoma
7.188 Metastatic tumours to the jaws occur most commonly where there may be residues of erythropoietic marrow (typically in the molar and retromolar regions of the mandible) and usually derive from primary lesions in the lung, breast, gastrointestinal tract and prostate. They are mostly osteolytic, as in this example originating from a primary carcinoma of the lung, in which there is a large, radiolucent lesion in the left ascending ramus of the mandible. The boundary of the lesion is irregular and not clearly defined, and involves the proximal part of the inferior alveolar canal. The lesion is not densely radiolucent, there being an overall granular radiopacity suggesting that it is centrally placed and still surrounded by cortical bone, a conclusion that was confirmed by other radiographs. PR

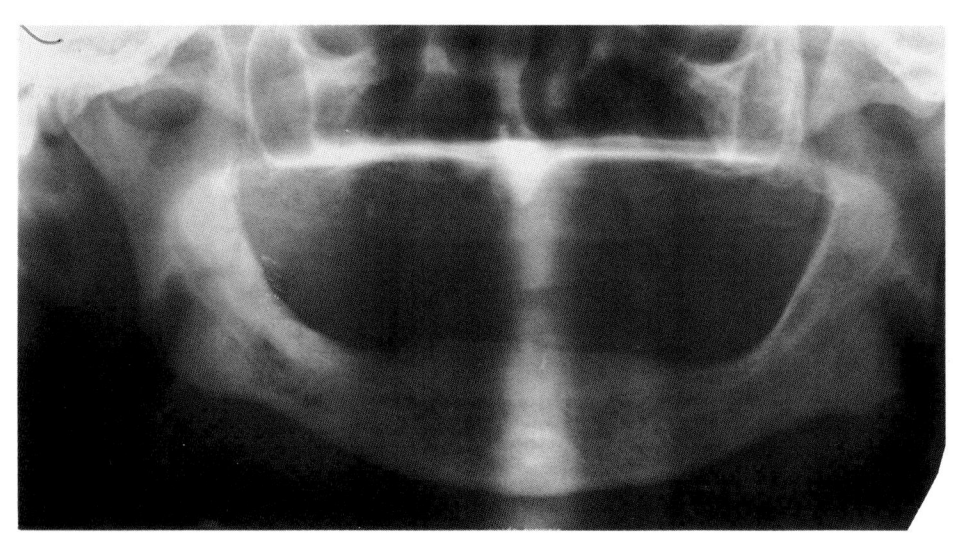

7.189 Another example originating from a primary hypernephroma of the kidney, where there is an irregularly shaped, poorly defined lesion of variable radiolucency in the inferior part of the molar region of the right mandible involving the inferior alveolar canal. PR

The Facial Bones 181

7.190 This metastatic carcinoma in the left body of the edentulous mandible has arisen from a primary tumour in the prostate. There is a poorly defined, radiolucent lesion with a 'moth eaten' appearance to the affected bone, in which numerous radiopaque, irregularly shaped trabeculae of reactive bone are also present. The latter are particularly well demonstrated within that part of the mass projected beyond the anatomical limit of the mandible, where there is a radiopaque, soft tissue swelling. Such metastases are described as osteoplastic and are a particular feature of carcinoma of the prostate. PR

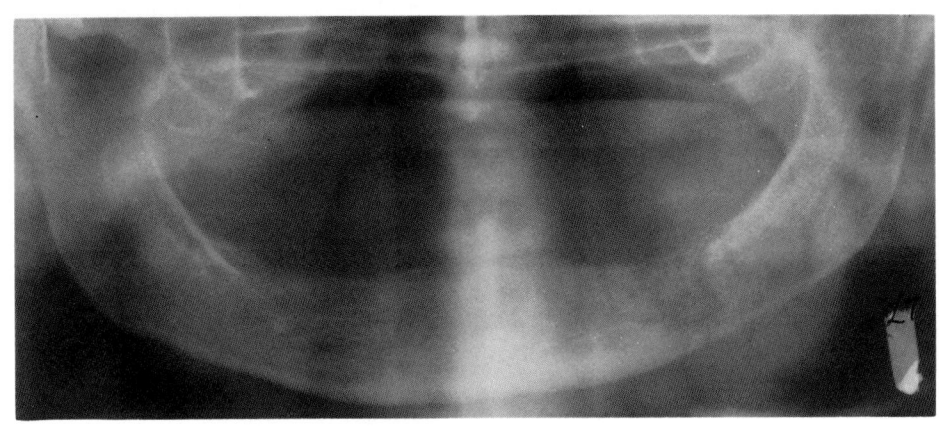

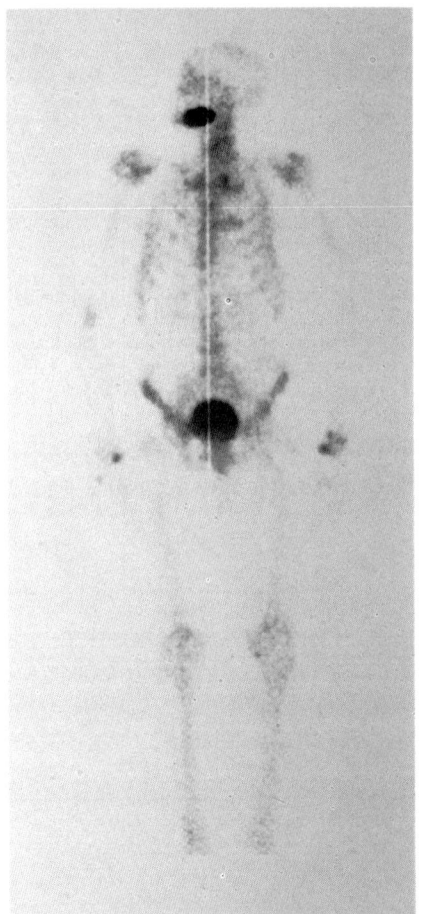

7.191 When metastatic tumours are suspected, bone scintiscans are a useful adjunct, since other unsuspected deposits may be revealed. In this patient, the dark hot-spot at the site of the jaw metastasis is prominent, although no other intra-osseous metastases were apparent. The circular hot-spot in the pelvic region is due to accumulation of radioactive material in the bladder. SC

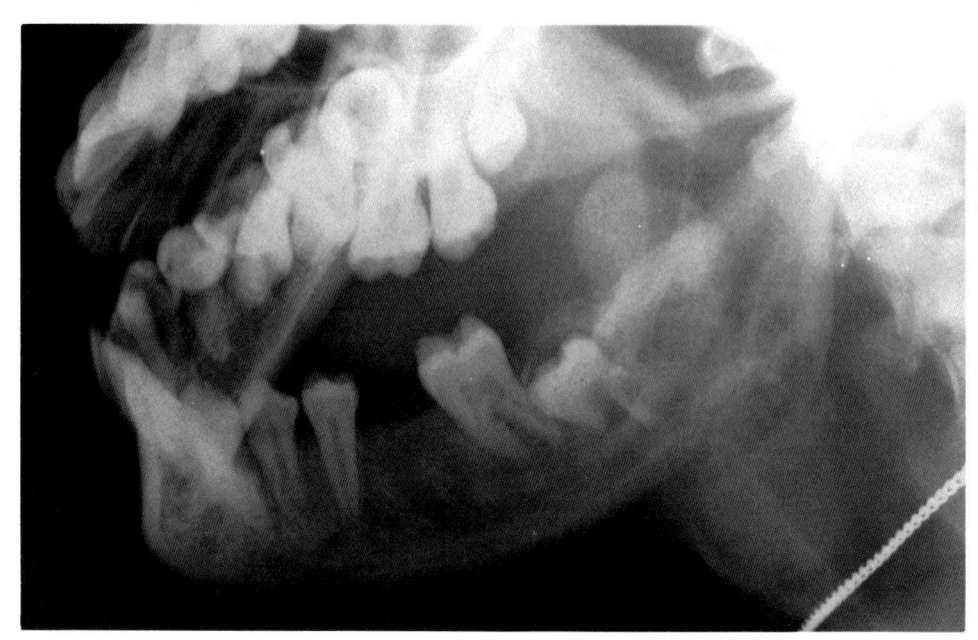

182   *A Radiological Atlas of Diseases of the Teeth and Jaws*

Osteogenic sarcoma

7.192 Osteogenic sarcomas usually arise centrally within the bone and rapidly destroy the overlying cortex. According to the degree of differentiation of the tumour cells, variable amounts of tumour bone may be deposited and thus a variable radiographical picture is obtained. Typically, the tumour bone is deposited in a radial, sun-ray pattern, beyond the original bony outline. In this lesion in a 16-year-old, there is an irregular radiolucency extending from the third molar region to the lower border of the mandible at the left angle, and upwards distal to the unerupted, partially formed, third molar into the lower part of the ascending ramus. The cortical bone at the inferior border of the mandible has been eroded and there are radiating spicules of tumour bone projecting inferiorly, giving the classical 'sun-ray' pattern. The image of the hyoid bone is superimposed upon the tumour, forming a radiopacity over the distal part of the third molar root. Note the recent extraction socket ̅6̅ with a small circular area of osteosclerosis apically to the distal root, which is an incidental finding, and a similar area close to the mesial root ̅7̅. OLM

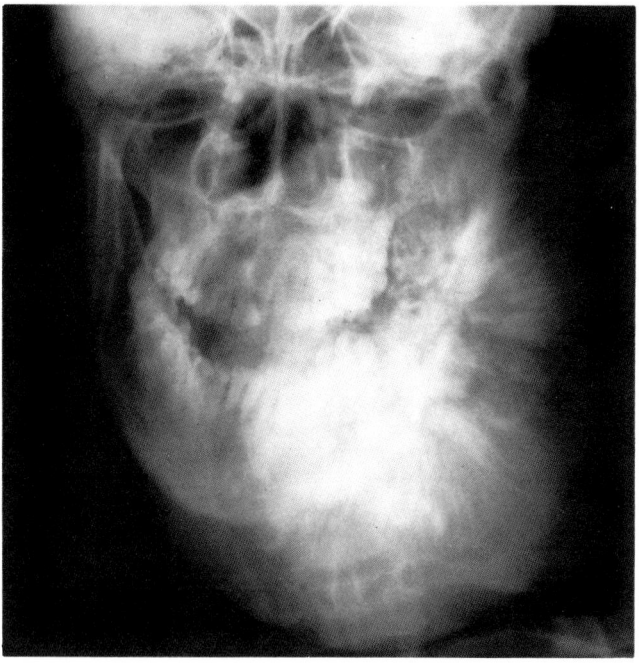

7.193 A huge lesion involving the whole of the left side of the mandible. The lateral aspect of the original bony outline of the mandible is still faintly discernible, and radiating from it in all directions are numerous, coarse, radiopaque trabeculations of tumour bone which become progressively thinner towards the outer surface of the tumour, which is covered by a thickened, soft tissue shadow inferiorly. The trabeculations of tumour bone show some variation in width and radiopacity according to their stage of development and the degree to which they are mineralised. Note that the air shadow of the pharynx, larynx and trachea is displaced to the right, indicating that the tumour has spread infero-medially to involve these structures. PA

The Facial Bones 183

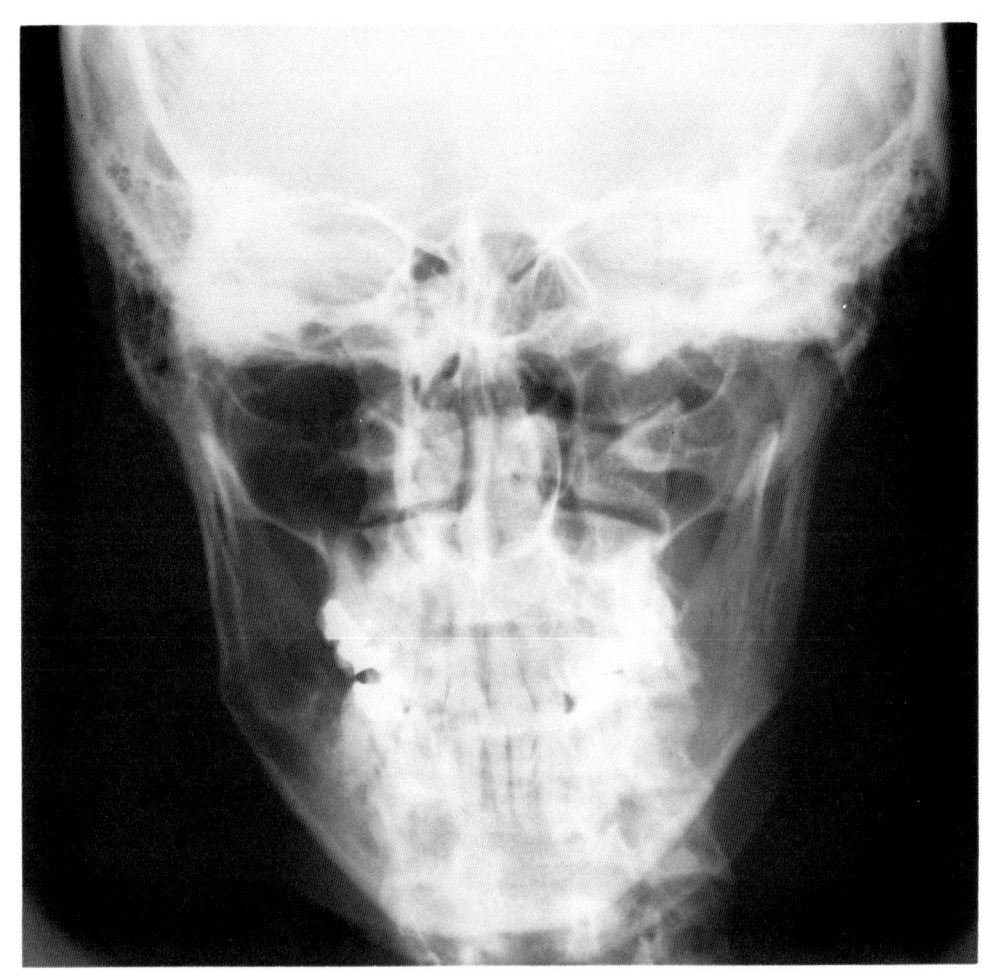

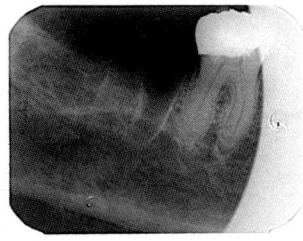

**Chondrosarcoma
7.194 (left) and 7.195
(above)** A lesion at the base of the right ramus of the mandible, forming a poorly defined, radiolucent area with indistinct margins, and thinning of the cortical bone at the inferior border. On the intra-oral film (Fig. 7.195), the loss of normal trabecular pattern in the body of the mandible can be determined, and contrasts with that around the roots 6̄|. Note the recent extraction socket of the mesial root 7̄| which is demarcated by a thin radiopaque lamina. PA & P

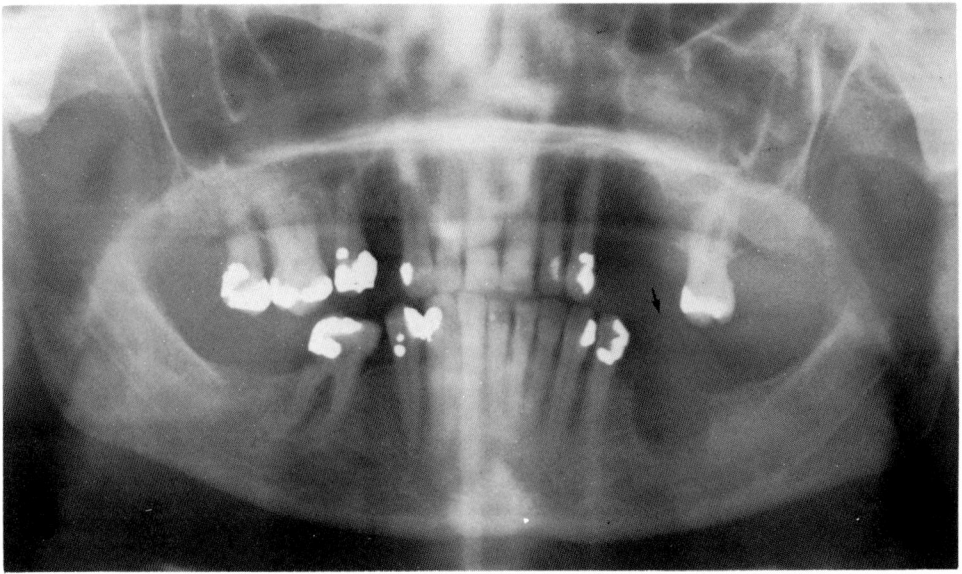

**Fibrosarcoma
7.196** A tumour in the left molar region of the mandible which grew into the socket |6̄ a few months after the tooth had been extracted. There is a poorly defined, radiolucent area with ragged, ill defined margins except mesially, where remnants of the lamina dura of the mesial wall of |6̄ socket are still present. The dome-shaped, soft tissue mass onto which |7̄ was occluding, can just be seen above the bony defect (arrow). PR

7.197 A larger tumour of the right body and ramus of the mandible, extending from the premolar region anteriorly to the base of the coronoid process posteriorly. The radiolucent lesion has resulted in considerable bone destruction and its boundary is more clearly defined buccally than lingually, where more of the cortical bone has been eroded. Note the calcified pineal gland projected in the middle of the frontal sinus. PA

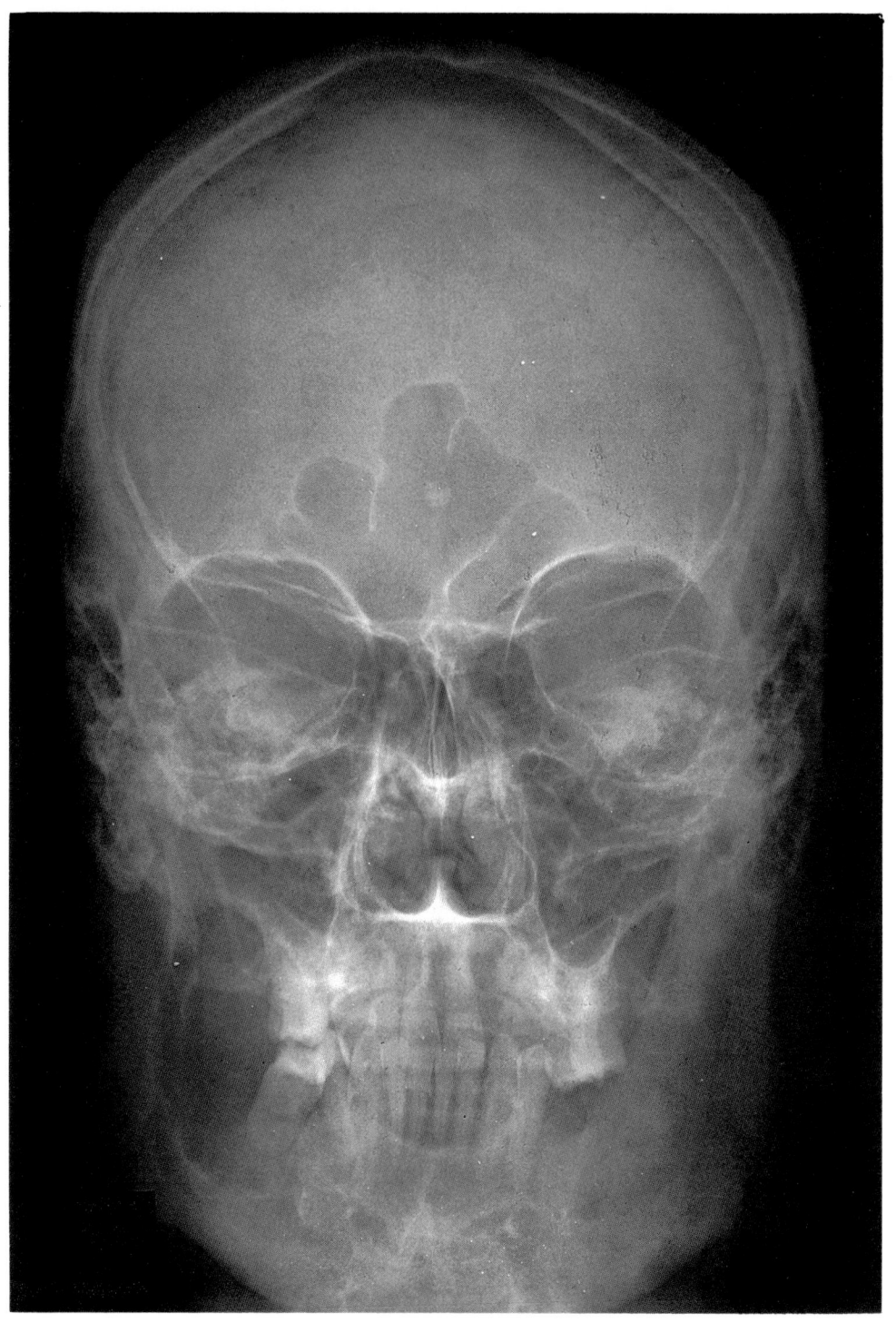

Multiple myelomatosis 7.198 (right) 7.199 (far right) and 7.200 (below right) This condition is characterised by the presence of multifocal osteolytic tumour deposits which may involve the jaws. It is, however, unusual for the jaws to be affected before other bones. In this example, there are multiple irregularly loculated, radiolucent areas of bone destruction with ill defined outlines, affecting predominantly the alveolar bone extending from ⌐3–6, around which the lamina dura has been destroyed. Areas of bone resorption are superimposed upon the apical halves of the roots of these teeth, causing an appearance that may be confused with root resorption. There is, however, resorption of the apex ⌐4, as indicated by its shortened, irregularly concave outline. In addition, there are often multiple radiolucent defects scattered throughout the vault of the skull and elsewhere in the skeleton. In this example, the skull lesions (Fig. 7.200) are of varying size, shape and density, most of them being clearly defined giving the characteristic 'punched out' appearance. P & L

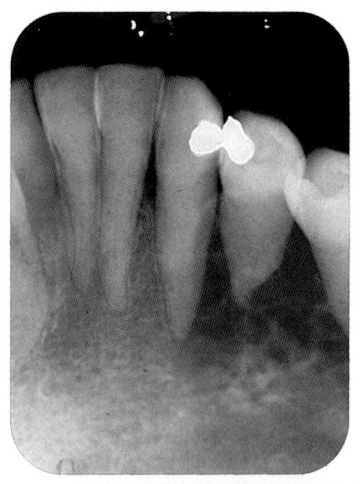

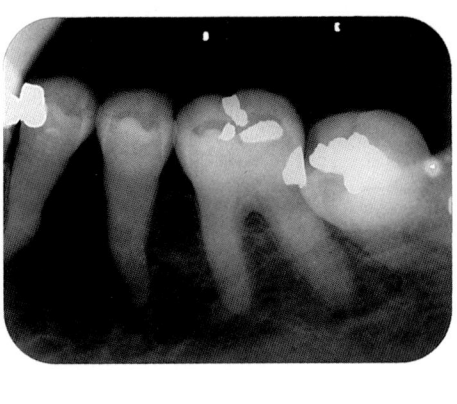

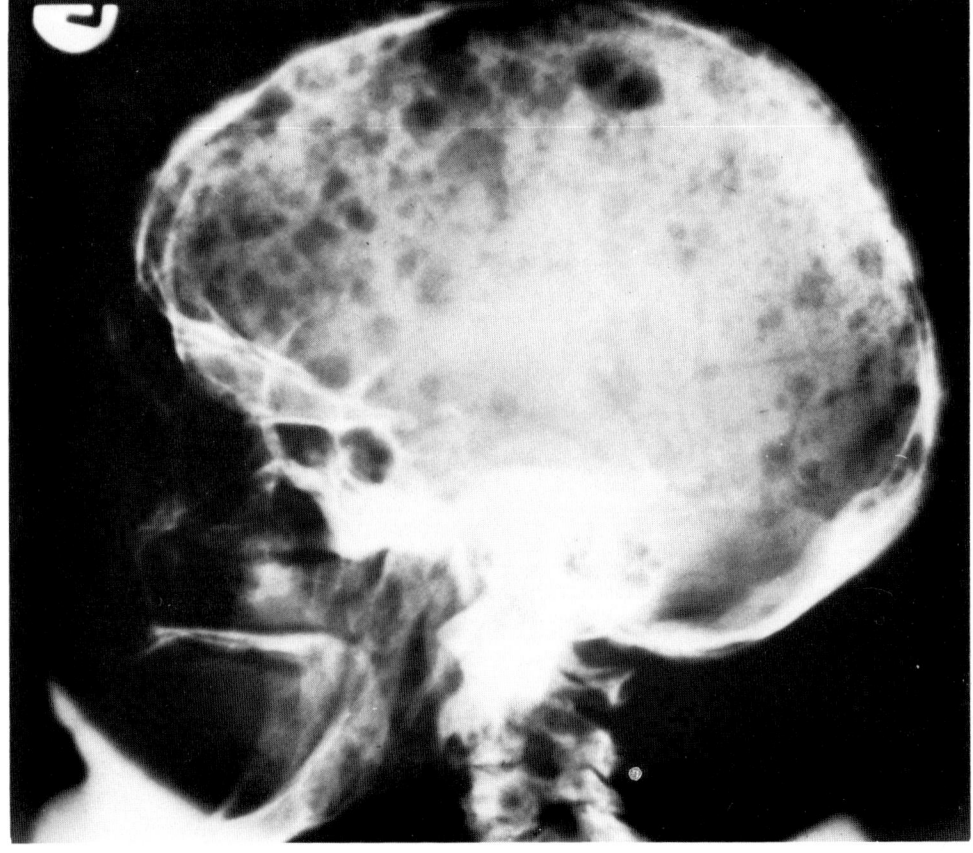

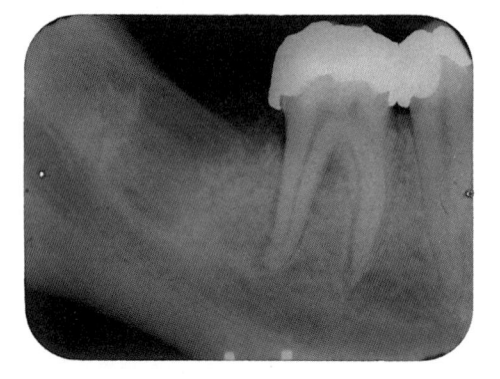

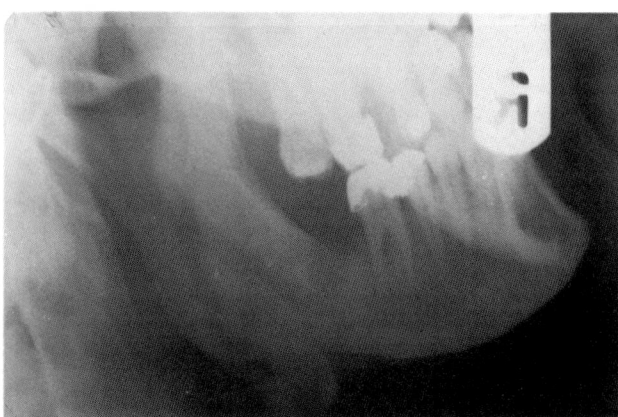

Malignant lymphoma
7.201 (top) and 7.202 (bottom) A centrally arising lymphoma of the follicular centre cell type in the 654⏋ region in a 35-year-old. There is a poorly defined radiolucency of variable density within which the trabeculations show an abnormal pattern. The periodontal ligament space 6⏋ is irregularly widened with loss of most of the lamina dura around its distal root. Although 7⏋ was extracted only a few weeks previously and its radiolucent socket persists, the lamina dura is absent and it is surrounded by some osteosclerosis. The extent of the lesion, occupying predominantly the periapical region of the bone, can be more readily determined on the extra-oral film (Fig. 7.202). P & OLM

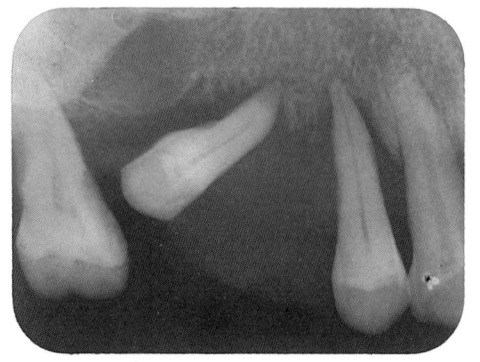

Malignant melanoma
7.203 A tumour arising in the right maxillary premolar/molar region in a patient with long-standing chronic periodontitis, as a result of which there is advanced loss of alveolar bone around the standing teeth. The tumour has arisen in the gingival mucosa and the soft tissue swelling is clearly displayed. The bone deep to the mass, particularly in relation to 5⏌, exhibits increased radiolucency with an ill defined, deep margin and loss of surface cortical lamina, due to invasion by the infiltrating tumour. 5⏌ has been displaced by the lesion and the radiopaque lamina outlining the floor of the antrum is incompletely defined anteriorly, suggesting early destruction. P

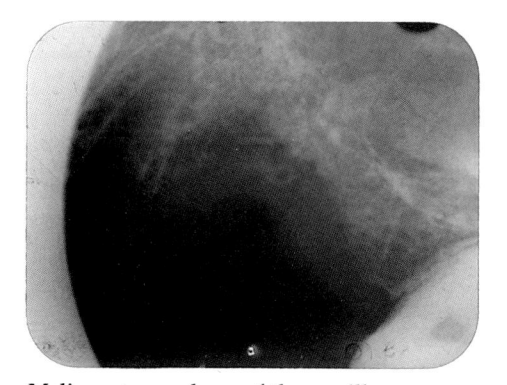

Malignant granuloma of the maxilla
7.204 A lesion affecting the edentulous, left maxillary ridge extending from ⌊4 socket to the mesial aspect ⌊7. The bony architecture in the affected area is indistinct, but particularly noticeable is the lack of definition of the radiopaque lamina of the floor of the antrum, only part of which can be determined. The margins of the lesion are ill defined. Bone destruction is more advanced on the edentulous ridge where, in most parts, the cortical bone has been completely destroyed, and its surface is ragged and contains irregular, separate, radiopaque fragments of incompletely resorbed bone trabeculae. P

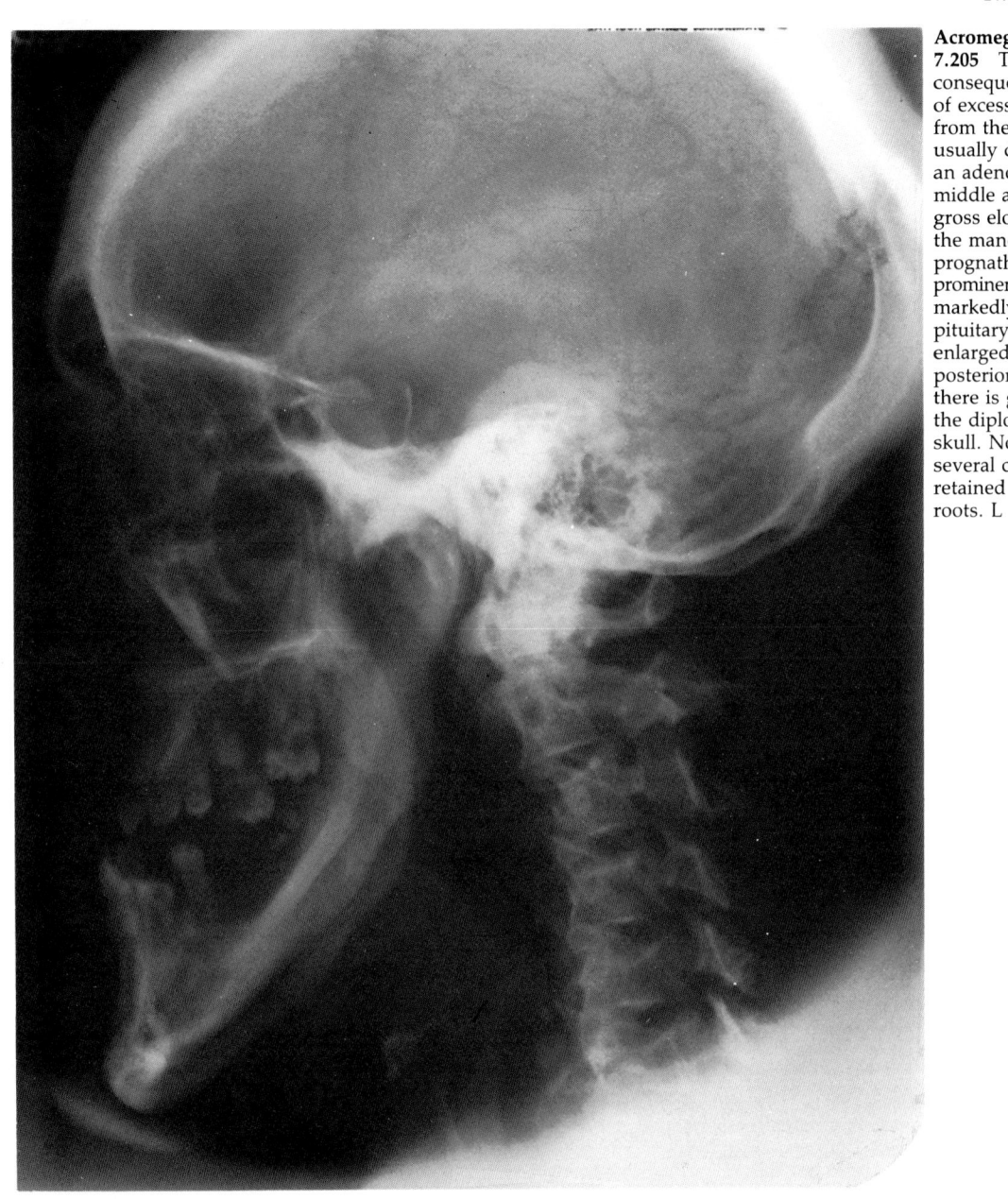

Acromegaly

7.205 This lesion is a consequence of the secretion of excess growth hormone from the pituitary gland, usually due to the presence of an adenoma, in adults. In this middle aged patient, there is gross elongation of all parts of the mandible with prognathism, an enlarged prominent mental process, and markedly obtuse angles. The pituitary fossa (sella turcica) is enlarged with thinning of its posterior wall. In addition, there is general thickening of the diploë of the vault of the skull. Note the presence of several carious teeth and the retained mandibular molar roots. L

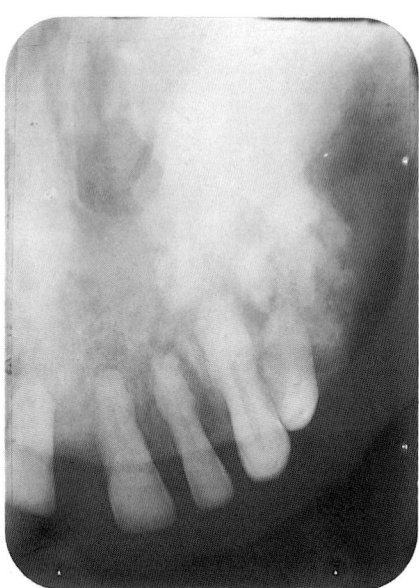

188 *A Radiological Atlas of Diseases of the Teeth and Jaws*

Paget's disease of bone (osteitis deformans)
7.206 (top), 7.207 (middle) and 7.208 (bottom) In this condition, there is disordered bone metabolism which is characterised in its early stages by resorption and subsequently by deposition of excessive amounts of increasingly dense bone. These progressive changes may occur at different rates in adjacent parts of the same bone, and thus a variable radiographical picture may be presented. In this example, the normal trabecular pattern of the maxilla is lost and has a diffuse granular appearance, and in several areas there are irregularly shaped radiopaque masses of varying size where bone sclerosis has occurred. These latter changes, which are particularly marked in the |34 region, contribute to the typical 'cotton wool' appearance of this lesion. The expansion of the maxilla has resulted in spacing of the teeth, most of which exhibit bulbosities of the apical part of their roots due to hypercementosis. The lamina dura around the roots of the teeth is in many areas obscured, as are the boundaries of the antrum and floor of the nose in the occlusal film. UOO & P

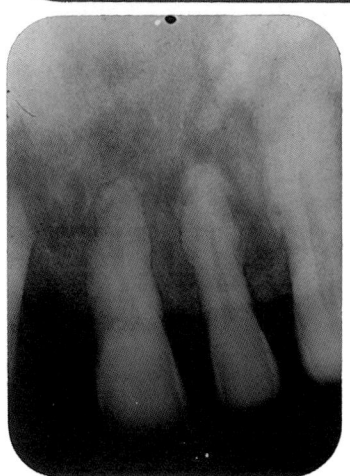

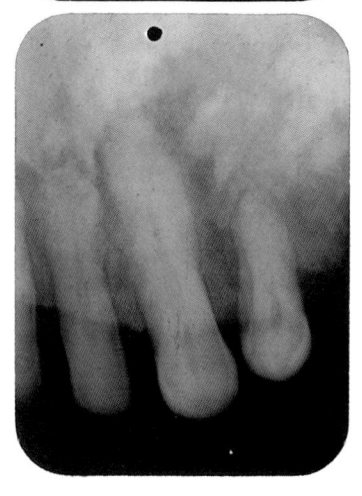

The Facial Bones 189

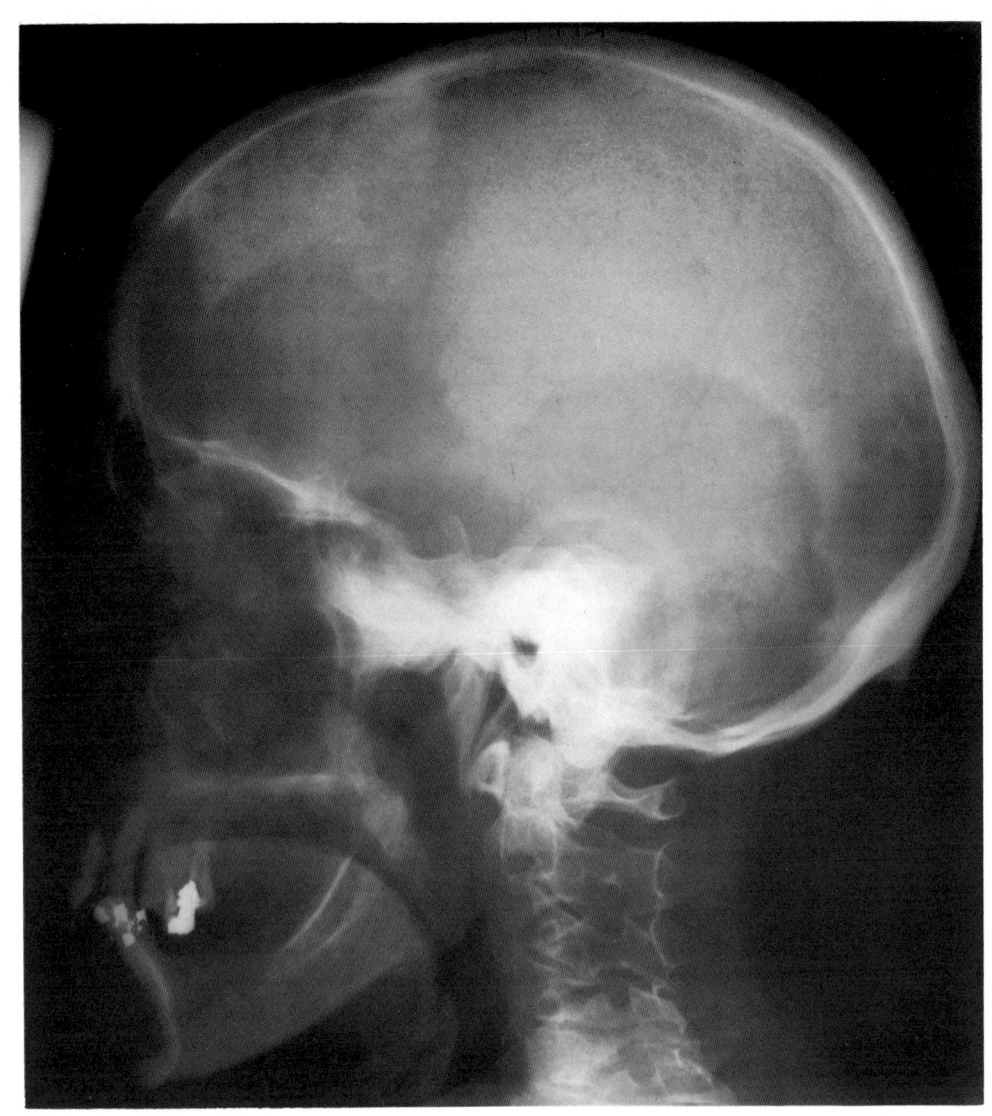

7.209 The early resorptive stage of the disease is particularly obvious in the vault of the skull. The resorption gives rise to confluent areas of radiolucency, usually starting anteriorly. In this example, the radiolucency extends across the lower part of the vault from front to back and has a scalloped superior margin, and is seen end on anteriorly as thinning of the diploë above the frontal sinus. This appearance is known as osteoporosis circumscripta. Note the oval outline of the pinna encircling the dense radiopaque image of the petrous part of the base of the skull. L

7.210 (top) and 7.211 (bottom) An edentulous patient at the later, osteosclerotic stage with involvement of the skull and maxilla. The bones in the vault of the skull show patchy radiopacities of varying size, shape and density, together with scattered, poorly defined, radiolucent areas forming the classical 'cotton wool' appearance. There is marked thickening and sclerosis of the diploë anteriorly and thinning in the basi-occipital region. The antra are both almost fully occluded by abnormal bone, and there is marked enlargement and thickening of the alveolar part of the maxilla which exhibits a more granular pattern of radiopacity in the panoramic radiograph (Fig. 7.211). The mandible is apparently unaffected. L & PR

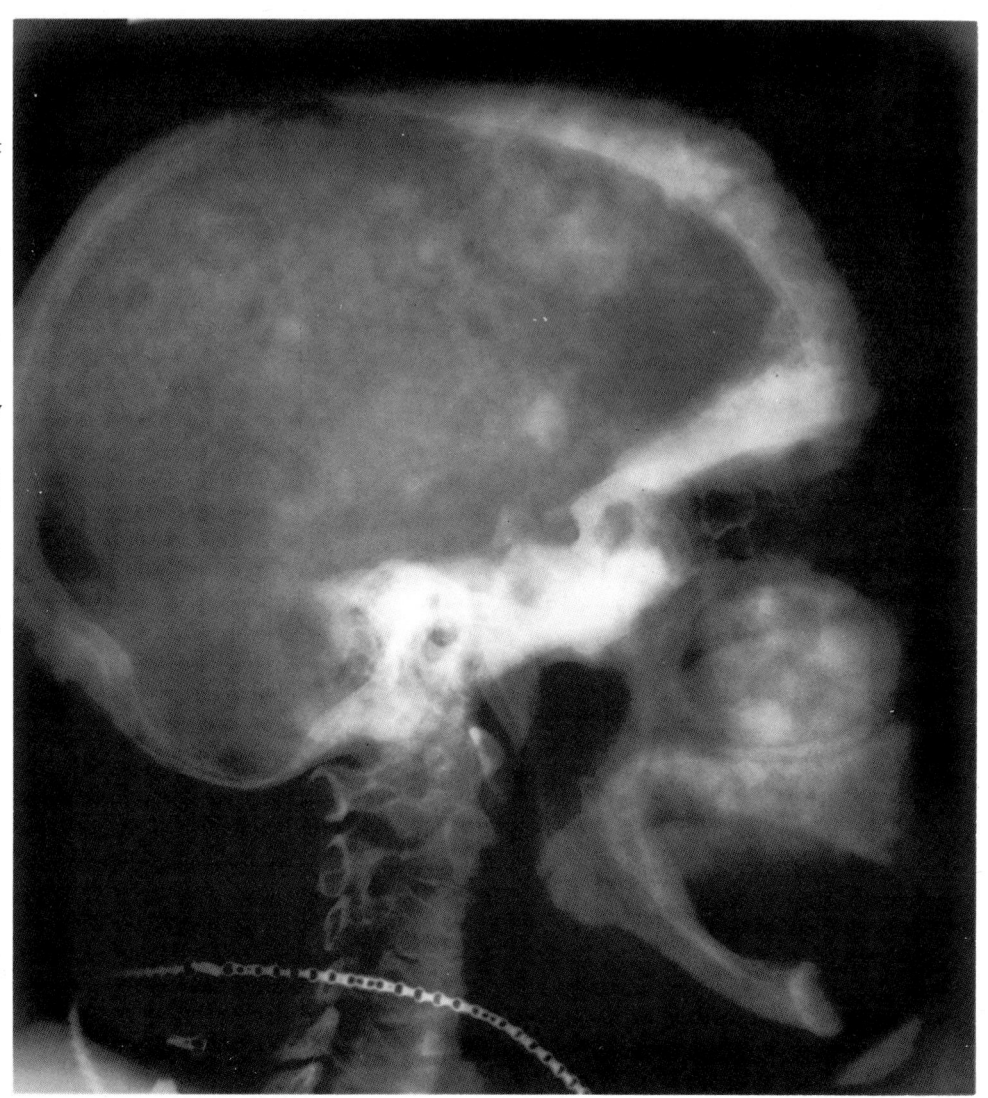

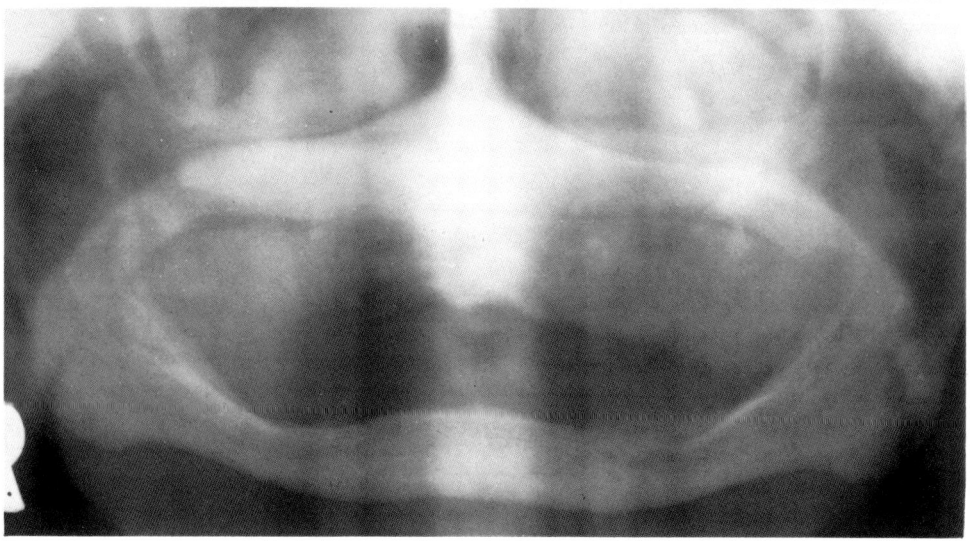

The Facial Bones 191

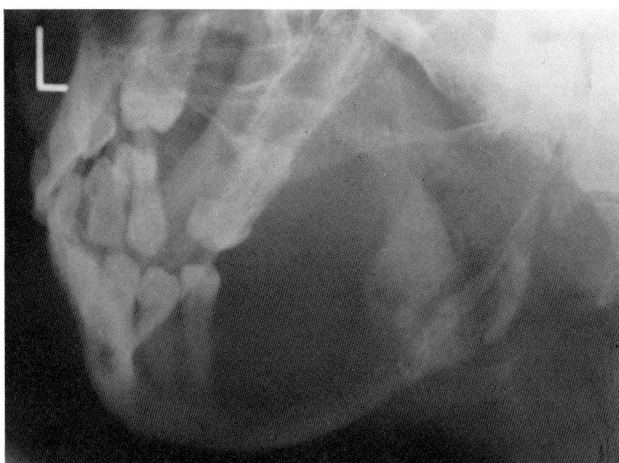

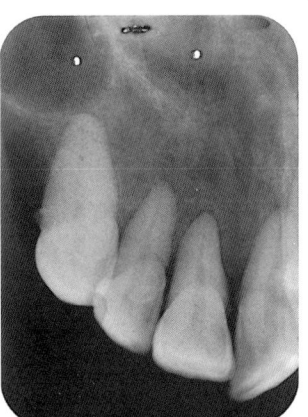

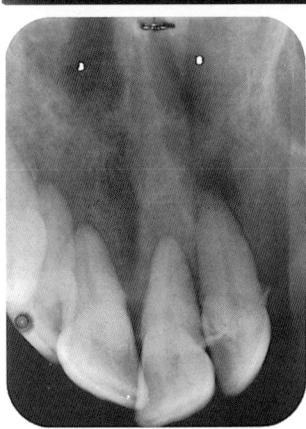

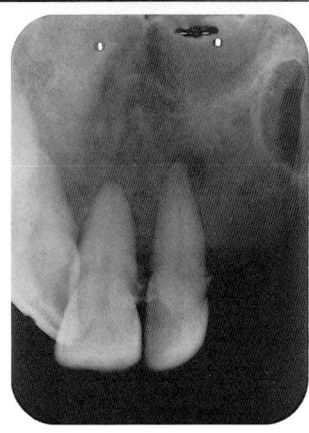

**Hyperparathyroidism
7.212 (top) and 7.213
(bottom)** As a consequence
of the secretion of excess
parathyroid hormone, mineral
is removed from the skeleton
as a result of bone resorption,
and these changes may first be
detected in the jaws. The bone
loss may be either focal in
pattern, in which case a
localised, radiolucent, cystic
area with clearly defined
margins may develop (Fig.
7.212), or diffuse, when the
changes affect all parts of the
jaws. In the latter, there is a
generalised loss of the lamina
dura (Fig. 7.213) with
osteoporosis, which is
manifested as an overall
radiolucency of the bone.
OLM & P

Chapter 8

The Temporo-mandibular Joint

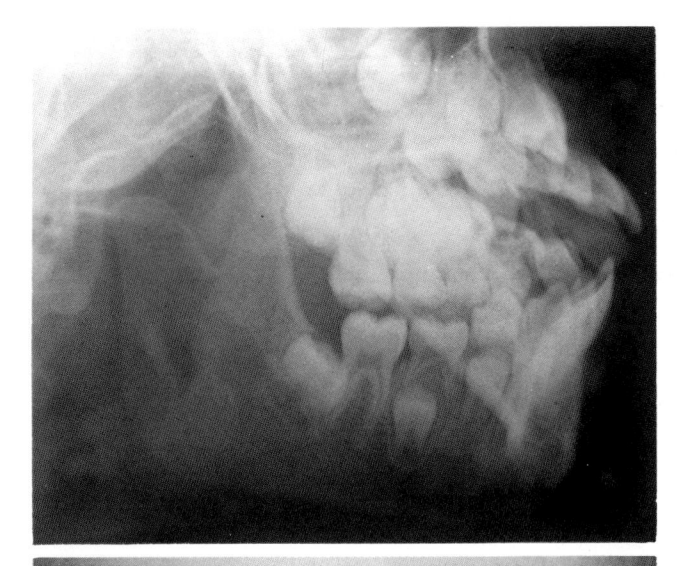

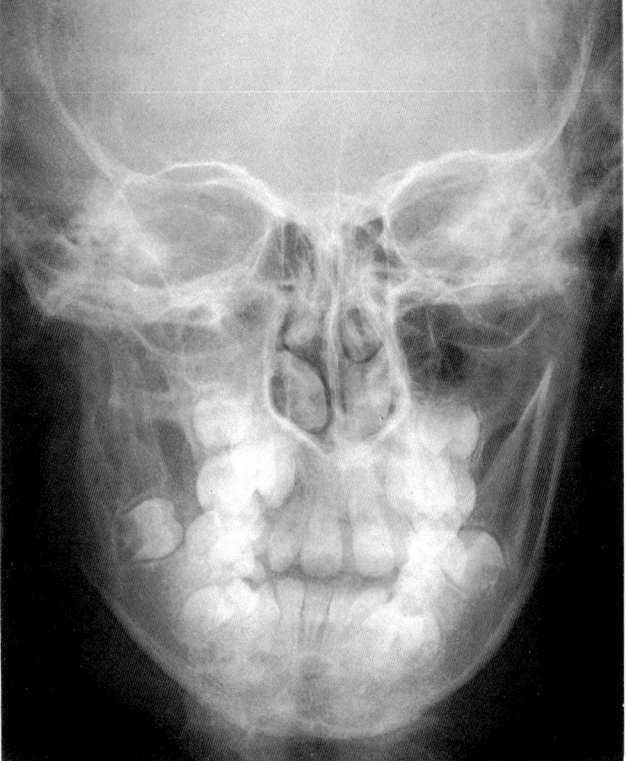

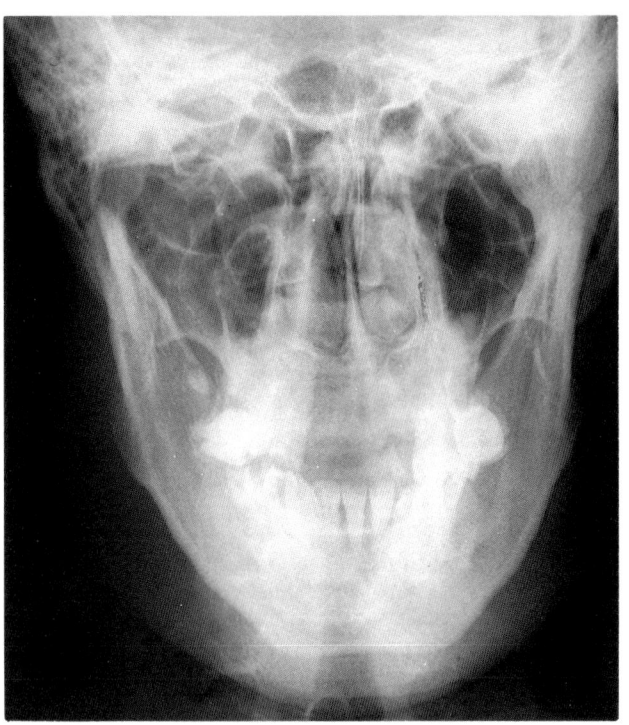

Condylar hyperplasia
8.3 In some instances, the hyperplasia affects predominantly the head of the mandibular condyle, as in this example, where there is gross enlargement of the left condyle, with thickening of the condylar neck. There is no obvious asymmetry or deviation of the midline of the mandible. Note the diminutive, unerupted, supernumerary tooth in the base of the right ramus. PA

Condylar hypoplasia
8.1 (top) and 8.2 (bottom) In this eight-year-old child, the right mandibular condyle is rudimentary, but its neck is widened antero-posteriorly with a deep, V-shaped sigmoid notch (Fig. 8.1). There has been underdevelopment of the right side of the mandible, the ramus of which is medially positioned relative to the other side, causing facial asymmetry (Fig. 8.2). No other developmental abnormalities were present. OLM & PA

196 *A Radiological Atlas of Diseases of the Teeth and Jaws*

8.4 In this example, the enlargement of the right condylar head, which projects antero-inferiorly, has resulted in downward displacement of the inferior border of the body of the mandible and of the occlusal plane on the right side. Note that all the mandibular teeth are tilted towards the affected side. PR

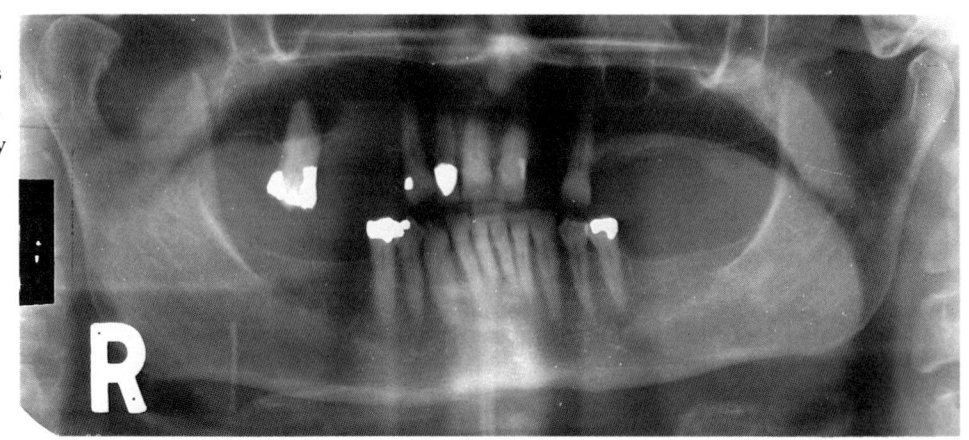

8.5 (right) and 8.6 (below right) Although the left condylar head is not so greatly enlarged in this patient, the hyperplasia has caused marked bowing of the inferior border of the mandible, with prominent, lateral open bite on the affected side, but only minimal displacement of the anterior midline of the mandible. The inferior alveolar canal is positioned closer to the inferior border of the mandible on the affected side, a feature often seen in this form of the condition.
PA & PR

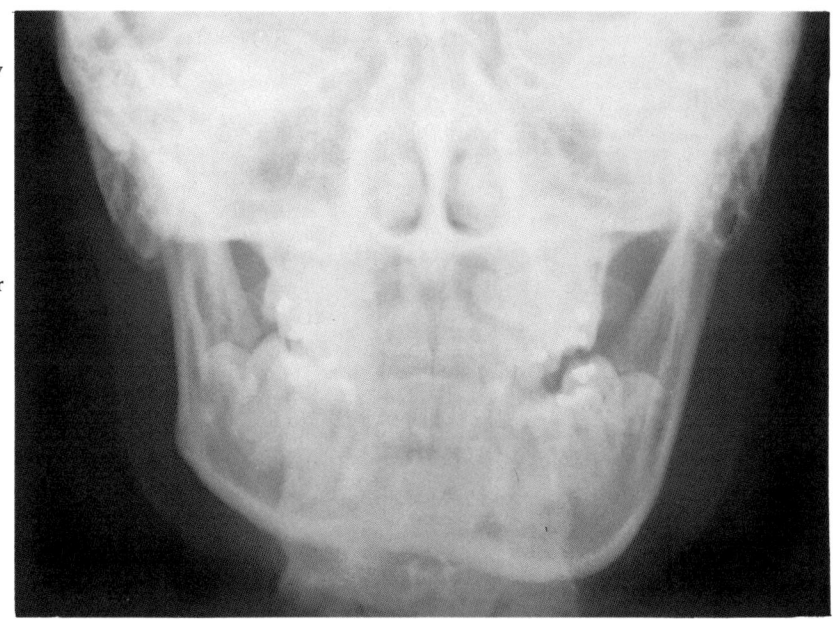

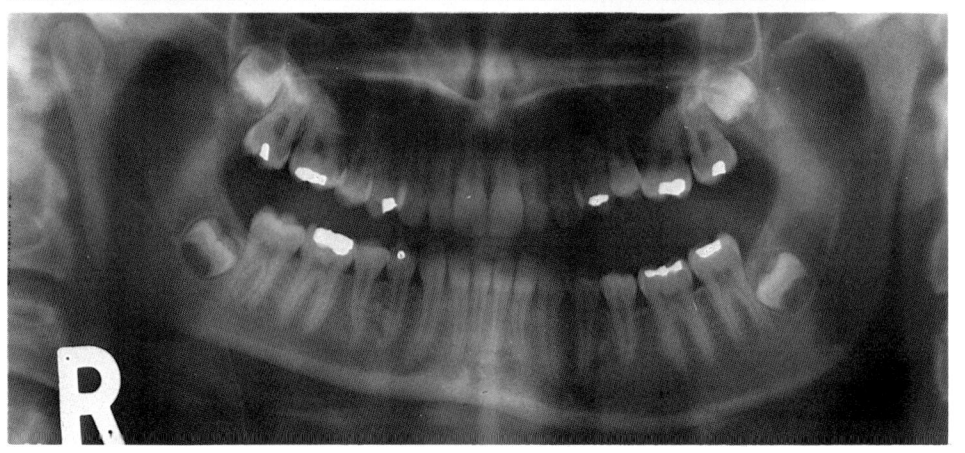

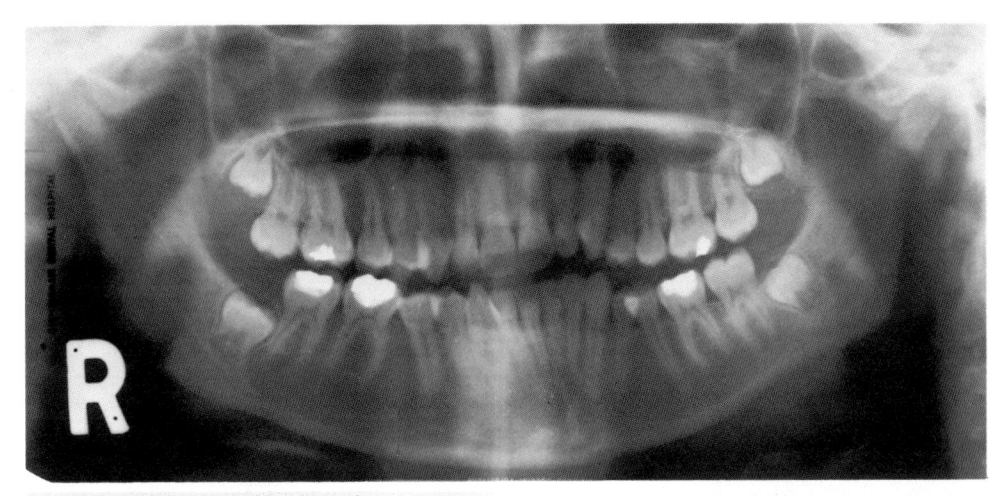

8.7 In other instances, the hyperplasia affects mainly the neck of the mandibular condyle, its head being approximately normal in size. In this example, the right side is affected, with an overall anterior displacement of the body of the mandible and shift of the midline away from the affected side. Note that the teeth remain in occlusion and there is no bowing of the inferior border of the mandible. PR

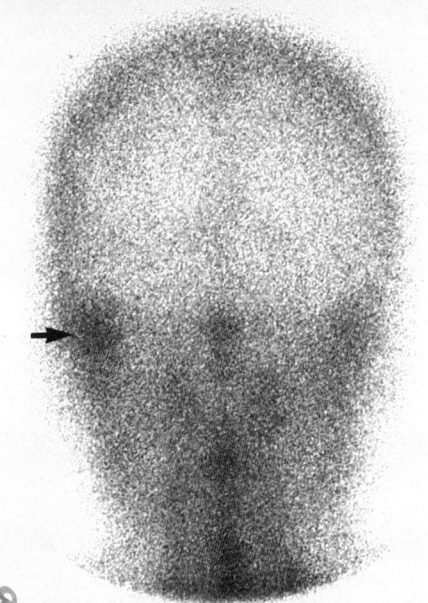

8.8 The overactivity of the mandibular condyle, despite the absence of enlargement of its head in this patient, is confirmed by a scintiscan. The area of increased uptake of radioisotope within the affected side is clearly demonstrated (arrow). SC

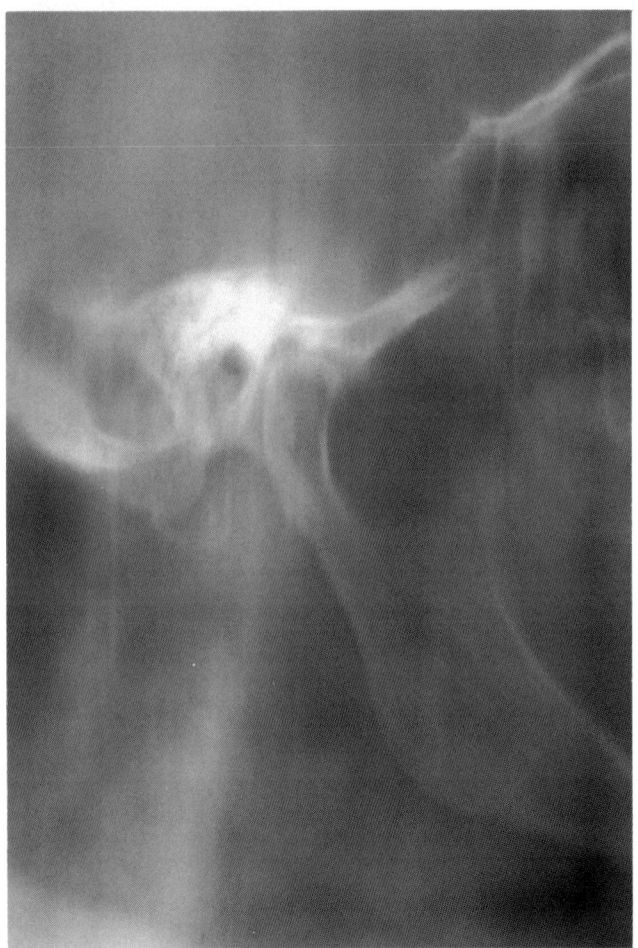

8.9 Another example, with marked elongation of the neck of the condyle. A tomogram in a lateral position is useful to demonstrate clearly the extent of the change. TG

Osteoarthrosis

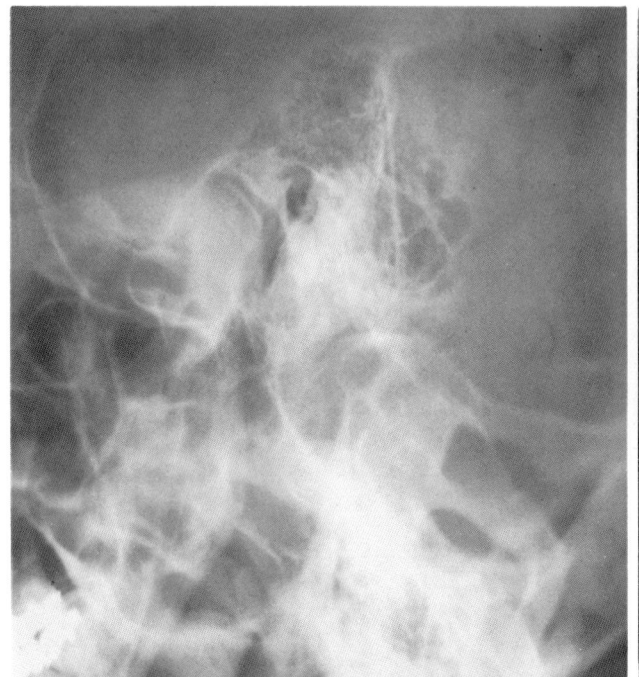

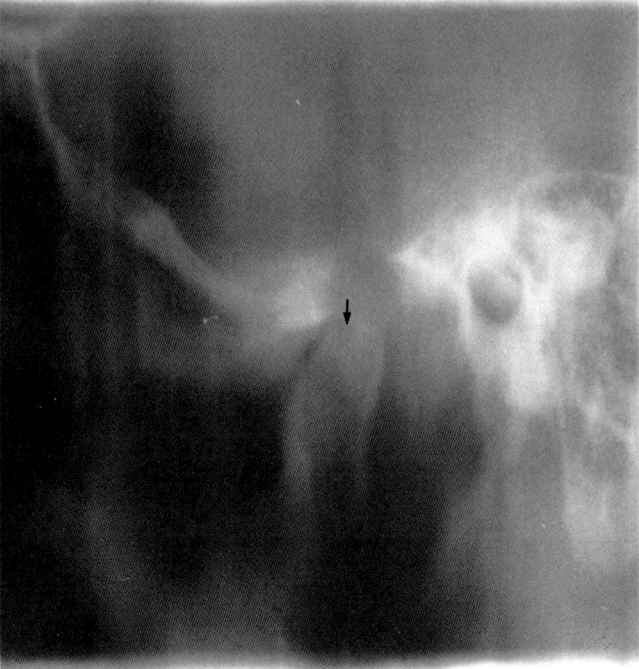

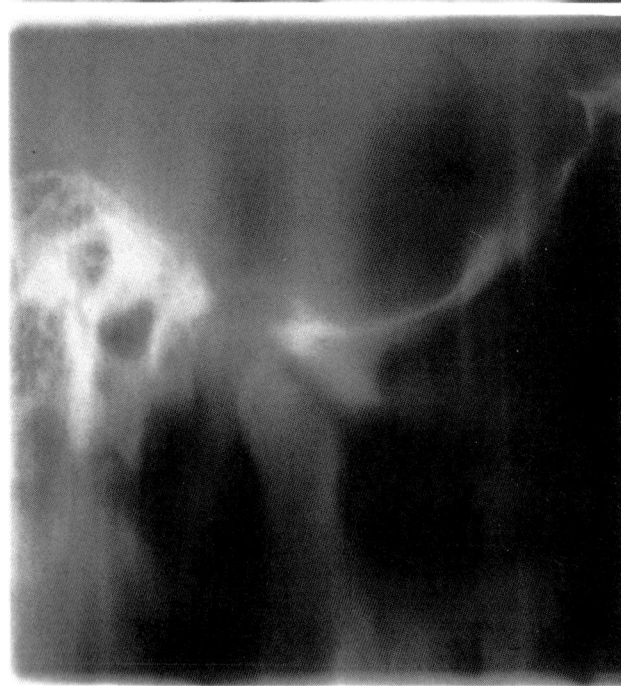

8.10 (top left), 8.11 (above) and 8.12 (left) On the standard transcranial radiograph (Fig. 8.10), the outline of the anterior aspect of the head of the left condyle is poorly defined suggesting that degenerative changes are present, although there is a normal cortical outline on the posterior aspect. There is also narrowing of the joint space anteriorly. A tomographic examination is helpful in confirming such changes and determining their extent. At the level of this tomograph (Fig. 8.11), an irregular, radiolucent crater is clearly visible, indicating erosion of the articular surface of the condyle (arrow). This condition is often bilateral, and the right joint is also affected (Fig. 8.12). The changes here are more advanced, and the erosion has involved most of the articular surface anteriorly resulting in flattening. TMJ & TG

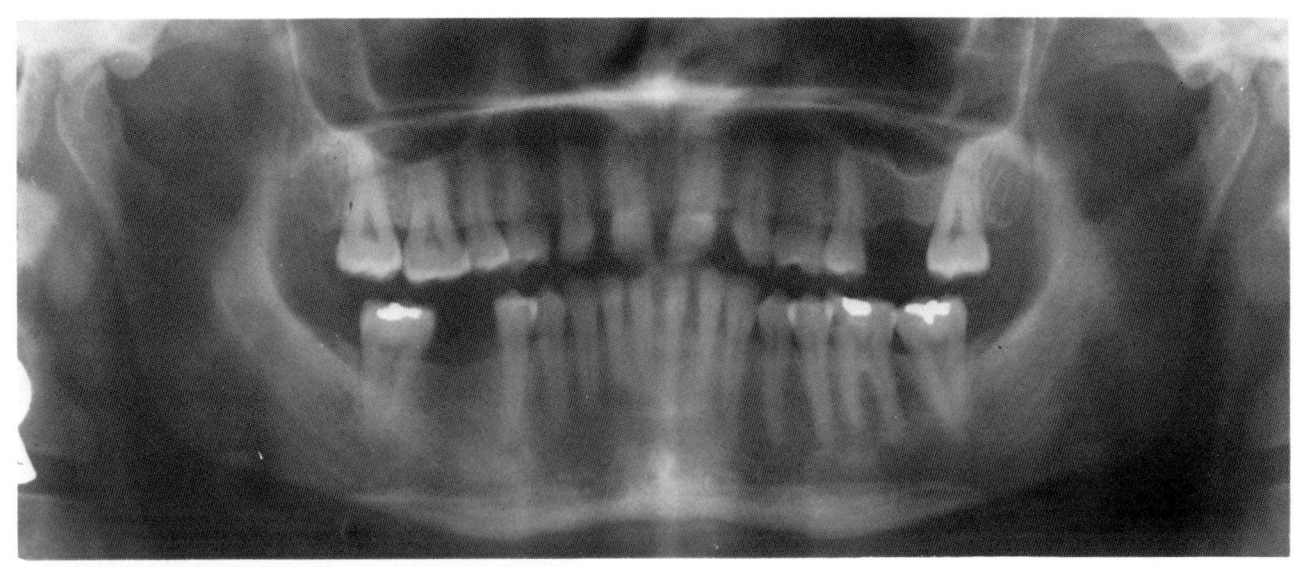

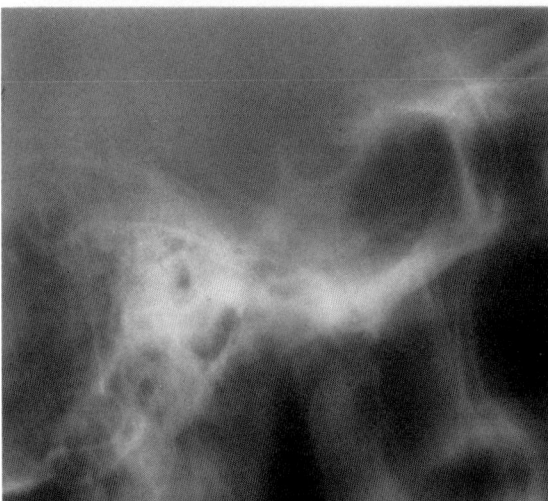

8.13 (above), 8.14 (left) and 8.15 (below left) Another example illustrating a less common pattern of erosion affecting predominantly the anterior aspect of the condylar heads. The condition is again bilateral, there being a clearly defined, irregularly shaped radiolucency together with a nodular bony protruberance on the anterior aspect of the condyles. The tomograms (Figs 8.14 and 8.15) confirm the presence and extent of these lesions, and indicate that the articular surfaces are also involved, there being radiolucent erosions on both sides. PR & TG

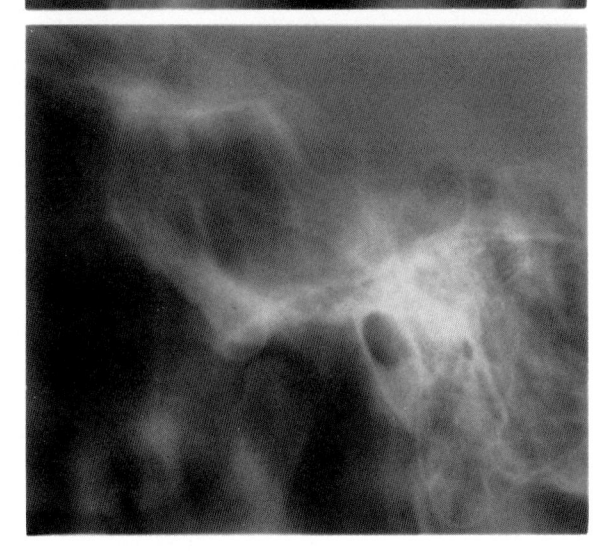

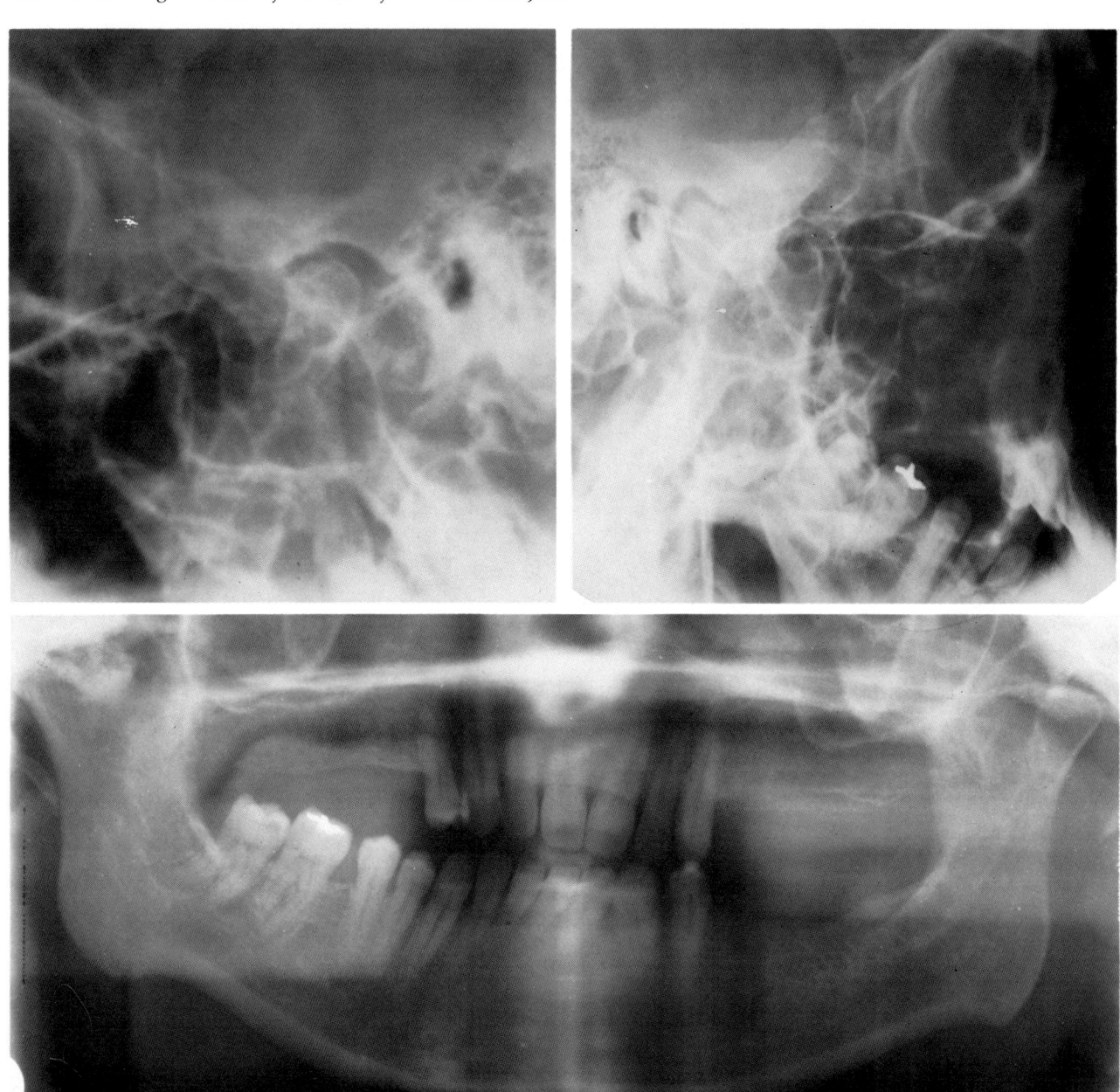

Rheumatoid arthritis
8.16 (top left), 8.17 (top right) and 8.18 (bottom) Juvenile rheumatoid arthritis (Still's disease), now 'burned out', affecting both temporo-mandibular joints in a 25-year-old. On the left side (Fig. 8.16), the articular surface of the condyle is uneven, and two small, circumscribed radiolucent areas of cystic osteoporosis are present just beneath its surface. A radiopaque, mineralised body is present in the joint space, which is slightly reduced in width anteriorly. On the right side (Fig. 8.17), there is bony continuity between the head of the condyle anteriorly and the articular eminence and wall of the glenoid fossa, together with an absence of the joint space on this aspect, indicating that bony ankylosis has occurred. Elsewhere, the condylar head is blunted in shape and the joint space reduced in width. Note that the right side has been examined with the patient attempting to open the mouth, confirming the lack of movement of the condylar head. In addition to the joint changes (Fig. 8.18), there is pronounced antegonial notching on both sides of the inferior border of the mandible, and the coronoid process on the right side is enlarged due to altered muscle activity. The mass of excessive bone in the ankylosed right joint is clearly demonstrated. TMJ & PR

The Temporo-mandibular Joint 201

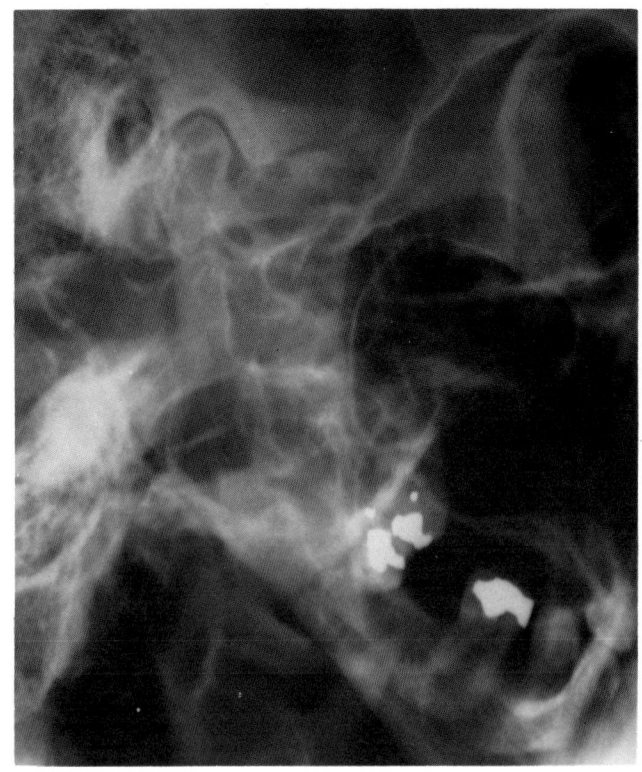

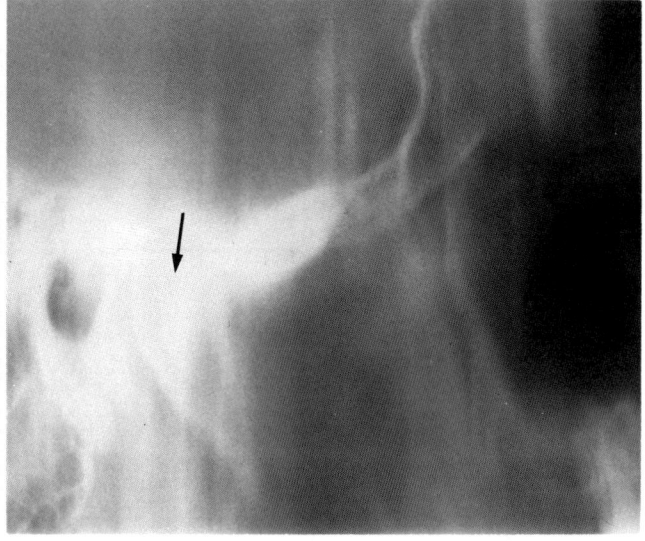

8.19 (left) and 8.20 (above) Active lesions in a 40-year-old, with involvement of many joints throughout the body. The transcranial view (Fig. 8.19) of the right temporo-mandibular joint shows no obvious irregularity of the condylar surface, but an irregularly oval radiolucency in the condylar head and narrowing of the joint space suggests that disease may be present. Again, tomograms (Fig. 8.20) confirmed this to be so and the condylar head is flattened with an irregular surface (arrow). TMJ & TG

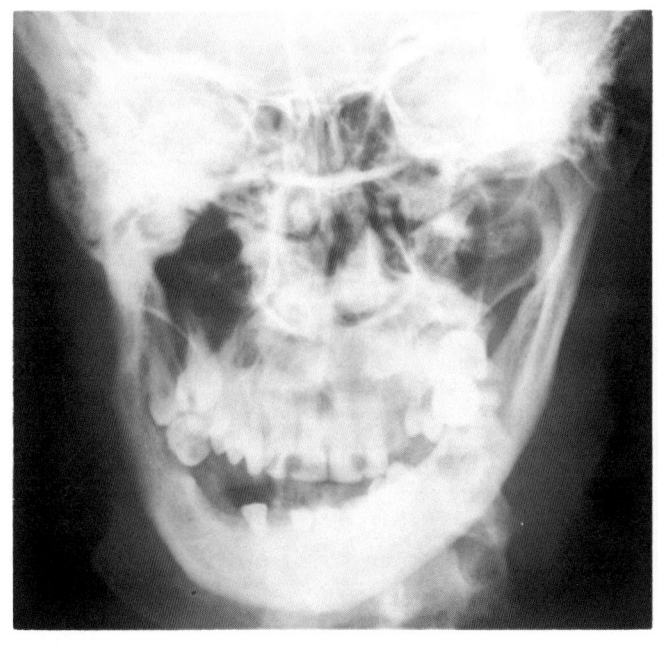

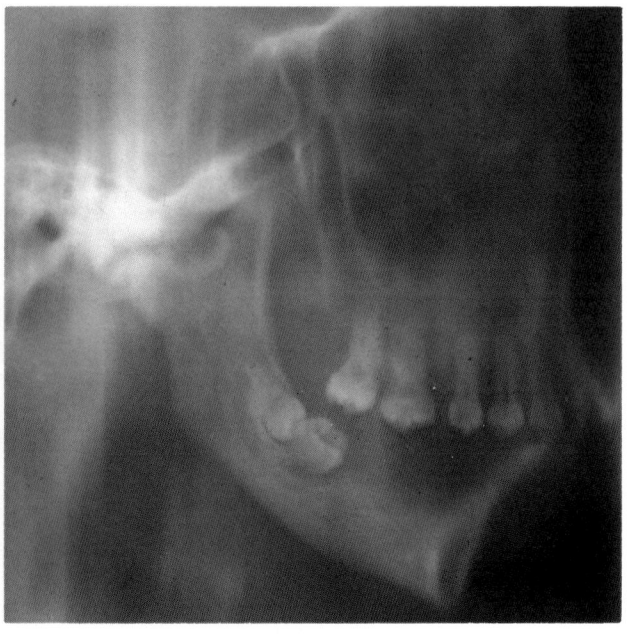

Ankylosis
8.21 (left) and 8.22 (right) Ankylosis of the right mandibular condyle to the temporal bone following osteomyelitis at age 12, as a consequence of which the condylar head has been destroyed. The right side of the mandible is underdeveloped and there is deviation of the midline to the affected side. The glenoid fossa has been obliterated with sclerotic bone (Fig. 8.22) and an irregular radiolucent zone of fibrous tissue separates the condylar stump from the sclerosed fossa. There is also sclerosis of the irregularly shaped condylar stump and margin of the sigmoid notch, and pronounced underdevelopment of the mental process. Note the horizontally impacted 8|. PA & TG

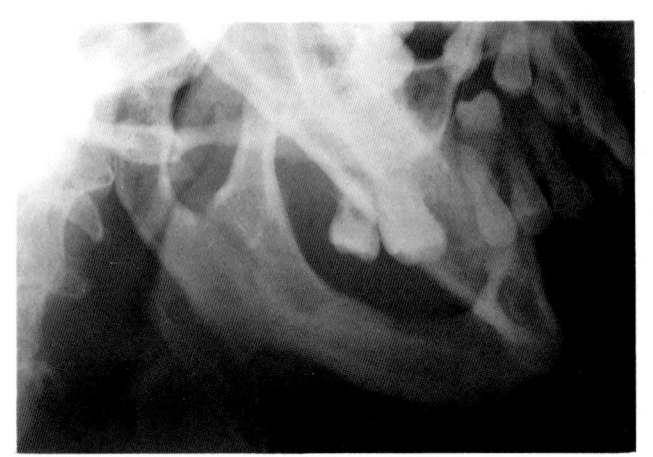

8.23 Ankylosis of the right temporo-mandibular joint in an adult following osteomyelitis and destruction of the cartilaginous growth centre in the mandibular condyle in childhood. As a consequence, there is mandibular micrognathism and osseous continuity between the condyle and the temporal bone, with absence of the joint cavity. There is elongation of the coronoid process and prominent antegonial notching on the inferior border of the mandible due to the muscle pull of the temporalis and masseter muscles, respectively. The deep, V-shaped sigmoid notch has been caused by the limited development of the mandible and the inferior alveolar canal opens into it. Note that the mandibular teeth have all been removed on the affected side. OLM

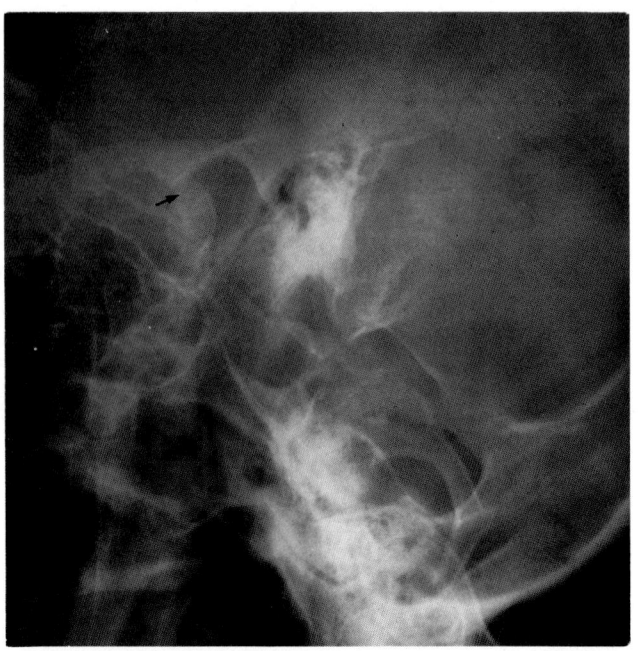

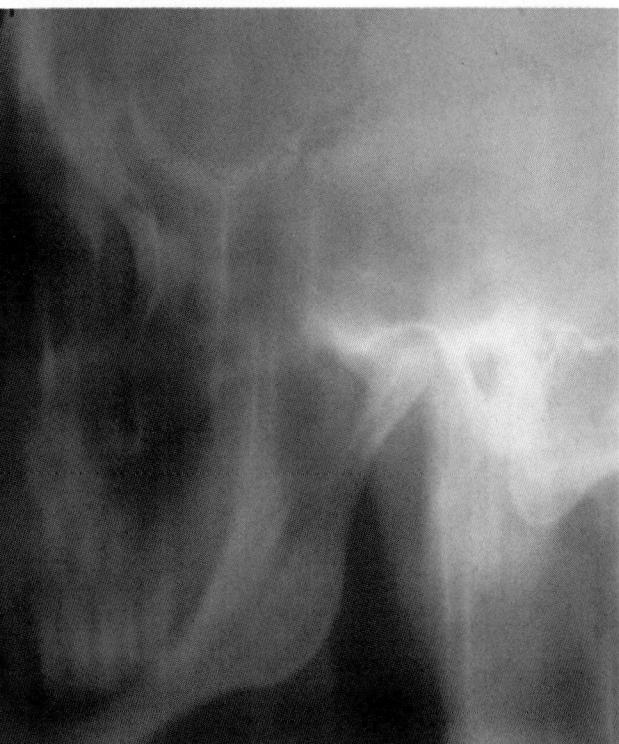

Synovial osteochondromatosis
8.24 (top) and 8.25 (bottom) In this unusual condition, seen here in an elderly patient, the articular surface of the left condyle (Fig. 8.24) appears notched with a continuous layer of cortical bone. Several radiopaque bodies (arrow) are present above and anterior to the condylar head occupying part of the widened joint space. These findings are confirmed on the tomograph (Fig. 8.25). TMJ & TG

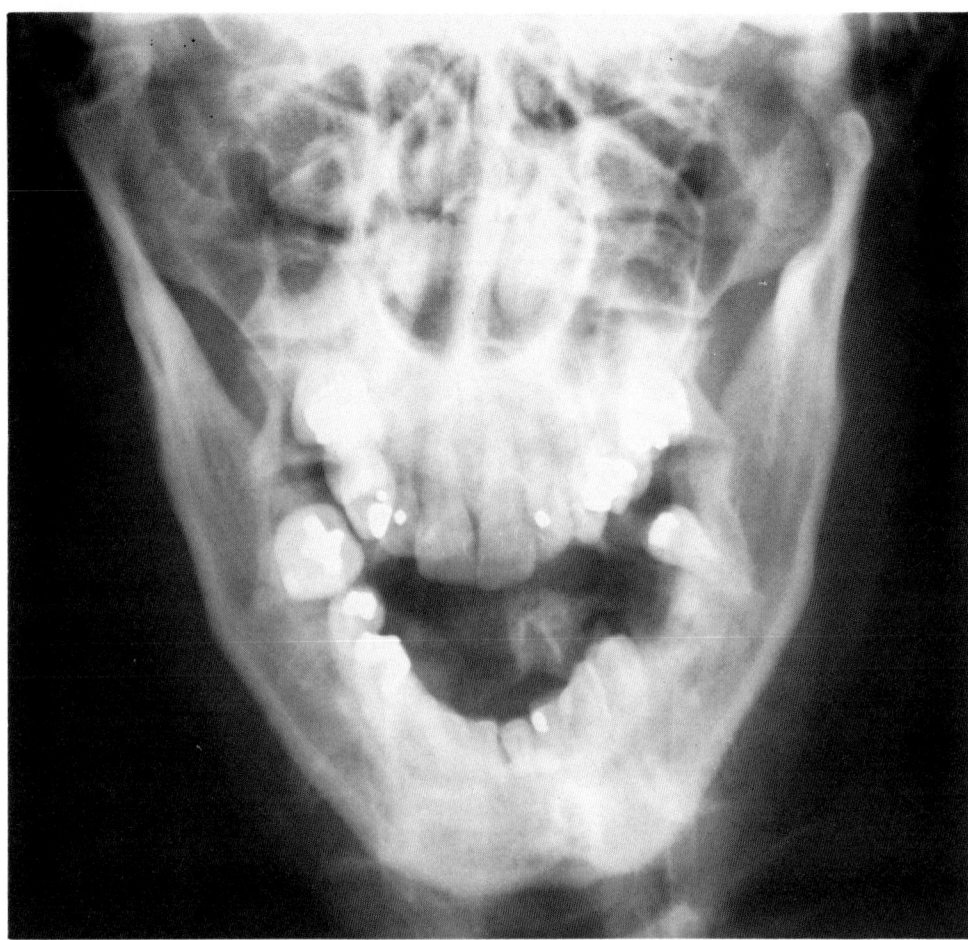

Fracture of the mandibular condyle

8.26 (top) and 8.27 (bottom) Abnormality of the left mandibular condyle following trauma during infancy. The lateral half of the condylar head has been displaced (Fig. 8.26) and lies (arrow) just anterior to the remainder of the condyle (Fig. 8.27). The body and ramus of the left mandible are underdeveloped compared with the opposite side, and there is deviation of the midline to the left on opening (Fig. 8.26). Note that ⌐5 has drifted a long way distally and its apex is curved mesially.
PAC & PR

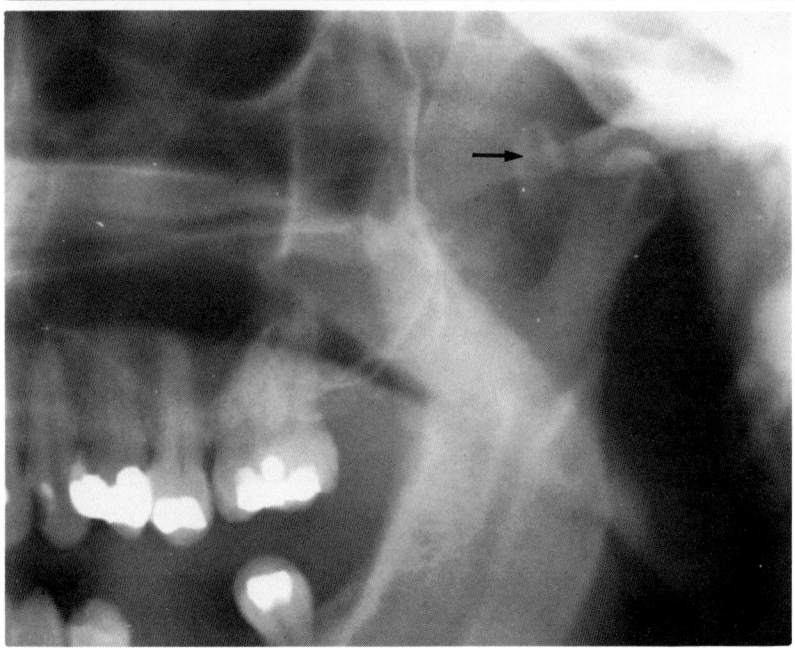

8.28 Bilateral fractures of the necks of the mandibular condyles following a blow to the chin. The radiolucent fracture lines are irregular and run approximately horizontally. On the left side, the condylar fragment has been only minimally displaced medially, whereas on the right side the medial displacement is greater. T

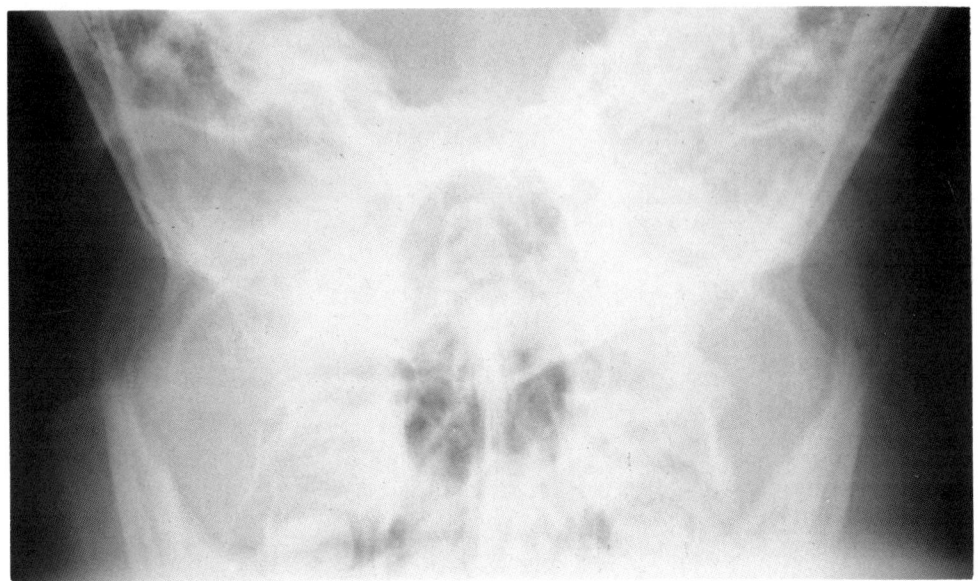

8.29 A fracture of the neck of the left mandibular condyle with marked displacement of the head of the condylar fragment medially due to pull of the attached lateral pterygoid muscle. T

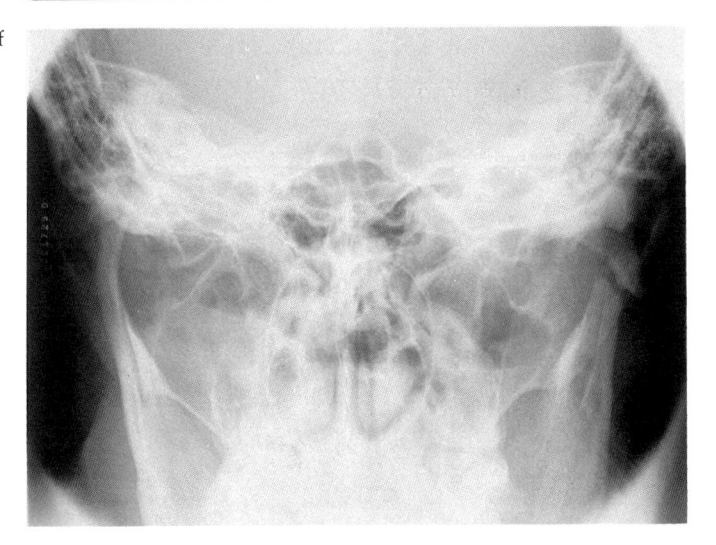

The Temporo-mandibular Joint 205

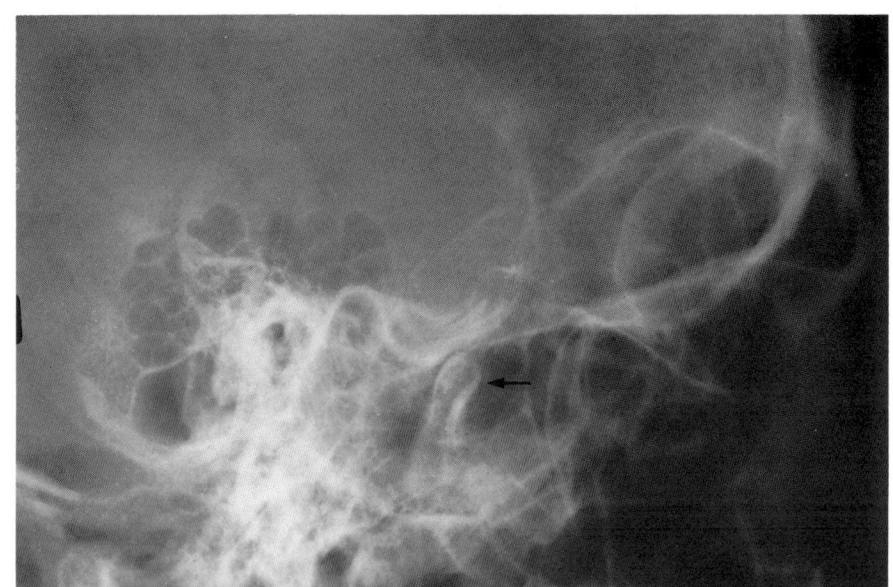

Dislocation of the mandibular condyle
8.30 Dislocation of the right mandibular condyle, the head of which (arrow) is lying anterior to the articular eminence. As a consequence, the glenoid fossa appears empty. TMJ

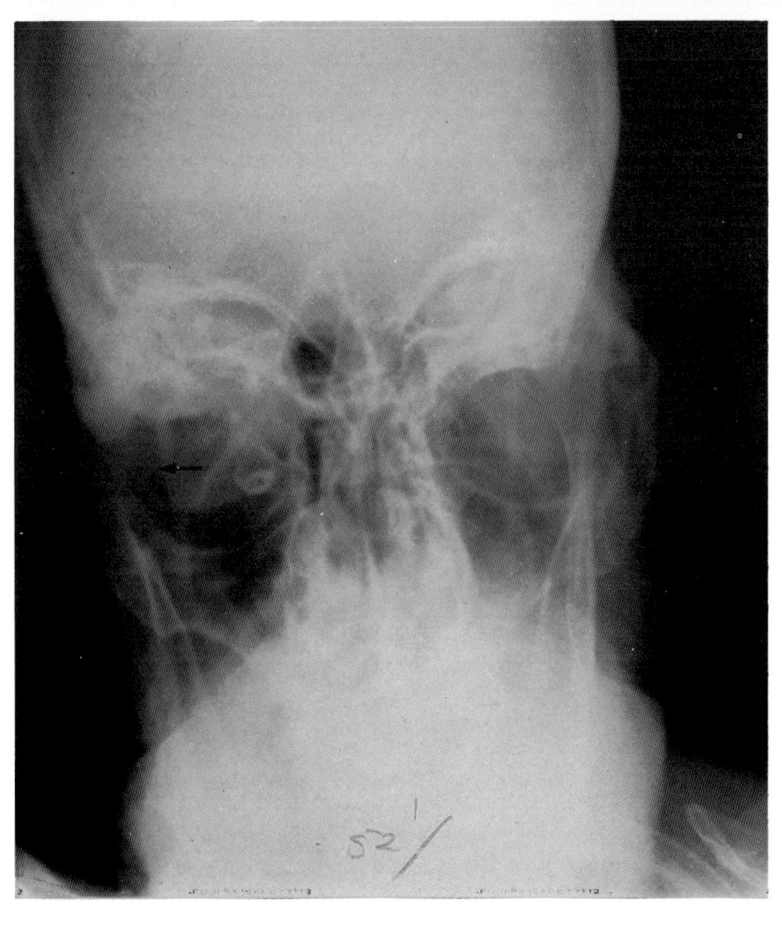

Metastatic carcinoma
8.31 A metastatic deposit of adenocarcinoma from a primary tumour in the colon. Compared with the normal side, the cortical outline of the right condyle is missing, particularly on the medial side (arrow) and the condyle itself has an irregularly radiolucent, 'moth-eaten' appearance. T

Chapter 9

The Soft Tissues including the Salivary Glands

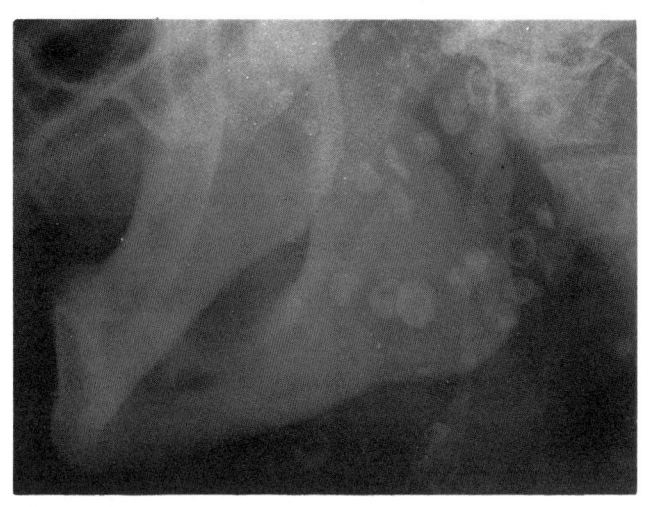

Haemangioma

9.1 A large lesion of the left side of the face, in an elderly person, containing numerous foci of dystrophic mineralisation (phleboliths) which are mostly superimposed over the ramus of the mandible. Phleboliths form by deposition of successive concentric layers of mineral around a focus of degenerative tissue or thrombus, and are thus approximately circular in outline and exhibit considerable variation in size. They are not densely radiopaque, some of them having radiolucent centres. OLM

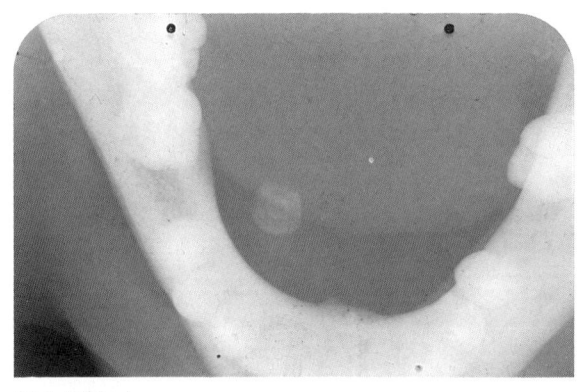

Sialolithiasis

9.2 Salivary stones (calculi) occur most commonly in the submandibular salivary gland and may be sited at any point along the duct system. Since such stones are formed by the deposition of successive layers of mineral upon a central nidus, they often appear as a series of concentric layers which are alternately radiopaque and radiolucent. In this example, there is an approximately circular stone in the anterior part of the duct of the right submandibular salivary gland, showing the typical structure. It is relatively poorly mineralised and the film was deliberately underexposed to make the stone more visible. As a consequence, the outline of the tongue, which runs across the stone, is also clearly demonstrated. LTO

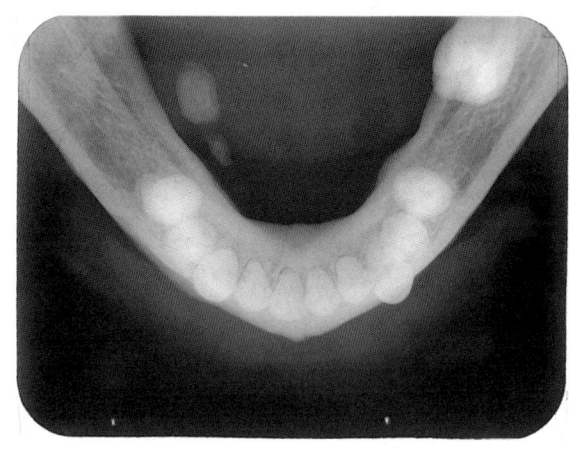

9.3 In this example, there are two oval-shaped stones of different size in the duct of the right, submandibular salivary gland. Once again, their lamellated pattern is clearly demonstrated. LTO

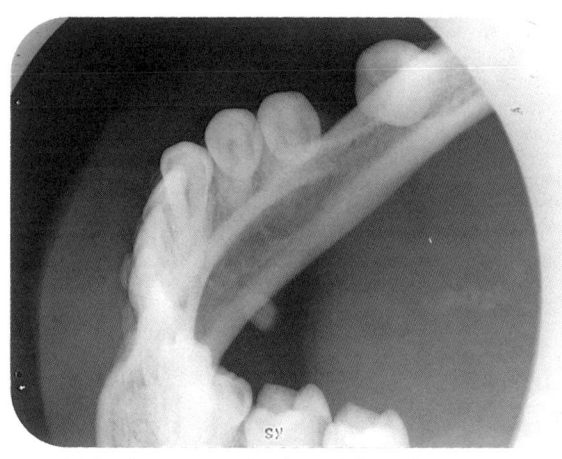

9.4 Multiple stones in the duct of the right, submandibular salivary gland. There is a discrete, circular, radiopaque stone close to the opening of the duct in the floor of the mouth, and several smaller stones of more irregular shape in the posterior part of the duct. Because of the oblique angle of this view, the shadow of the anteriorly placed stone is partly superimposed on the mandible. LOO

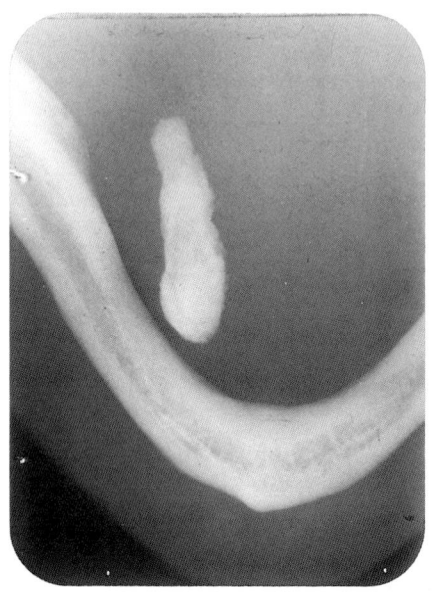

210   *A Radiological Atlas of Diseases of the Teeth and Jaws*

9.5 A particularly large, elongated, radiopaque stone in the duct of the right, submandibular salivary gland in an edentulous patient. It is wider anteriorly, where the mass originated, and tapers posteriorly. It is of variable radiodensity and has an irregular outline. LTO

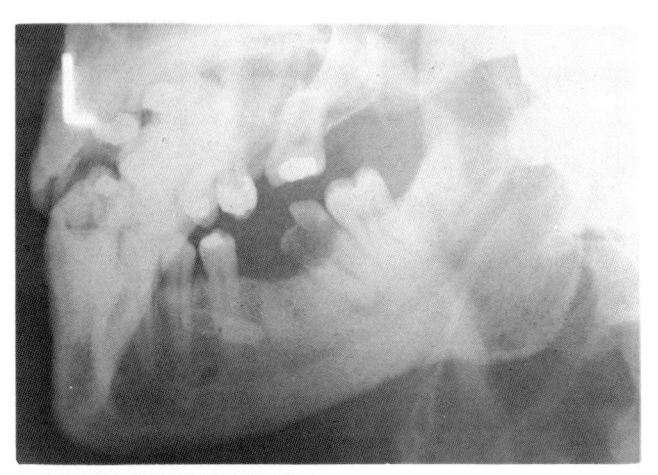

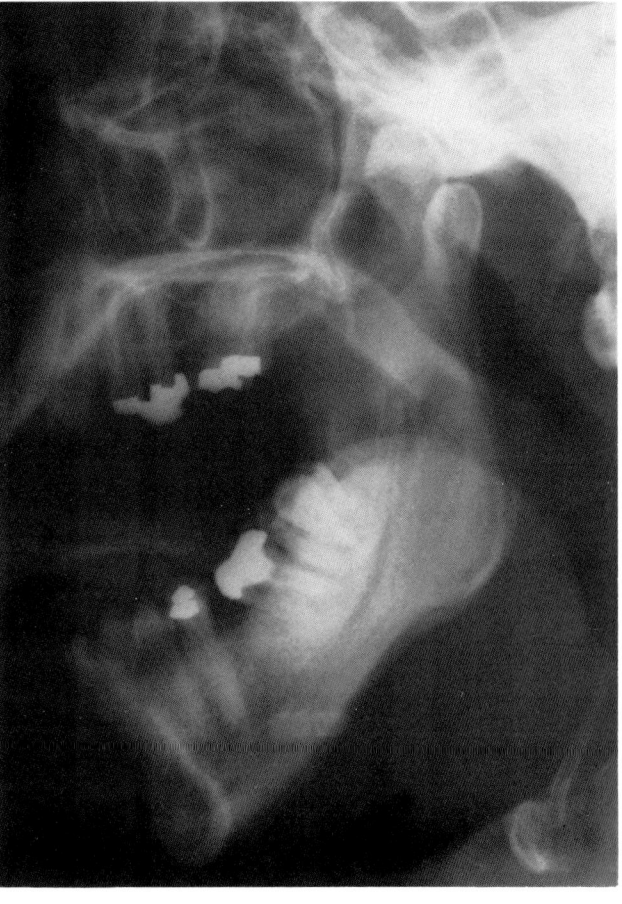

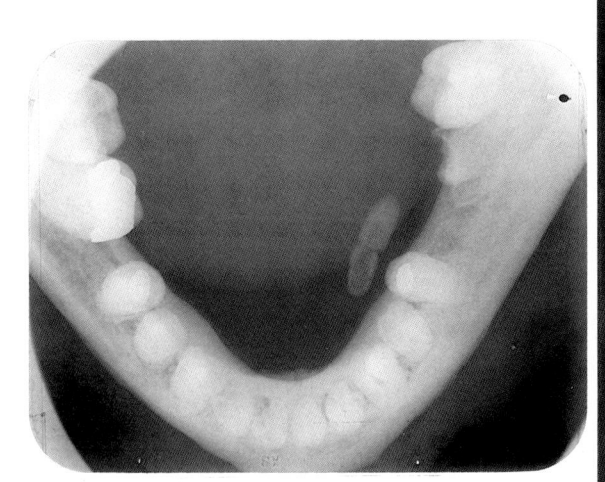

9.6 (above), 9.7 (top right) and 9.8 (bottom right) Two separate ovoid stones in the duct of the left, submandibular salivary gland, each of which has a more radiolucent core. In extra-oral films, the image of such stones may be superimposed upon other structures. In this example, they overlie the roots $\overline{45}$ in the lateral oblique mandible view (Fig. 9.7). By asking the patient to depress the floor of the mouth with the fingers, the image can be displaced to a more favourable position in a true lateral film where, as in this example (Fig. 9.8), it is superimposed upon the inferior border of the mandible. Note the large carious lesion $\overline{7}$ and periapical radiolucency on its mesial root. LTO, OLM & L

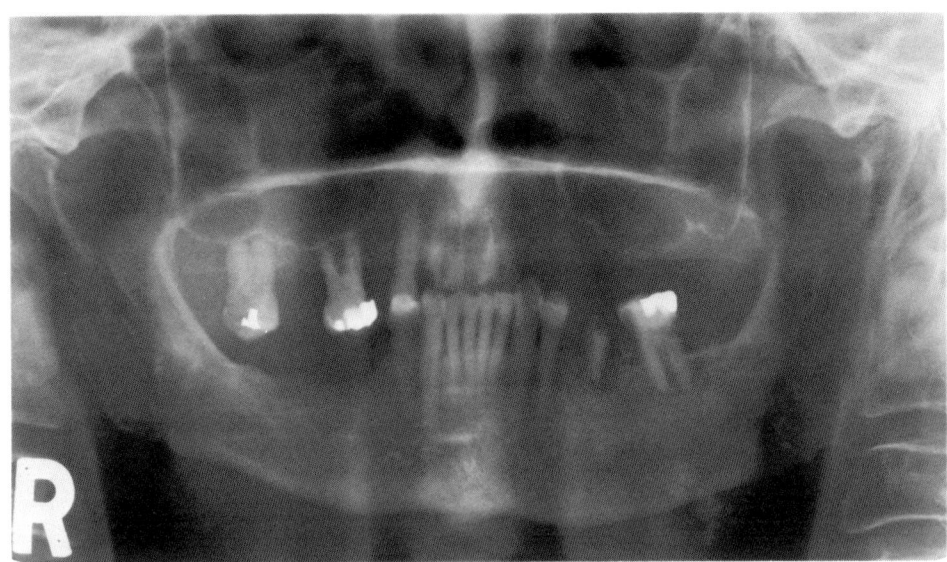

The Soft Tissues including the Salivary Glands 211

9.9 At least three stones are present within the intra-glandular part of the duct of the left, submandibular gland. The radiopaque stones are of granular appearance, the image of the supero-anterior one being superimposed upon the lower part of the mandible. Together they form a 'comma'-shaped pattern, which is typical of stones forming in the duct as it loops around the posterior border of the mylohyoid muscle. Note also the generally poor state of the dentition in this elderly patient, and the flattening of the condylar heads, particularly of the left side, suggestive of degenerative change. PR

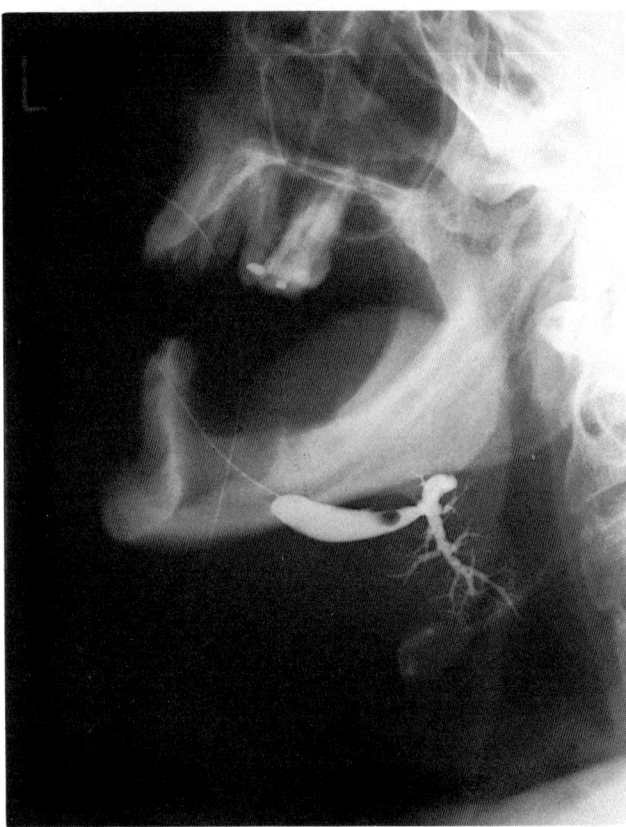

9.10 A sialogram of a submandibular gland with gross dilatation of the main duct and the intra-glandular part of the duct system, due to obstruction at its oral end, probably by a radiolucent stone. The ovoid radiolucency within the dilated duct is an air bubble, its position in the upper part of the duct indicating that, with the patient in the upright position, it has risen to the top of the injected fluid. Confirmation of this can be obtained on a repeat sialogram. Note the looped outline of the canula filled with contrast medium leading into the opening of the duct, which is relatively posterior in position due to retrusion of the tongue, the outline of which can be clearly seen. L

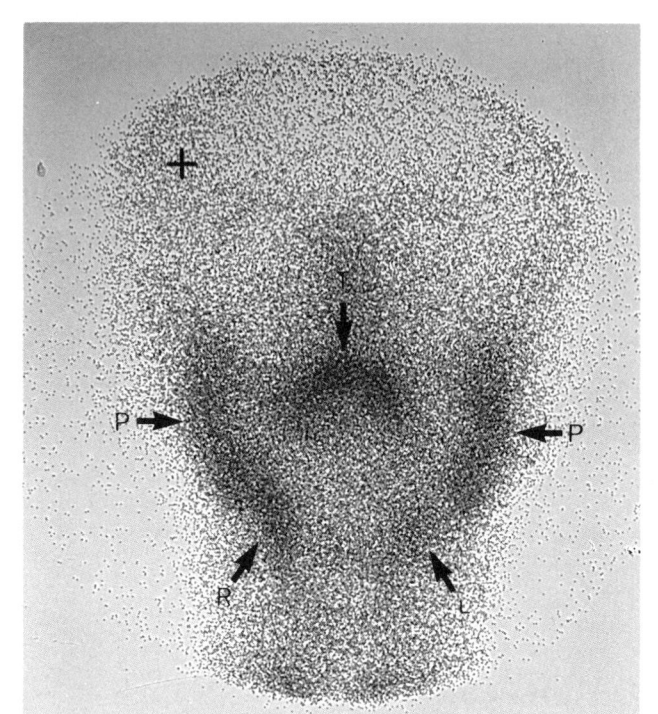

212 A Radiological Atlas of Diseases of the Teeth and Jaws

9.11 Obstruction of the salivary gland duct over a long period of time is accompanied by a reduction in its secretory output due to atrophy of the acinar cells. A scintiscan following the injection of technetium pertechnetate (^{99m}Tc) demonstrates any change in glandular activity. This scan in a patient with sialolithiasis of the left, submandibular gland, demonstrates the normal uptake of isotope in the two parotid glands (P), the right submandibular gland (R) and the accessory salivary glands of the palate and tongue (T), but the greatly reduced uptake in the left submandibular gland (L). SC

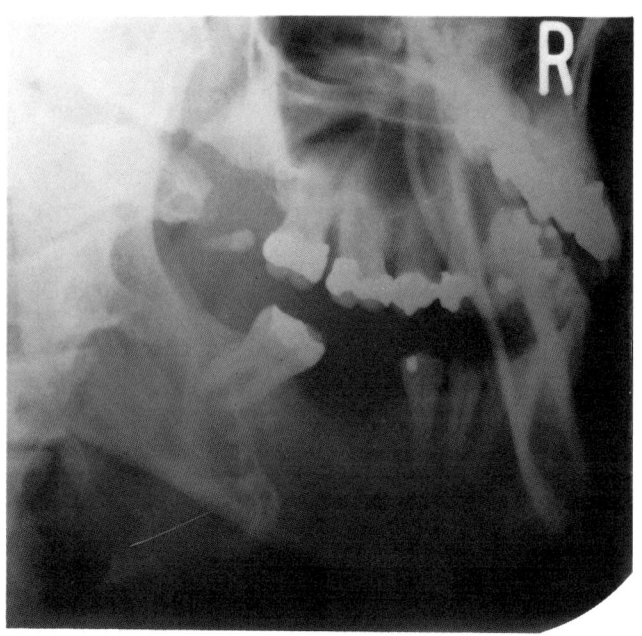

9.14 Stones in the ducts of the parotid gland are very much less common than in the submandibular gland, and when they occur are commonly close to the ampulla of the main duct. As a consequence, their image may be superimposed upon that of the dentition as in this example, where a radiopaque ovoid stone appears just distal to 7|. Note the fragments of amalgam within the 6| socket. OLM

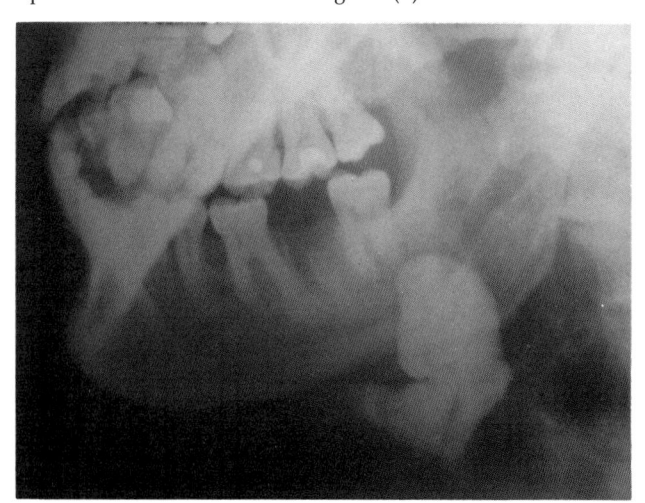

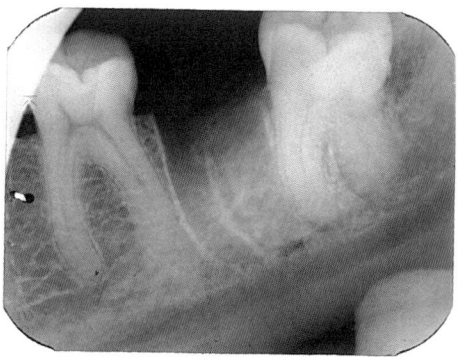

9.12 (left) and 9.13 (above) Extensive mineralisation of the left, submandibular gland involving both its superficial and deep parts. The deep groove on the anterior margin of the radiopaque mass represents the posterior border of the mylohyoid muscle, forming the boundary between the two parts of the gland. This patient was originally X rayed because of a painful |7 socket (Fig. 9.13), and the mass was discovered as an incidental finding. OLM & P

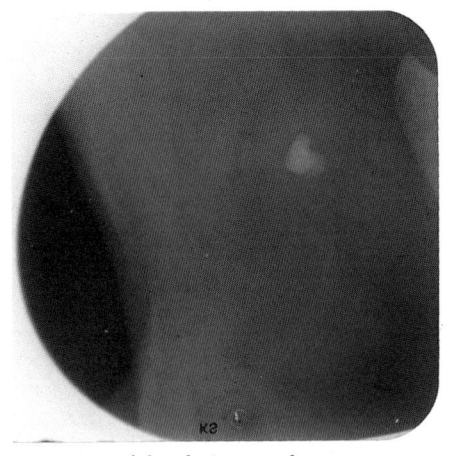

The Soft Tissues including the Salivary Glands 213

9.15 A useful technique to demonstrate parotid stones in the region of the ampulla is to place an occlusal film in the oral vestibule. Using a soft tissue exposure, the stones may be clearly displayed, as in this example. Note the head of the coronoid process. S

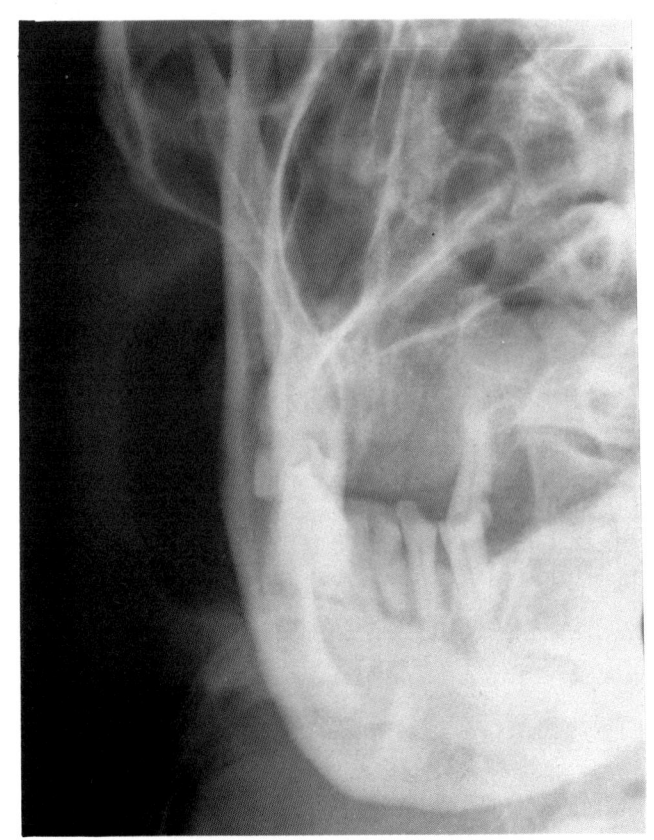

9.16 The presence of parotid stones is also well demonstrated on a rotated postero-anterior film taken with the cheek inflated. The radiolucent, air-filled vestibule is clearly demonstrated, bounded laterally by the slightly radiopaque shadow of the soft tissues of the cheek which are bulging outwards. The circular, radiopaque stone stands out clearly close to the mucosal surface in the upper part of the vestibule. RPA

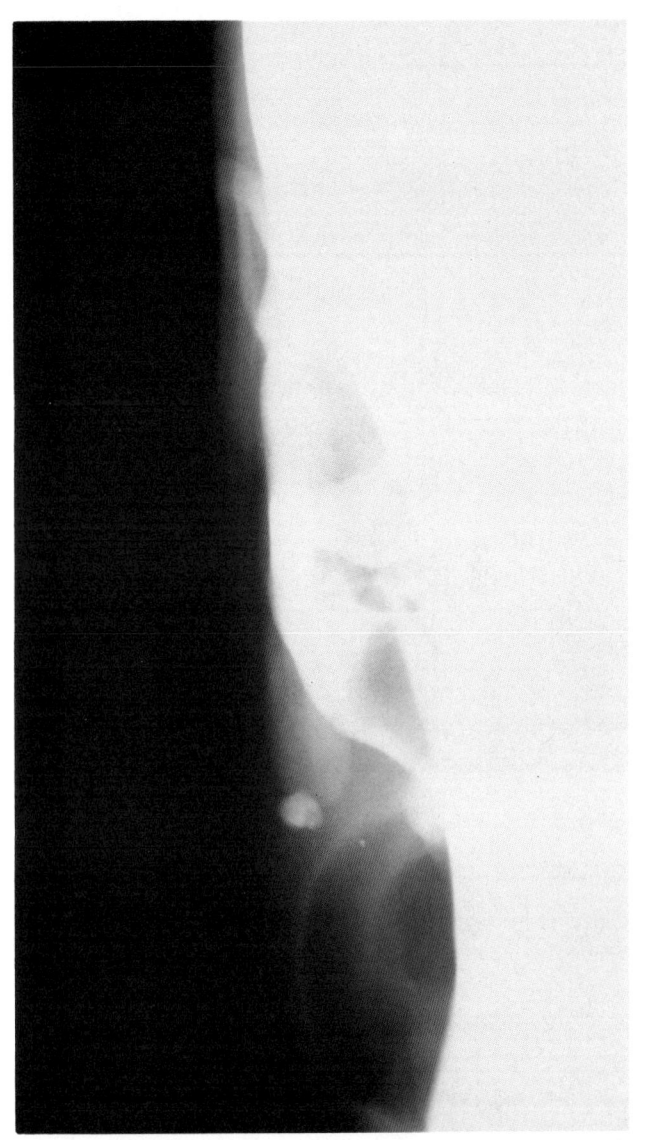

9.17 Since parotid stones are often poorly mineralised, better definition may be obtained by underexposure of the film, as in this example. The stone is highlighted lying close to the mucosal surface of the air filled, radiolucent vestibule. In such films, the detail of the mineralised parts of the skeleton is lost. RPA

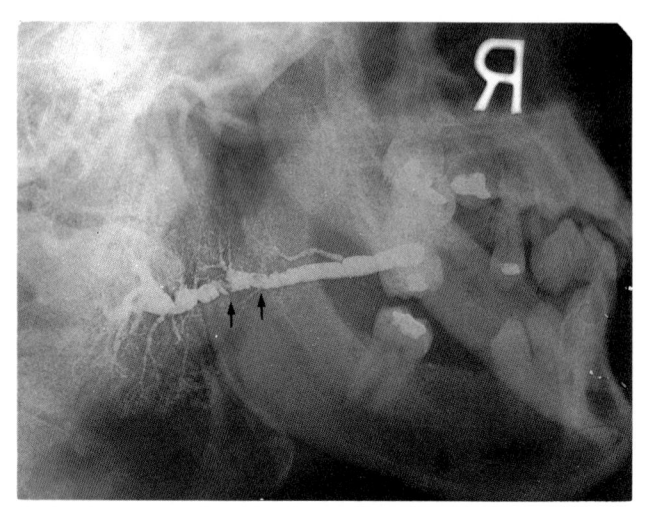

9.18 Approximately 40% of parotid stones are poorly mineralised and are therefore radiolucent. Under these circumstances, a sialogram is very helpful, as in this gland where there is a partial obstruction of the opening of the duct into the oral vestibule. The main duct is dilated and has a segmental outline, and there are two radiolucent stones (arrows) within it, shown by the rounded, radiolucent filling defects. OLM

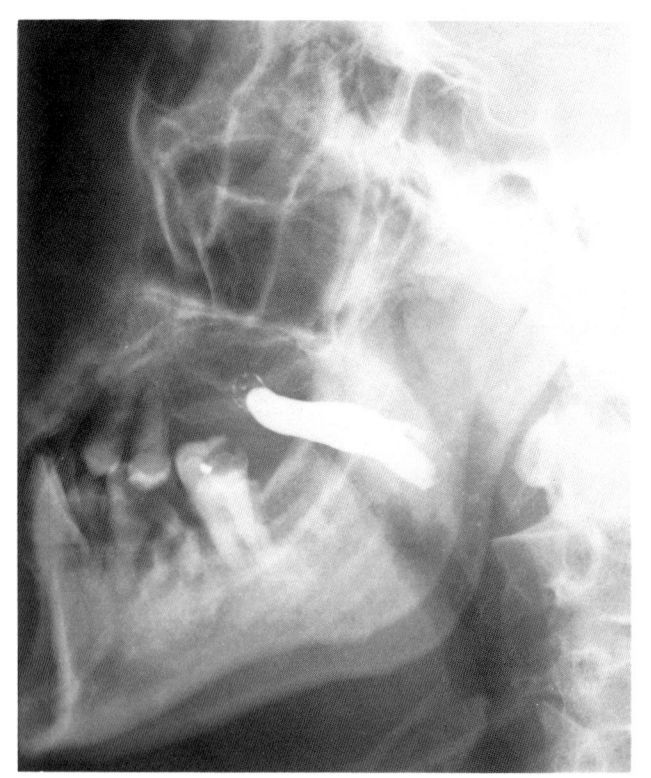

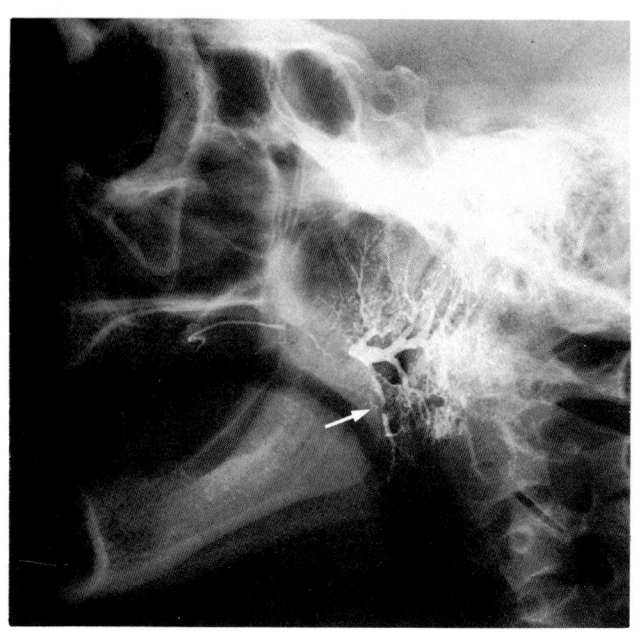

9.20 A parotid sialogram demonstrating a radiolucent stone in the middle part of the main duct, where there is an interruption in the continuity of the column of contrast medium. The anterior portion of the duct is of normal diameter and exhibits the characteristic hook-shape where it penetrates the buccinator muscle. Posterior to the obstruction, the main ducts are dilated, but still retain a branching pattern. There is also a discontinuity of the medium (arrow) in the first inferior branch which may also be due to the presence of a small radiolucent stone. L

9.19 A parotid sialogram showing marked dilatation of the duct due to the presence at its ampulla of a rounded radiolucent stone, which has been outlined by a halo of contrast medium. The normal amount of contrast medium introduced into the duct system has been insufficient to fill its finer ramifications due to the gross dilatation. L

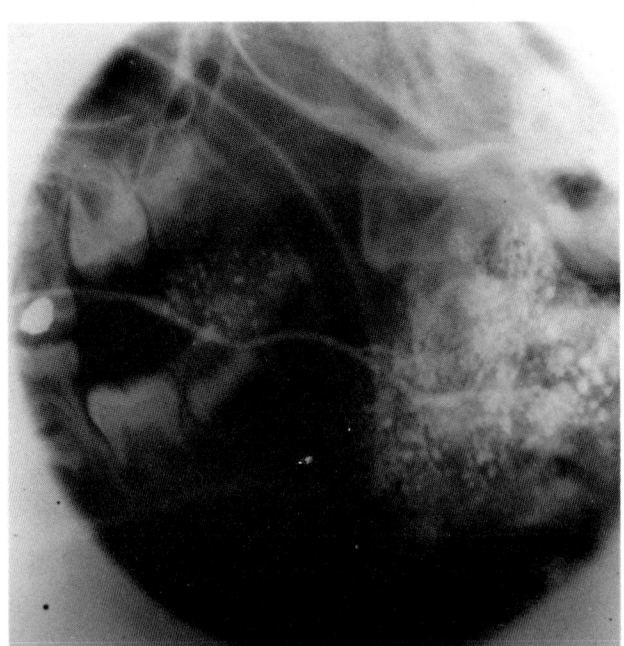

The Soft Tissues including the Salivary Glands 215

Recurrent parotitis

9.21 A parotid sialogram in a five-year-old with a history of recurrent swelling of the gland. The main duct is of normal outline and diameter, but the branches arising from it are poorly demonstrated and there are numerous globular foci of contrast medium (sialectasis) of variable size in a generally hazy background occupying the substance of the gland. A similar appearance is present in the accessory lobule of the gland which is unusually anteriorly placed. Note the outline of the endotracheal tube arching down between the two parts of the gland. OLM

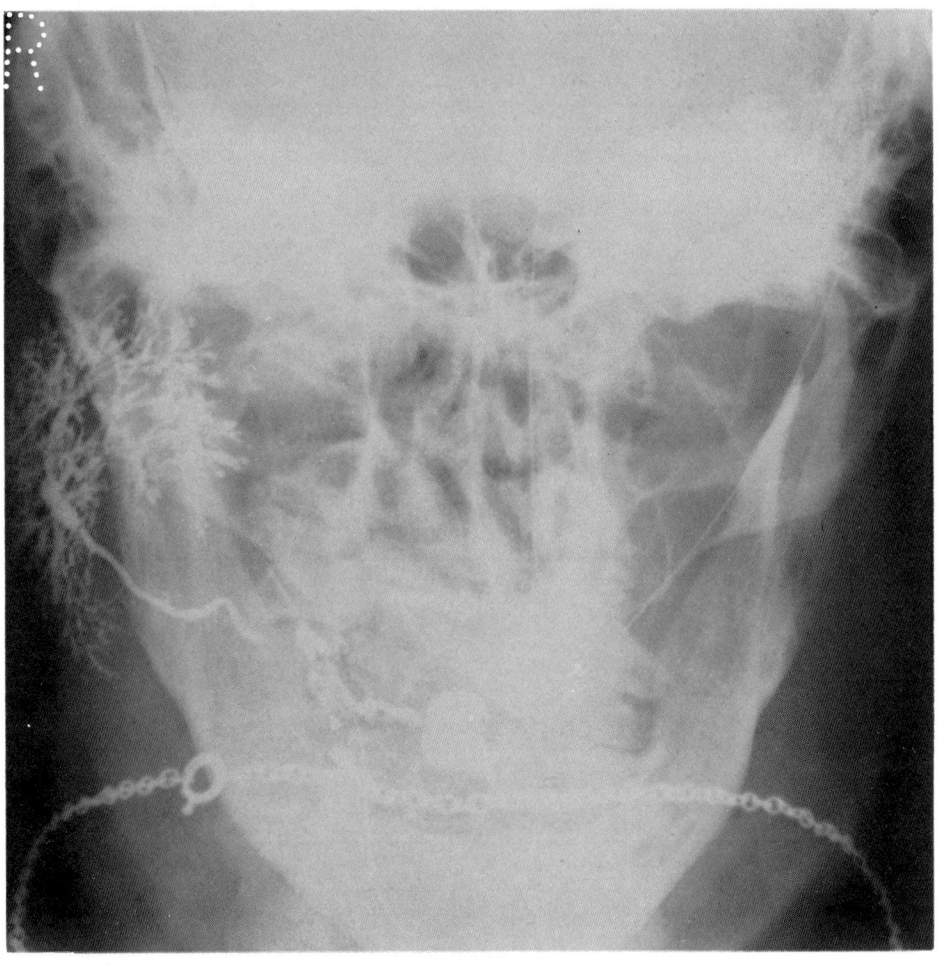

9.22 A parotid sialogram in a middle-aged adult exhibiting mild sialectasis. The proximal part of the main duct is dilated, suggesting that it is partially obstructed at the anterior border of the gland, as are some of the minor ducts, many of which exhibit terminal globular dilations characteristic of sialectasis. As a consequence, since there is no obvious reduction in the number of terminal ramifications, the overall opacity of the image of the duct system is greater than normal. Note the looped outline of the contrast medium within the cannula, which is superimposed upon the facial skeleton, and the exotic necklace! PA

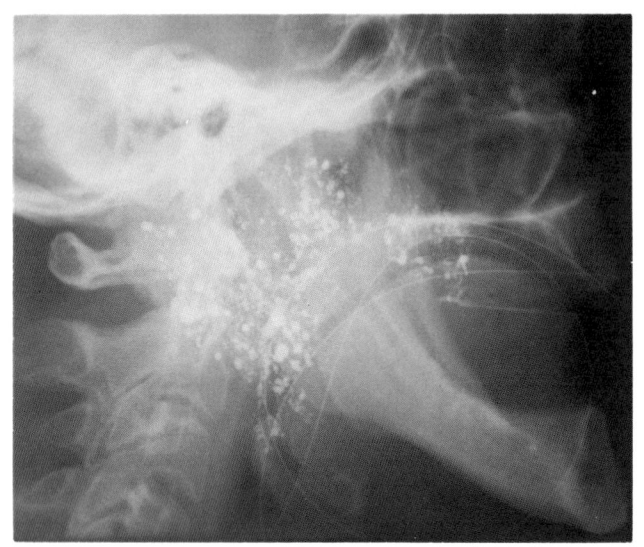

Sjogren's disease
9.23 In this auto-immune disease, which predominantly affects elderly females, there is swelling of the major salivary glands accompanied by progressive destruction of the normal glandular architecture, often with weakening of the walls of the finer ducts. In this parotid sialogram, the main ducts and many of the smaller ones are not well demonstrated. Where they are present, many of them end in fine globular dilatations. Elsewhere in the gland, there are larger, apparently discrete foci of contrast medium, probably a consequence of its extravasation into the glandular tissue through the weakened duct walls at the time of injection. The separate accessory lobule of the gland shows similar changes. When extravasation of contrast medium occurs, it may persist in the gland for some months. Note residual contrast medium in the looped cannula. L

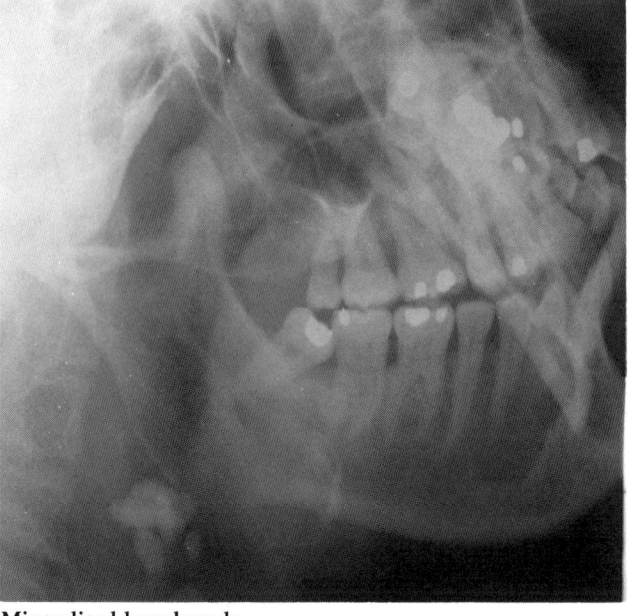

Mineralised lymph node
9.24 Such mineralisation occurs as a consequence of chronic inflammation of the nodes, most commonly in tuberculosis. In this example, several mineralised nodes are present in the upper part of the deep cervical chain of the right side of the neck. They are of uniform radiopacity, of variable size and shape with irregular outline, and lie just below the angle of the mandible. The relatively posterior position of the masses, their multiplicity, uneven surface, and lack of lamellations all contra-indicate a diagnosis of salivary calculus. OLM

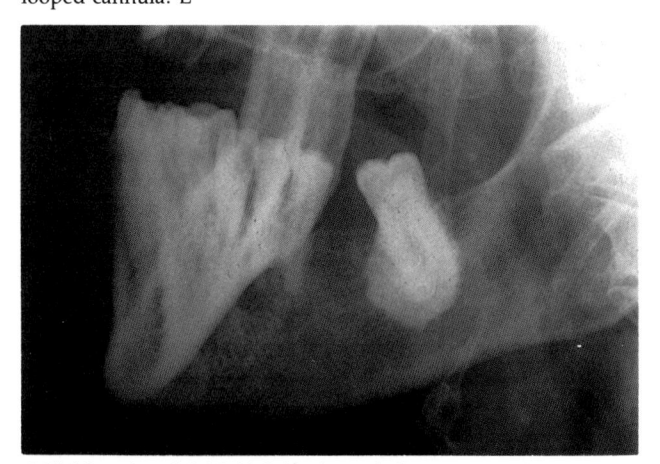

9.25 (above) and 9.26 (right) A single large, mineralised node in the upper end of the right, deep cervical chain. In this view (Fig. 9.25) of the left side of the mandible, the radiodense image of the mass has been projected upon the second molar. On first examination, this appearance may suggest osteosclerosis or cementoblastoma, but closer examination reveals an absence of radiolucent capsule and radiopaque lamina around its periphery, and that the mass is pear-shaped and continues up into the crown of the tooth. Its true position is confirmed by the lateral view (Fig. 9.26), which shows it to lie posterior to the angle of the mandible. The mass is uniformly radiopaque with an irregular outline. OLM & L

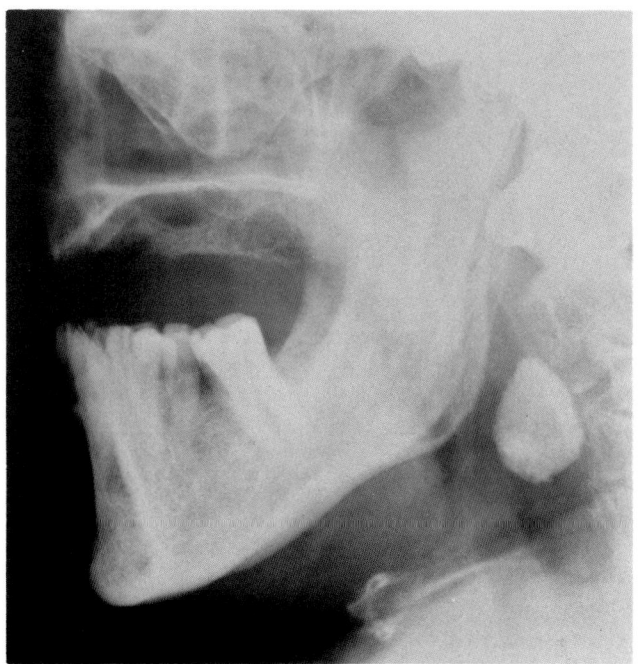

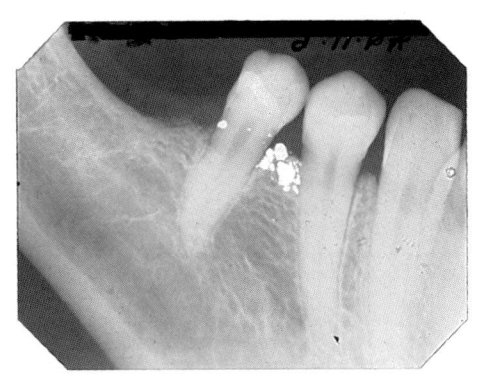

The Soft Tissues including the Salivary Glands 217

Foreign bodies
9.27 A wide range of foreign bodies may find their way into the soft tissues either iatrogenically or as a result of accidental trauma, in many instances being quite symptomless. In this way, particles of amalgam may cause discolouration of the mucosa, an amalgam tattoo. In this tattoo of the gingival mucosa, there are numerous, approximately circular, densely radiopaque granules superimposed predominantly over the interdental crest $\overline{54|}$, and partly over $\overline{5|}$ cervically. The dense radiopacity indicates the metallic nature of the material. P

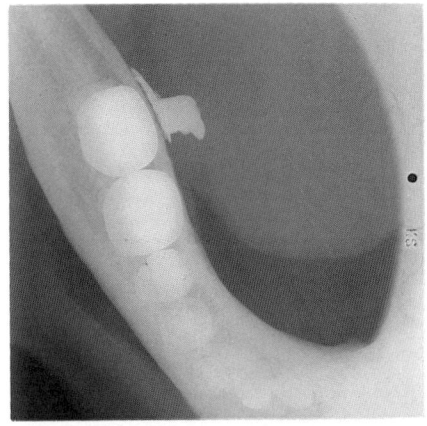

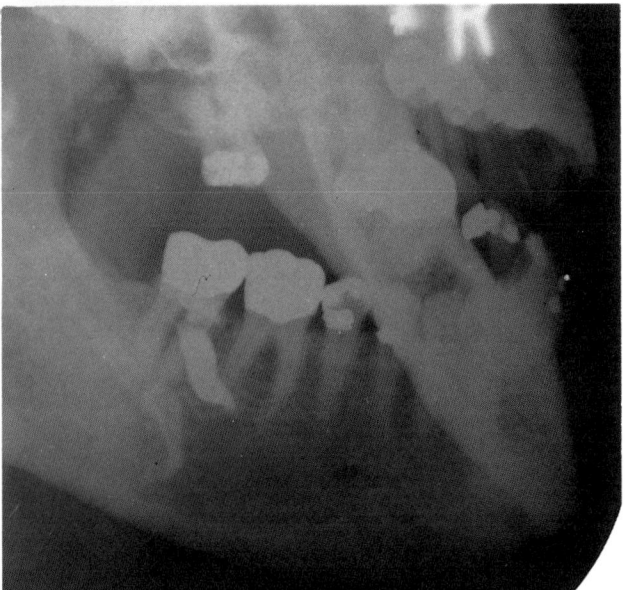

9.28 (top) and 9.29 (bottom) In this example, excess radiopaque rubber base impression material has been introduced into the lingual soft tissues following an impression of $\overline{7|}$ for a full veneer gold crown. The accident was unnoticed at the time, and when the patient subsequently returned in discomfort, the radiographs were taken. At least two views, approximately at right angles, have been taken to provide sufficient information concerning the size, shape and position of the foreign body. LTO & OLM

218 *A Radiological Atlas of Diseases of the Teeth and Jaws*

9.30 An air gun pellet lodged apparently over the right ramus of the mandible in the region of the sigmoid notch. The dense radiopacity and distinct outline of the foreign body indicate its metallic nature, and its shape is characteristic of an air gun pellet. A PA radiograph confirmed its position just medial to the ramus. Note the presence of taurodontism $\overline{7|}$ which forms the distal abutment to a fixed gold bridge. Note also the cantilever bridge replacing $\underline{|2}$ and the many root filled teeth. PR

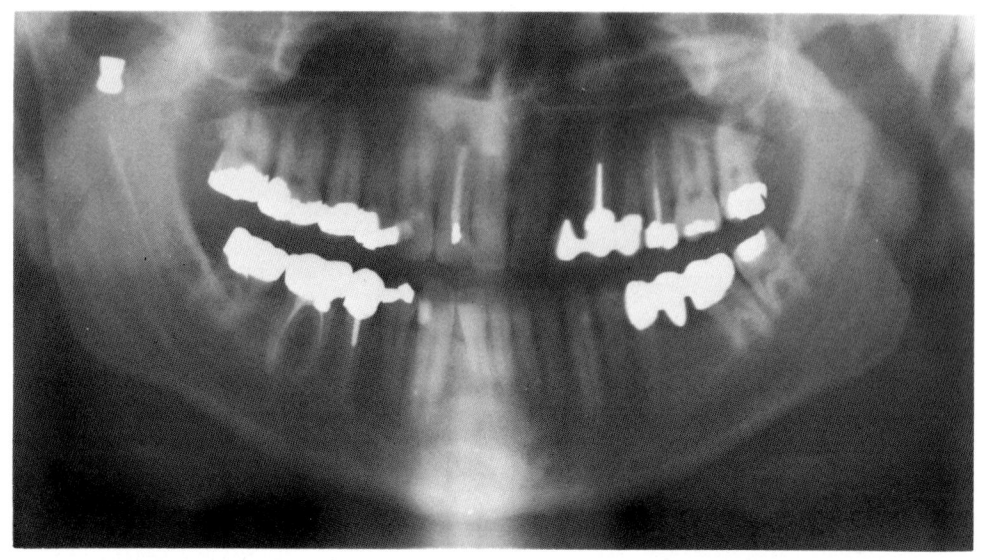

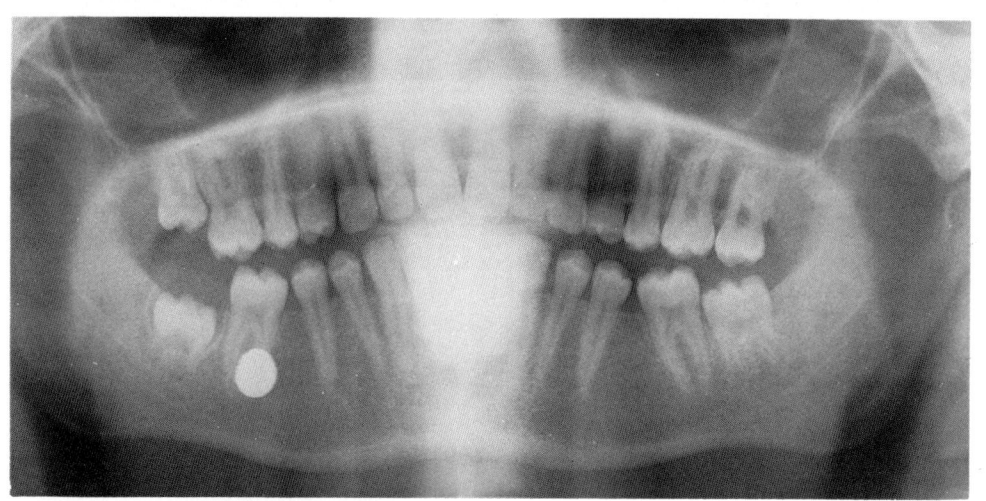

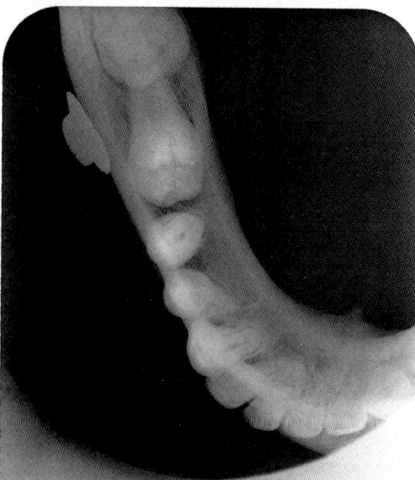

9.31 (above) and 9.32 (left) An air gun pellet which has flattened against the lateral surface of the body of the mandible in the $\overline{6|}$ region. The radiopaque foreign body is ovoid in shape and fuzzy in outline as a consequence of its distortion on impact with the bone. Its position lateral to the mandible and its gross distortion is confirmed on the occlusal film (Fig. 9.32). PR & LTO

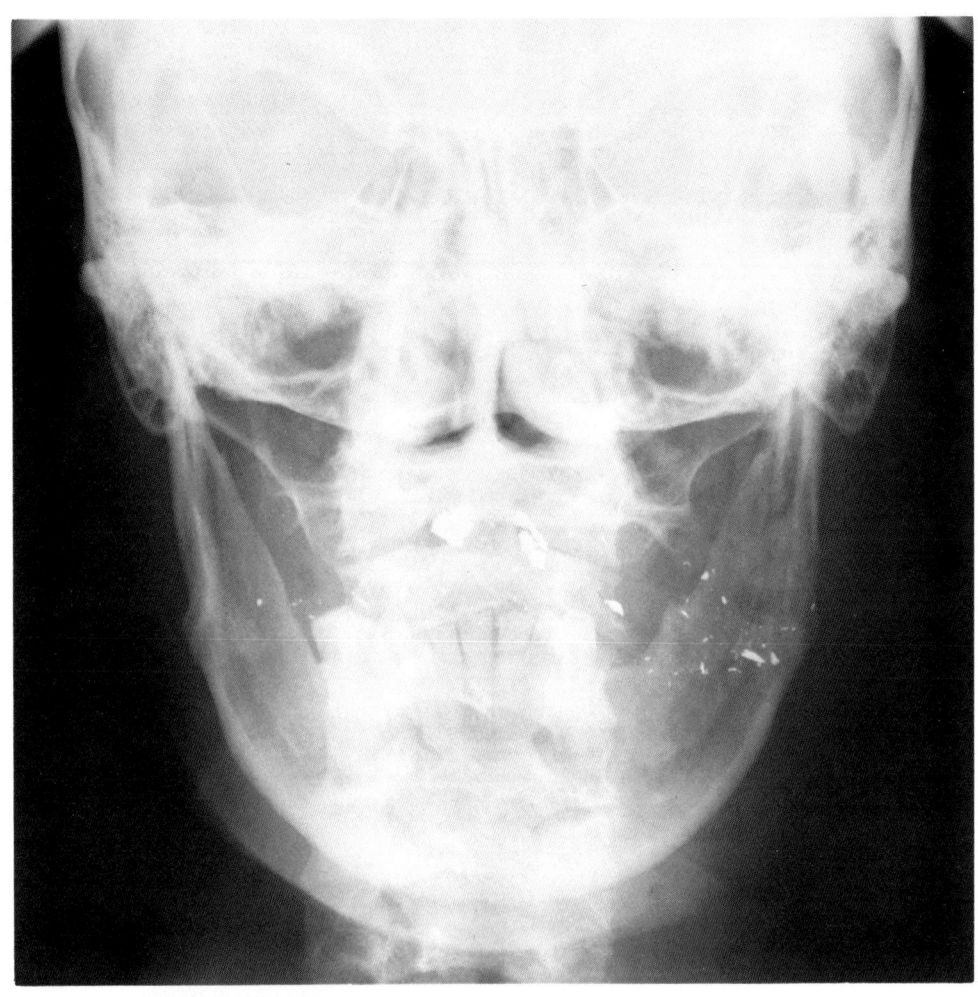

9.33 In this patient who was shot with a handgun, the low velocity bullet entered the right cheek, and after fracturing the edentulous maxillary anterior alveolar ridge, shattered in the tongue where the major fragments can be seen. Thereafter, it left through the left side of the neck, the pathway of the exit track being demonstrated by a number of small, radiopaque fragments which are superimposed over the mandible, which was not involved. PA

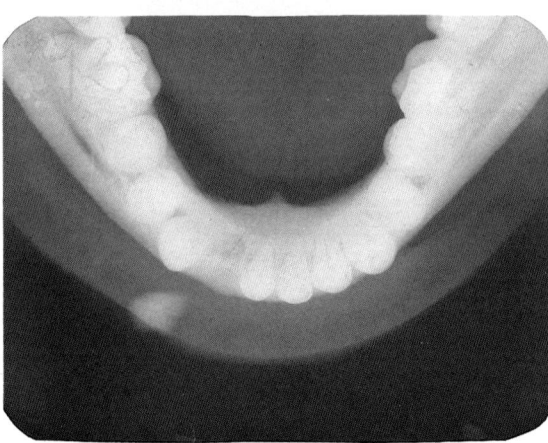

9.34 Fragments of glass embedded within the lower lip following a road traffic accident. They are only slightly radiopaque, the largest having an irregular, angular outline. The smaller fragments lie postero-laterally. LTO

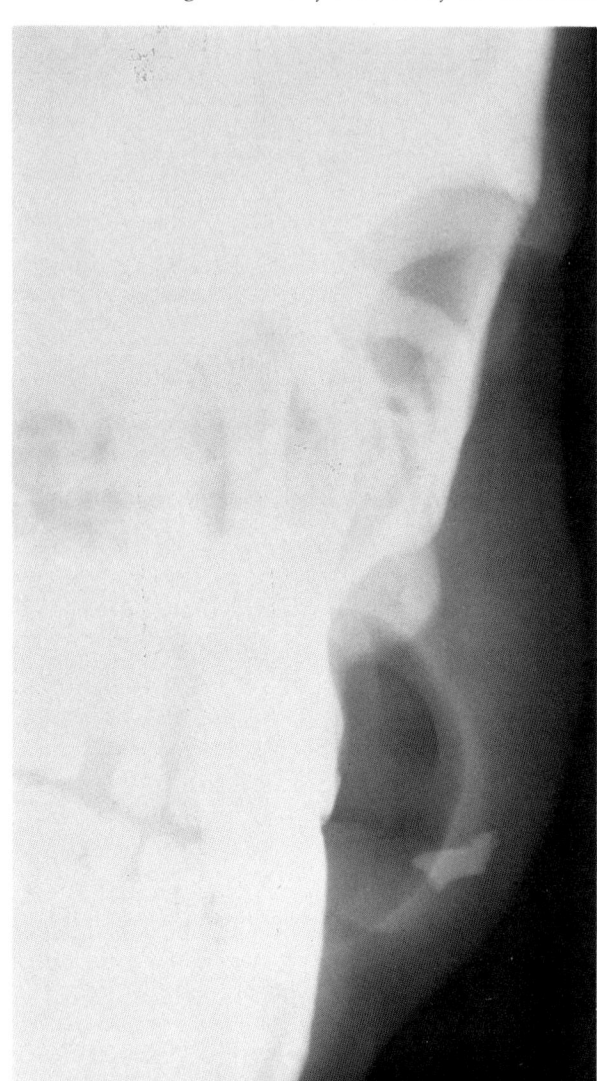

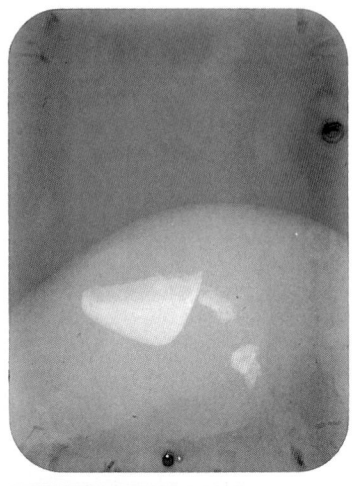

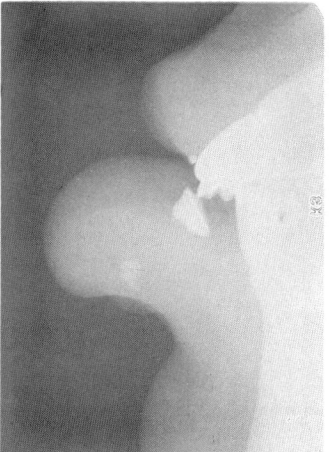

9.36 (left) and 9.37 (below left) Fragments from the crowns of fractured maxillary incisors embedded within the lower lip. At least three fragments are present, one of which is derived from an oblique fracture through the crown of a central incisor. The second film (Fig. 9.37) again emphasises the importance of taking more than one view, and demonstrates a significant difference in the antero-posterior position of the fragments, not apparent in the first film. It also demonstrates the swelling of the lower lip. S

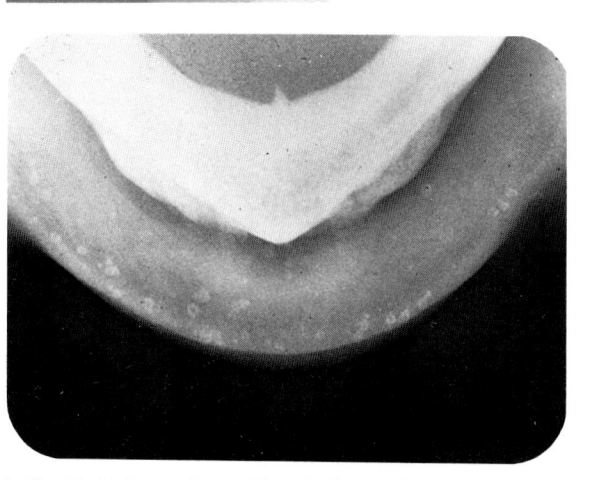

9.35 A fragment of windscreen glass embedded within the soft tissues of the cheek following a road traffic accident. Its features are similar to those exhibited in Fig. 9.34. The foreign body has been displayed more clearly by underexposing the film and by the slight rotation of the head and blowing out of the cheek. RPA

9.38 Multiple small particles of silica within the skin of the lower lip and chin of a machine polisher. The particles are faintly radiopaque, variable in size, and of approximately circular outline, some of them having radiolucent centres. The outline of the everted vermilion part of the lip is projected beyond the main soft tissue contour. Note the crestal part of the edentulous incisal ridge projected anteriorly to the inferior border of the mandible which has a more dense cortical outline. LTO

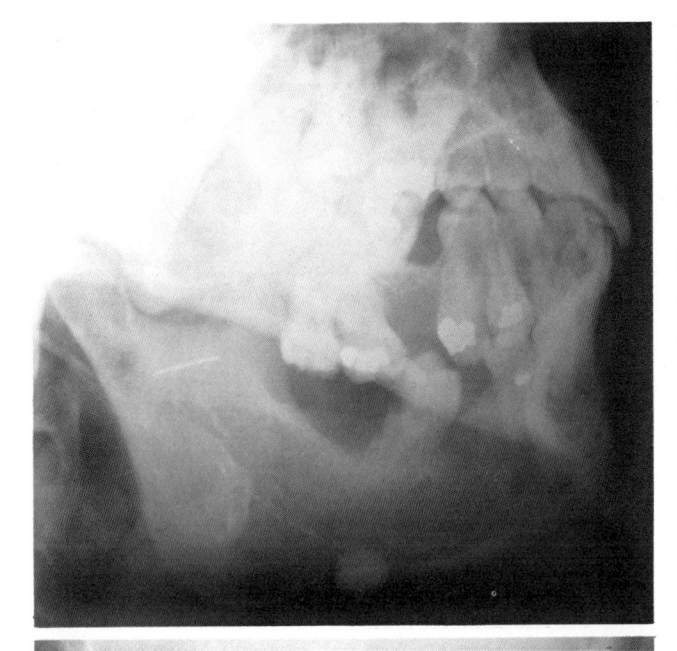

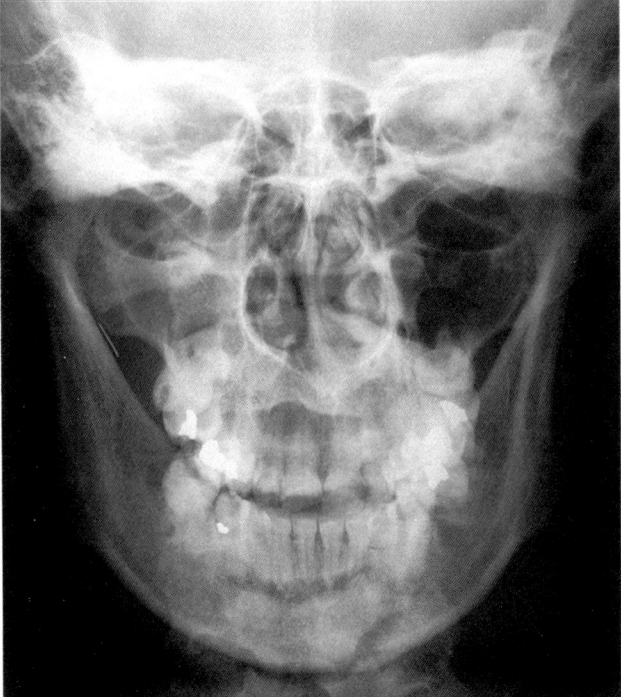

The Soft Tissues including the Salivary Glands 221

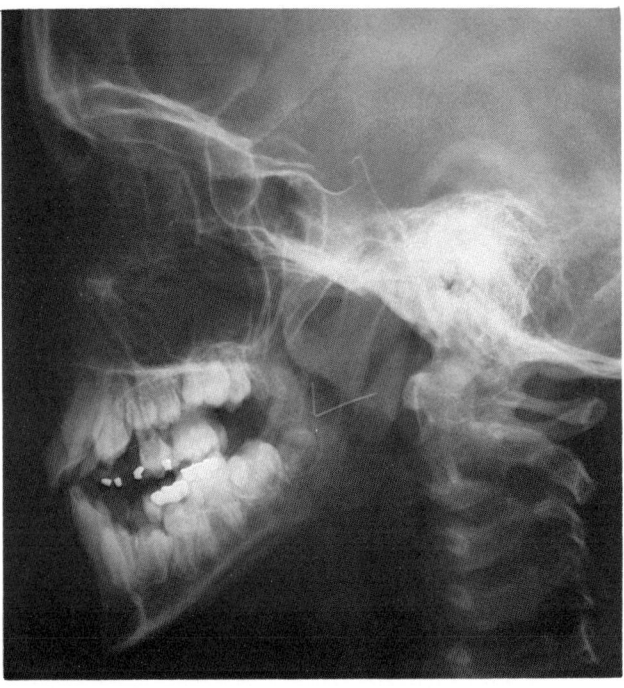

9.41 A needle fractured during the administration of an inferior alveolar nerve block and retained in the tissues in a ten-year-old. The needle has broken at the hub and is bent upwards approximately a third of the way along its length. It is shown superimposed upon the ramus of the mandible. L

Fractured needle
9.39 (top) and 9.40 (bottom) Part of a local anaesthetic needle fractured during administration of a right inferior alveolar nerve block and retained in the pterygo-mandibular space. Its position medial to the ramus of the mandible is clearly demonstrated (Fig. 9.40). OLM & PA

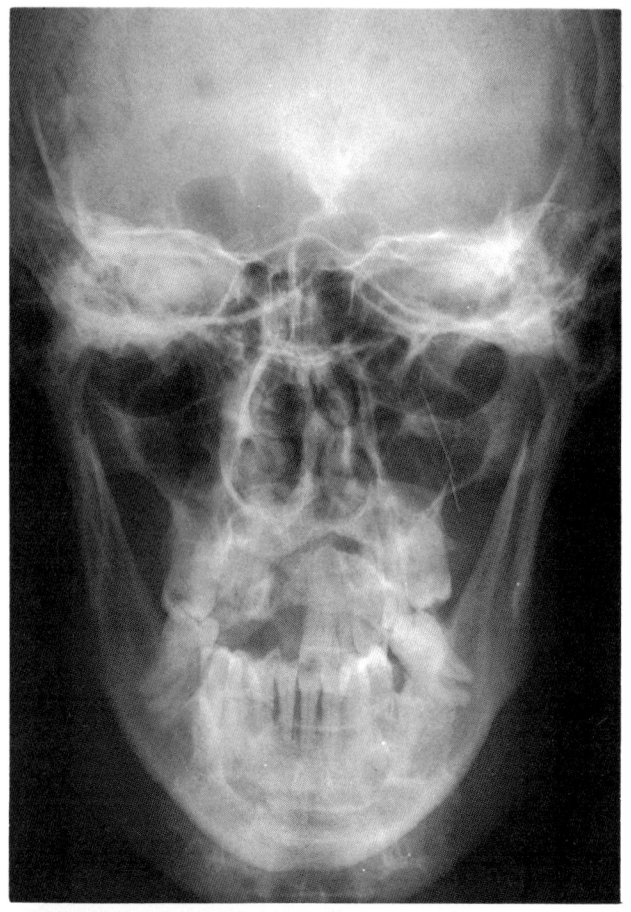

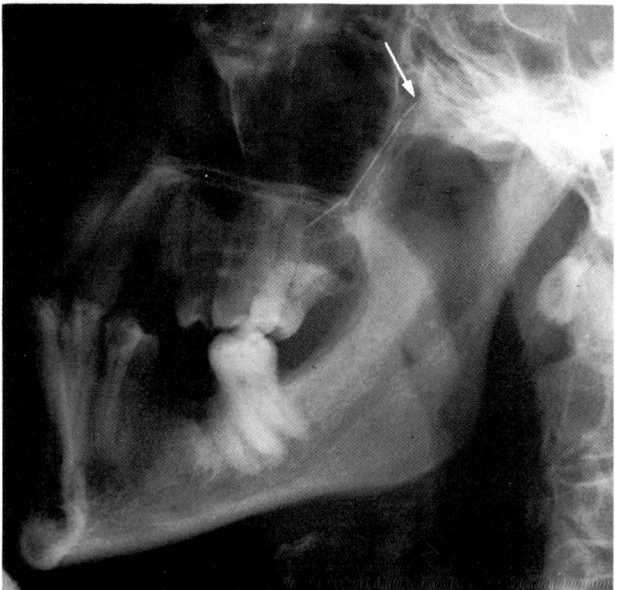

222 *A Radiological Atlas of Diseases of the Teeth and Jaws*

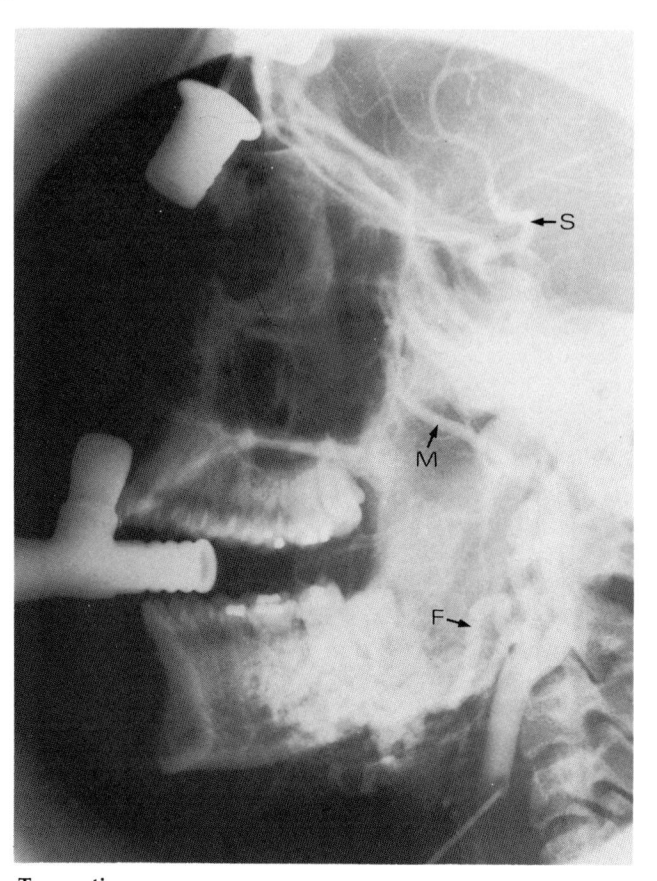

Traumatic aneurysm
9.44 A carotid angiogram of a lesion of the left cheek into which radiopaque medium has been injected through the external carotid artery. The facial artery (F) loops downwards over the posterior part of the ramus of the mandible to its lower border, from which point a complex mass of tortuous vessels is displayed overlying the body of the mandible. The maxillary artery (M), running obliquely upwards and forwards to the posterior boundary of the maxilla from the region of the neck of the condyle, and the superficial temporal artery (S) and its ramifications spreading over the temporal region are also clearly displayed. Note the connectors for the airway for the general anaesthetic. L

9.42 (top) and 9.43 (bottom) A needle broken into three separate pieces during the administration of a left posterior superior alveolar nerve block. The three fragments are displaced slightly, the smallest one at the distal end of the needle (arrow). PA & L

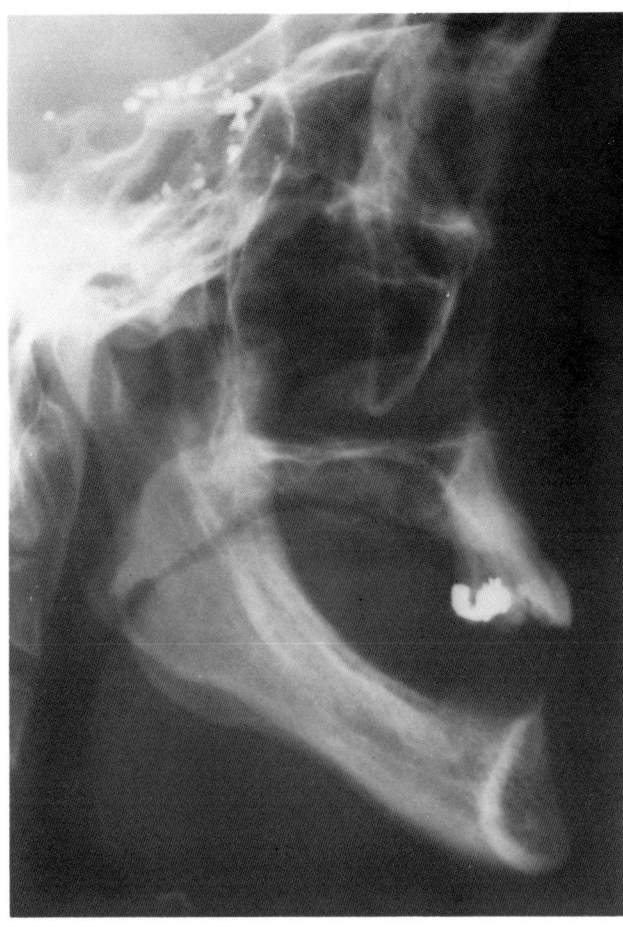

The Soft Tissues including the Salivary Glands   223

Retained contrast medium
9.45   Globules of radiopaque dye (Myelodil) persisting in the basilar system in the region of the middle cranial fossa, several years after a myelogram. The radiopaque globules are of varying shape and size, and might arise as an incidental finding in radiographs taken for dental purposes, as in this example. L

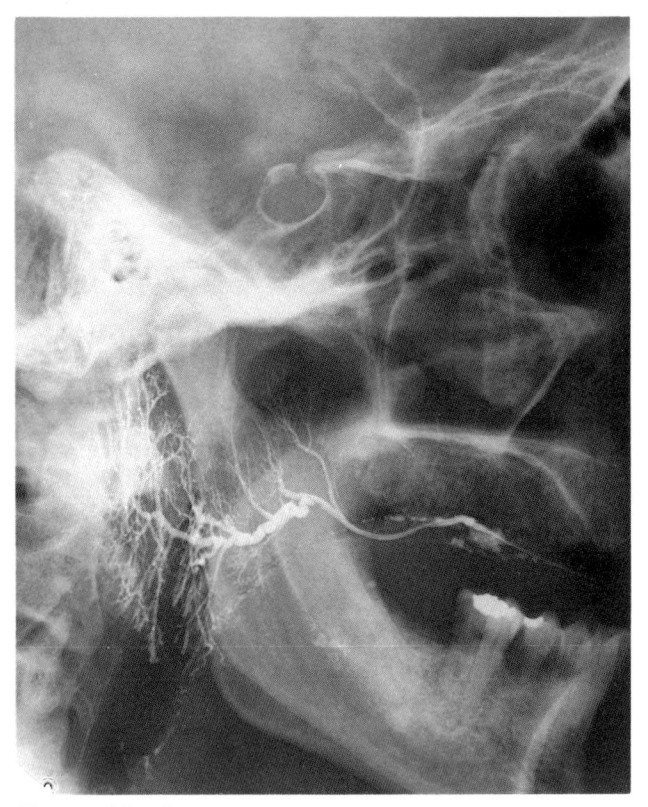

Pleomorphic adenoma
9.46   A sialogram of a parotid gland with a neoplasm in the accessory lobe. This expansile, benign tumour has displaced the main duct inferiorly, which describes a gentle downward curvature in its anterior part. Proximal to the mass, the main duct is dilated due to its partial obstruction by the tumour, although there is no obvious abnormality of the finer ramifications of the duct system. The posterior and inferior margins of the tumour are outlined by a thin, radiopaque line, probably as a consequence of the extravasation of contrast medium from the distorted acini at the periphery of the mass. Note the image of the surface of the dorsum of the tongue outlined by granular residues of the contrast medium which have escaped into the mouth. L

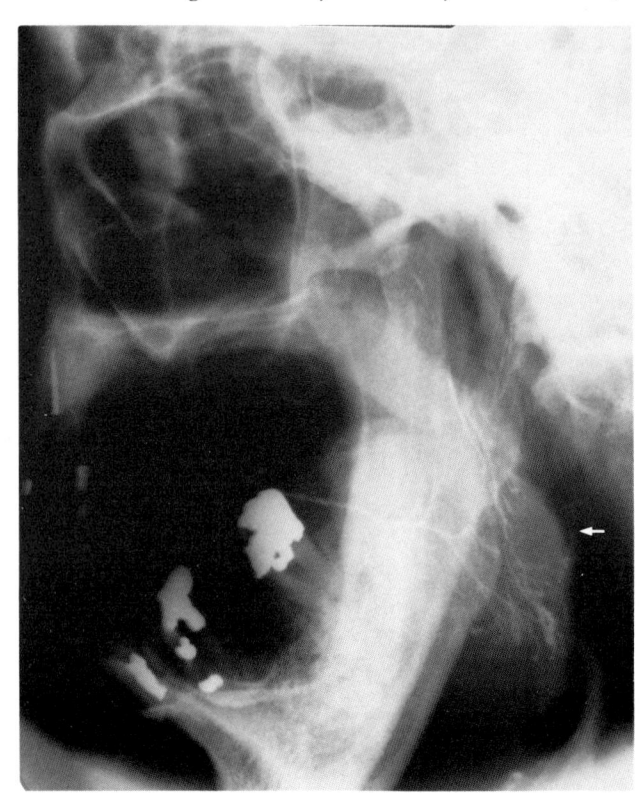

9.47 A tumour within the lower half of the main part of the parotid gland, close to its posterior margin. The sialogram reveals that the outline of the main duct is normal and that the branching architecture inferiorly and superiorly is present, although there is some evidence of sialectasis inferiorly. However, the tumour has caused marked filling defects of many of the ducts in the central part of the gland with displacement of others, although some finer ducts (arrow) are filled even over the posterior aspect of the mass. Note the shadow of the epiglottis clearly displayed postero-inferiorly to the gland, and the root filling in a maxillary incisor. L

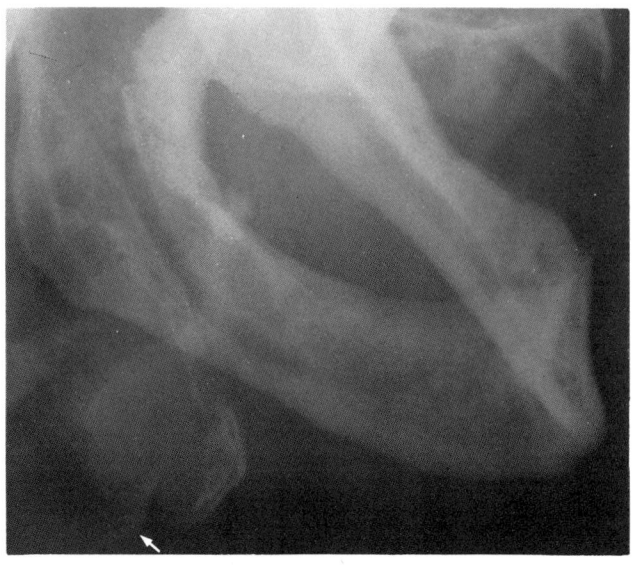

Dystrophic mineralisation
9.48 Mineralisation of the thyroid cartilage of the larynx in an elderly, edentulous patient. A large part of the outline of the cartilage can be determined, although it is more obvious posteriorly and anteriorly. Posteriorly, there are irregular, patchy radiopacities projected beneath the angle of the mandible, running obliquely postero-inferiorly across the radiolucent shadow of the laryngeal air inlet. Anteriorly, the prominence (arrow) of the thyroid cartilage, which lies just posterior to the body of the hyoid bone, is clearly displayed. Note the root fragment in the right mandibular molar region. OLM

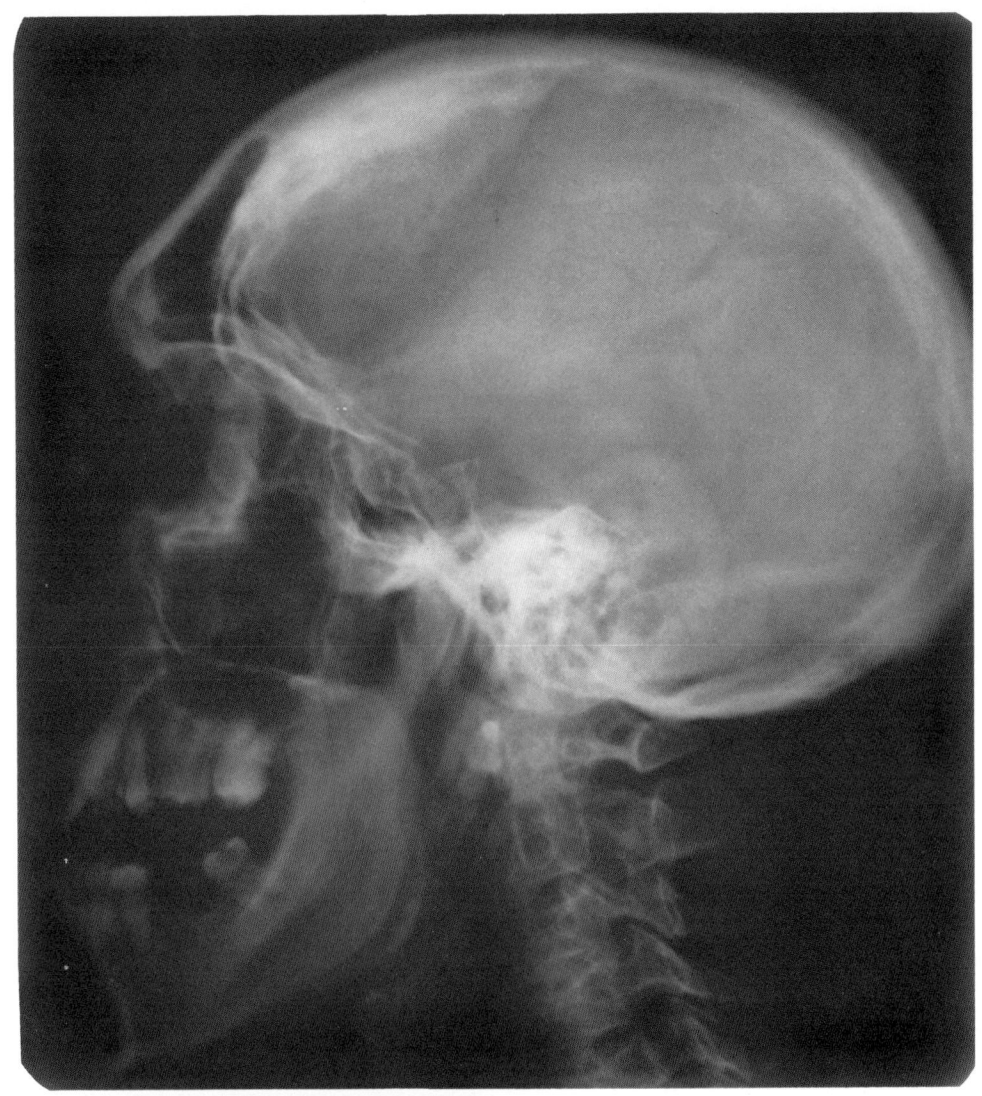

The Soft Tissues including the Salivary Glands 225

9.49 Mineralisation may also occur in the stylohyoid ligaments, becoming increasingly common with age. In this patient, there is bilateral involvement, the radiopaque segmentally mineralised ligaments running obliquely downwards just posterior to the rami of the mandible, from the base of the skull to the greater cornu of the hyoid bone. Note the shadow of the pinna of the ear and the occlusal cavity in the mandibular molar. L

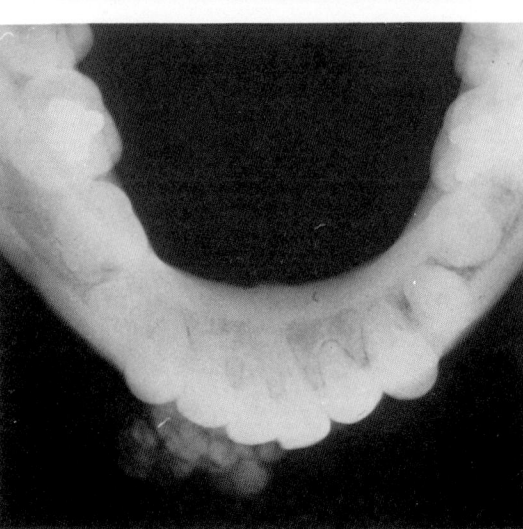

Calcinosis
9.50 In this condition, deposition of areas of dystrophic mineralisation commonly occurs within the dermis and occasionally also within the oral submucosa. In this example, numerous rounded radiopaque deposits are present within the soft tissues of the chin. LTO

Chapter 10

The Maxillary Antrum

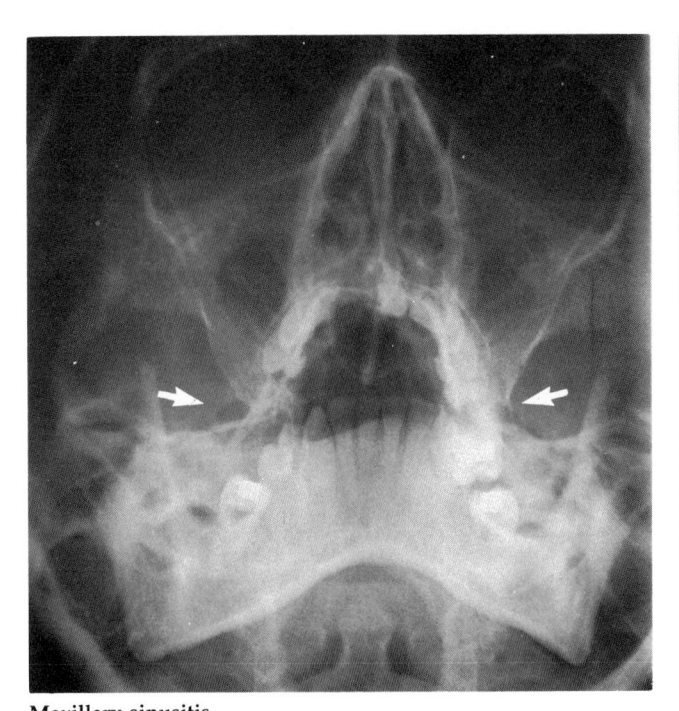

Maxillary sinusitis

10.1 Bilateral sinusitis is often a complication of inflammation of the upper respiratory tract and may be infective or allergic in origin. In this example, the soft tissue lining of both antra is markedly thickened forming a radiopaque contour which follows their bony outline. As a consequence, the radiolucent air shadows within them are greatly reduced in size. No fluid levels are present. Note that the foramen ovale is clearly displayed on both sides (arrows). OM

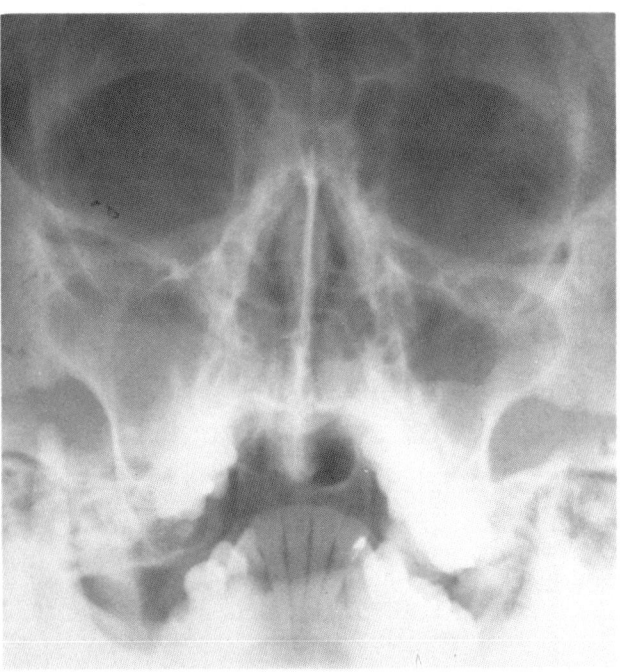

10.2 Bilateral sinusitis with an empyema of the right side, where a distinct, horizontal fluid level is present. The radiopaque fluid occupies most of the antral cavity and only a small air space remains superiorly. In the left antrum, there is gross thickening of the soft tissue which forms a thickened, radiopaque contour to the cavity and is dome-shaped inferiorly, suggesting the presence of a polyp. OM

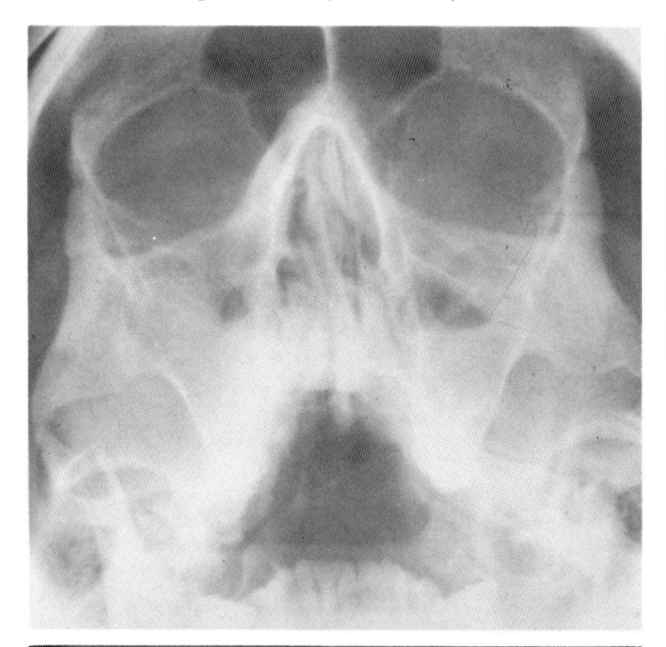

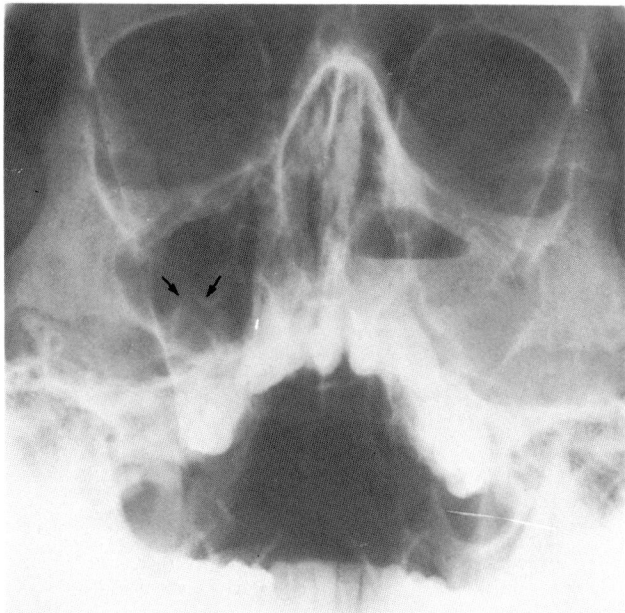

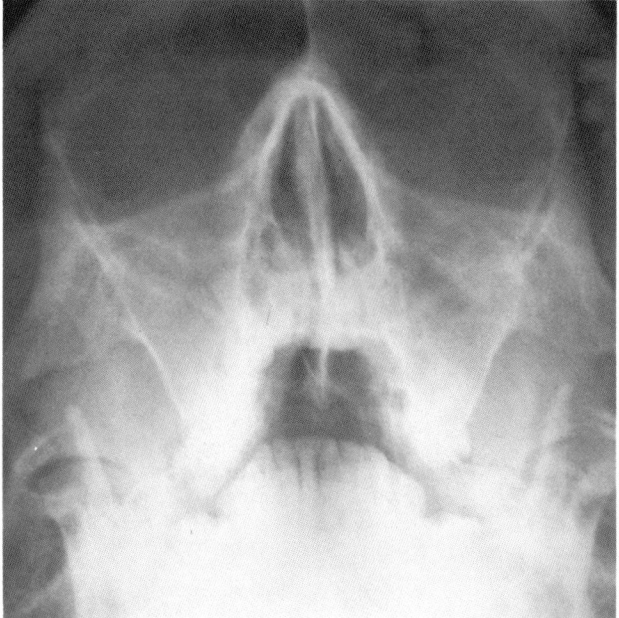

10.5 Unilateral sinusitis is often due to dental causes, as in this patient who had a non-draining oro-antral fistula. The left antrum is radiopaque in all but its superior portion, where it is bounded by a clearly defined, horizontal fluid level which is menisciform at its margins. All the other sinuses are normal, apart from a dome-shaped radiopaque mass (arrows) on the floor of the right antrum, suggesting the presence of a mucous cyst or polyp. OM

10.3 (top) and 10.4 (bottom) The fluid nature of maxillary empyema can be confirmed by examining the patient once in the erect position and then again either in the prone position or with the head tilted laterally, so inducing a change in the fluid level. These two films of the same patient with bilateral sinusitis were taken in the erect (Fig. 10.3) and prone (Fig. 10.4) positions. Whereas in the former, mucosal thickening and a fluid level is present in both antra with only a small radiolucent air space persisting, the change in the position of the patient through ninety degrees has resulted in complete radiopacity of both sides and loss of any fluid level, which would now be in the same plane as the film. Note that the nasal mucosa also appears thickened, with opacity of the nasal cavity, particularly on the erect film, although the frontal sinuses are clear. OM

The Maxillary Antrum 231

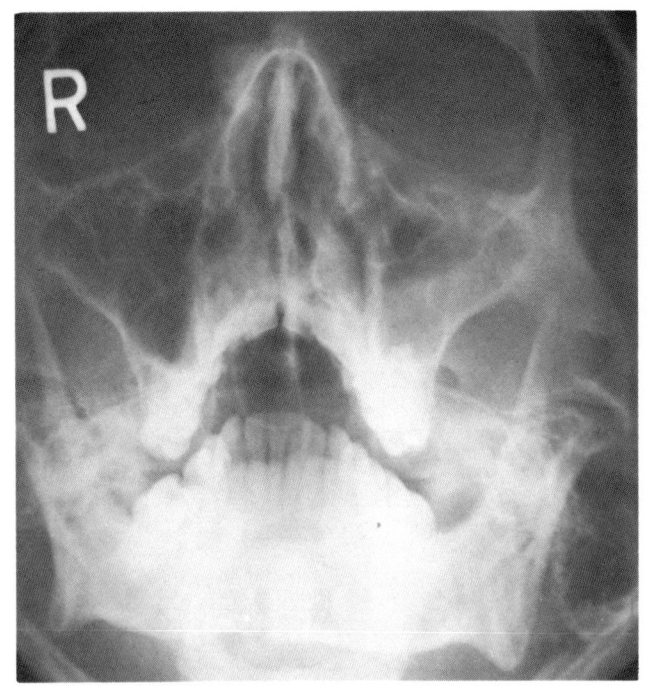

10.6 (above) and 10.7 (right) Unilateral sinusitis with radiopacity of the entire cavity of the left antrum and no obvious fluid level. Such an appearance is due either to gross thickening of the lining or to empyema with blockage of the ostium, so that the cavity has become fully occluded with pus and any residual air displaced. Note as an incidental finding the presence of a clearly defined, radiopaque mass with smooth outline in the region of the floor of the right frontal sinus. The lateral view (Fig. 10.7) suggests the mass, which is an osteoma, is present in the anterior ethmoid air sinuses. OM & L

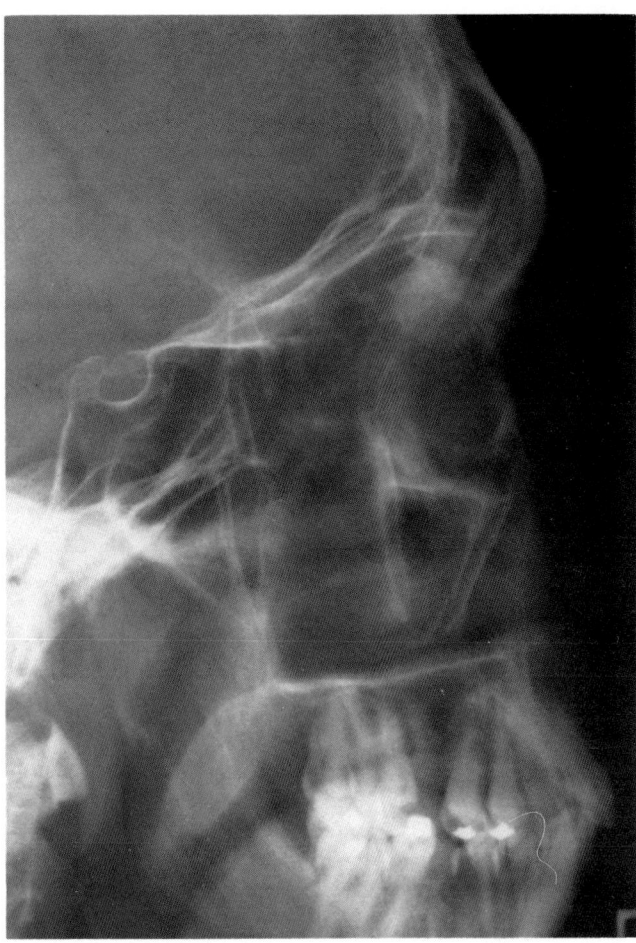

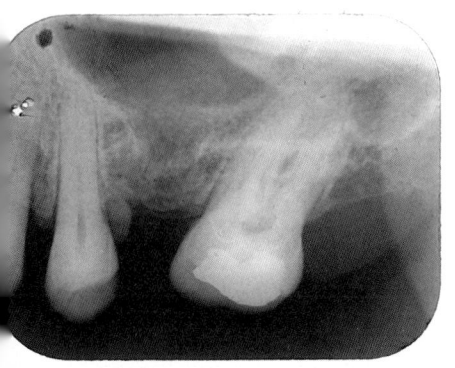

Antral polyp
10.8 This film, which was taken to confirm the presence of a small root fragment distal |5, also revealed a lesion in the floor of the antrum. The radiopaque lamina outlining the antral floor dips inferiorly between |5 7 above which there is a smooth, dome-shaped, radiopaque swelling projecting into the antral cavity and not separated from it by a bony margin, typical of an antral polyp. Note the coronoid process distally |7. P

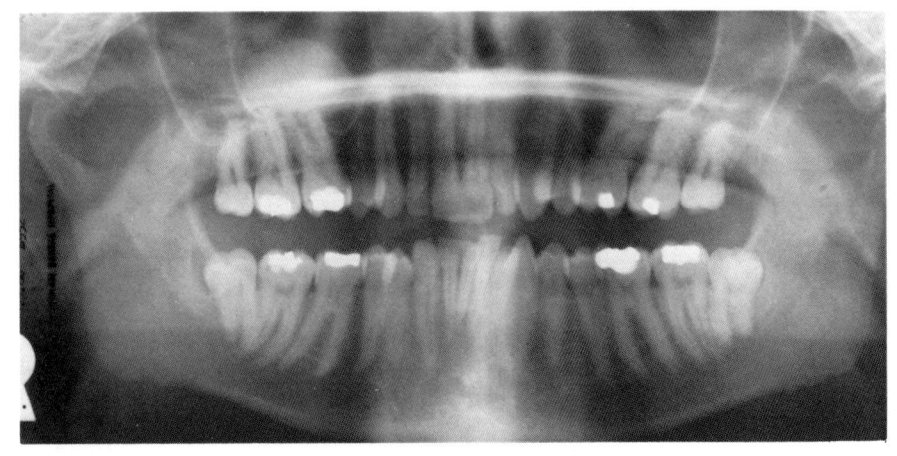

Mucous cyst
10.9 A large dome-shaped radiopaque lesion occupying the lower part of the right antrum. It has a smooth surface and is not separated from the antral cavity by a bony margin. The rest of the antrum appears normal. Note the abnormally shaped, hypoplastic right mandibular condyle which had not given rise to any asymmetry and was discovered as an incidental finding. Note also the bilateral, disto-angularly impacted mandibular third molars. PR

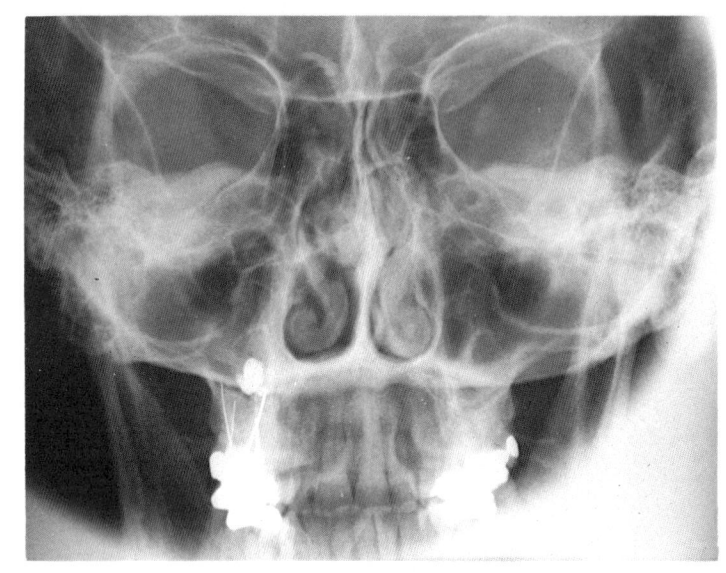

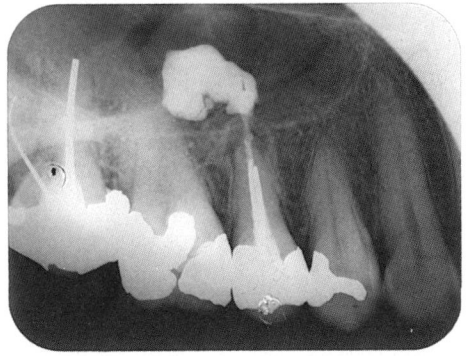

Foreign body

10.10 (above) and 10.11 (left) A mass of radiopaque root filling cement accidentally introduced into the antral cavity during endodontic treatment 5⌋ one week previously. 5⌋ is root filled and has a radiolucent periapical lesion, probably a granuloma, through which a tail of material passes from the tooth apex to the antral mass. The lamina dura is absent periapically, but a thin cortical lamina surrounds the periapical lesion and blends with that outlining the floor of the antral cavity. The position of the material within the antrum is confirmed in the extra-oral film (Fig. 10.11) which also shows no evidence of antral infection. Note the prominent inferior nasal conchae bilaterally. P & PA

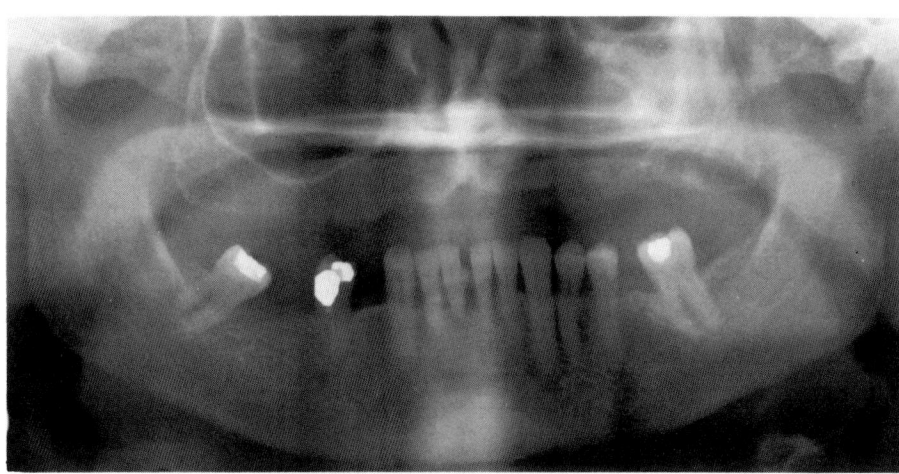

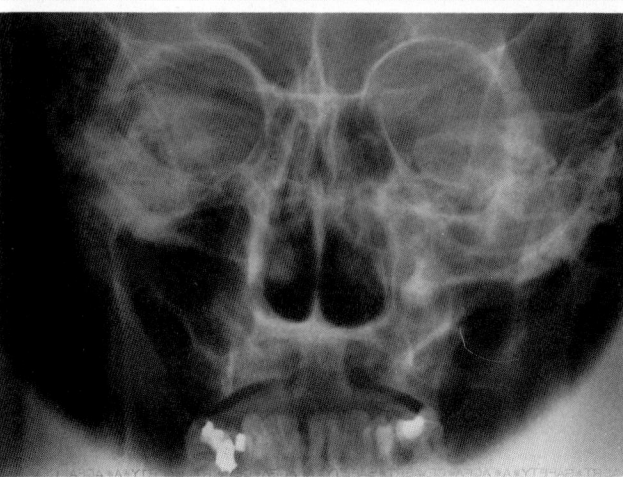

Antrolith

10.12 (left) and 10.13 (bottom left) Antroliths form by the deposition of mineral upon the surface of a suitable nidus, which may be degenerate tissue or a foreign body. In this example, a radiopaque antrolith of irregular outline is present in the left maxillary antrum. The antral cavity is also radiopaque and its bony outline is indistinct, particularly on its lateral aspect. The antrolith is in close relationship to the medial wall of the antrum. There is a root fragment in the ⌊7 region. Note the fractured spiral rotary paste filler in the root canal 5⌋ and the calculus deposits on the mandibular incisors. The foreshortened appearance of the roots of the latter is an artefact due to their apical parts being outside the focal plane of the film (Fig. 10.12). PR & PA

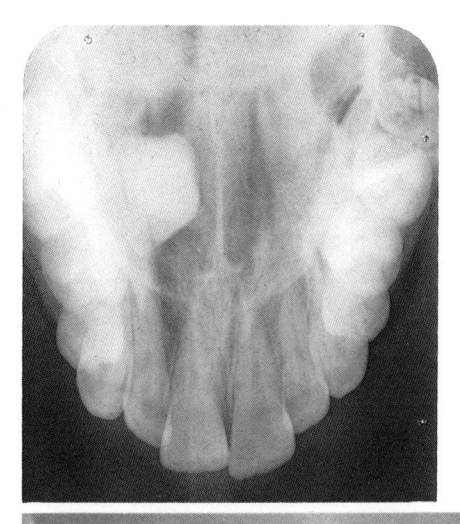

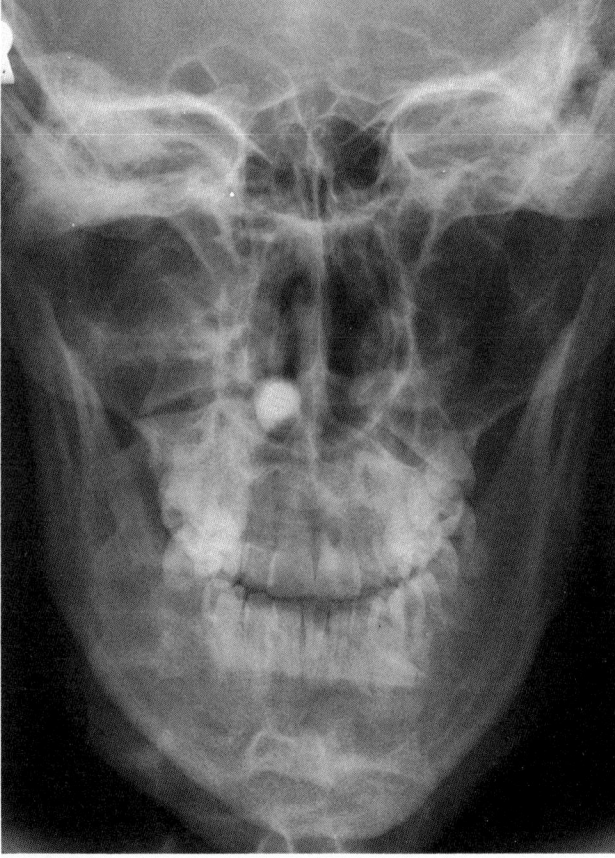

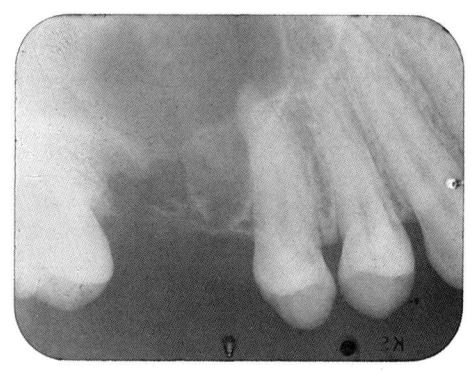

Oro-antral fistula

10.16 Oro-antral fistula is not an uncommon complication of molar extractions in the maxilla where the antral floor dips down around their roots and the resulting communication between the oral and antral cavities fails to heal. In this example, the fistula developed following extraction of 7⌋ some two weeks previously. The radiopaque lamina outlining the antral floor runs postero-inferiorly over the apical parts of the roots 54⌋ almost to the crest of the edentulous ridge, and is absent overlying the radiolucent tooth socket 7⌋, which is the site of the fistula, before continuing posteriorly over the root 8⌋. Note the absence of 6⌋, which may account for the low position of the antral floor. P

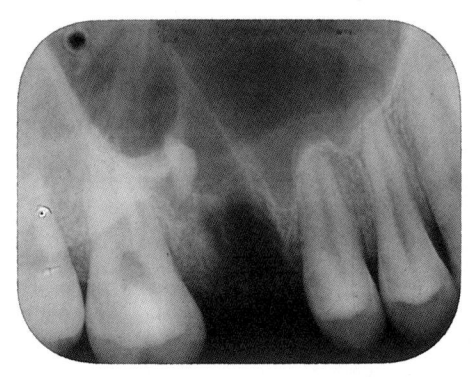

Displaced roots

10.17 Root fragments, most commonly the palatal roots of maxillary molars, may also be displaced into the antral cavity for the same reasons that lead to the formation of an oro-antral fistula. Following attempted extraction of 6⌋, a root fragment has been displaced into the antral cavity. It is inverted, its fractured surface facing superiorly, and has a distinct root canal, but it is not surrounded by a lamina dura or periodontal ligament space. In addition, a much smaller fragment persists in the distal part of the socket, in the apical parts of which the cortical lamina of the antral floor is breached. Note how the antral floor also dips around the apical parts of the roots 54⌋. P

Rhinolith

10.14 (top) and 10.15 (bottom) Rhinoliths arise in a similar manner to antroliths, except that they form in the nasal rather than the antral cavity. In this patient, there is an irregularly shaped, radiopaque mass in the floor of the right nasal cavity, the centre of which is more dense than its periphery. The pattern, together with the absence of a circumferencial cortical lamina and follicular space, excludes the possibility of its being an unerupted tooth, odontome or osteoma, and its position in the nasal cavity is confirmed on the postero-anterior film. USO & PA

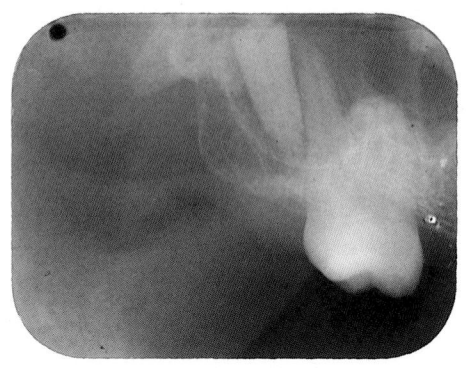

234 *A Radiological Atlas of Diseases of the Teeth and Jaws*

10.18 In this example following extraction of 6⏐, the palatal root has been displaced into the antrum and lies on its floor posterior to 7⏐. Again it is inverted, has an obvious root canal and there is no surrounding lamina dura. This film has been taken from a more posterior position than usual, with the X-ray tube angled anteriorly so that the palatal root 7⏐ is projected away from the buccal roots, which are foreshortened. Images of the zygomatic arch, pterygoid plate, pterygoid hamulus and coronoid process of the mandible are also present. P

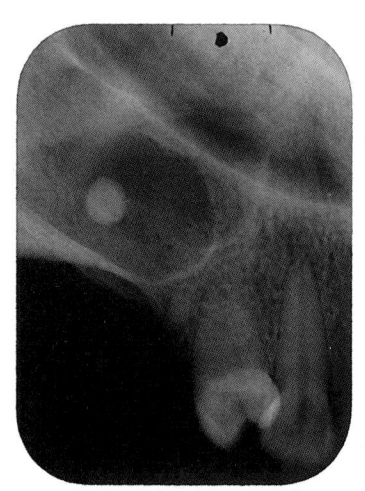

10.19 (left) The root fragment has been in the antral cavity for some time and is viewed 'end on'. A central root canal can just be determined and there is no surrounding lamina dura. A second smaller fragment is present in the alveolus distal to 4⏐. Note the thin, radiopaque lamina of the lateral part of the floor of the nose running obliquely across the upper part of the film. P

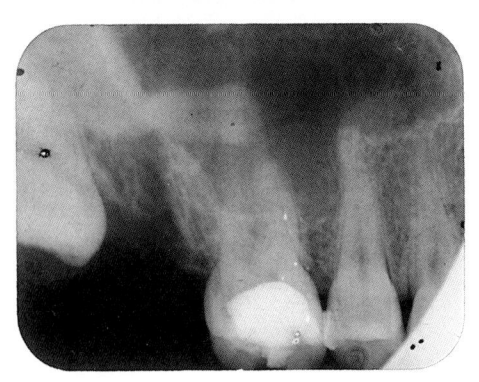

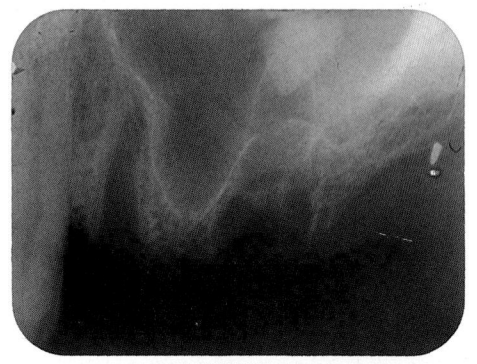

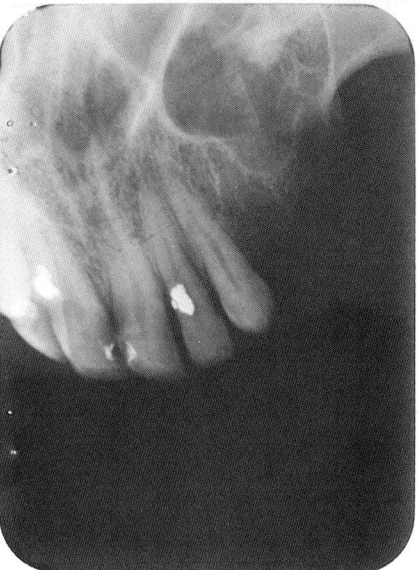

10.21 (top) and 10.22 (bottom) The palatal root ⏐6 displaced into the antrum, is tilted distally at 45° close to the apex of its socket. The lamina dura outlining the socket is partly superimposed upon the root and is closely related to the antrum, which dips down almost to the crest of the edentulous ridge mesial to it. The lateral limit of the antral floor in relation to the socket is displayed by the thin lamina running across the middle part of it. The socket of the recently extracted ⏐4 is also present. The occlusal film (Fig. 10.22) reveals a greater part of the antrum and may be particularly valuable in demonstrating the root fragment if it has been displaced away from the tooth socket. P & UOO

10.20 The palatal root 7⏐ has been displaced into the antral cavity and lies horizontally above the roots 6⏐. Again, the central root canal and absence of lamina dura are clearly displayed, and the cortical lamina outlining the floor of the antrum dips far down around the roots 65⏐. The outline of 7⏐ socket is indistinct and is partly obscured by superimposition of the root of the zygomatic arch. P

The Maxillary Antrum 235

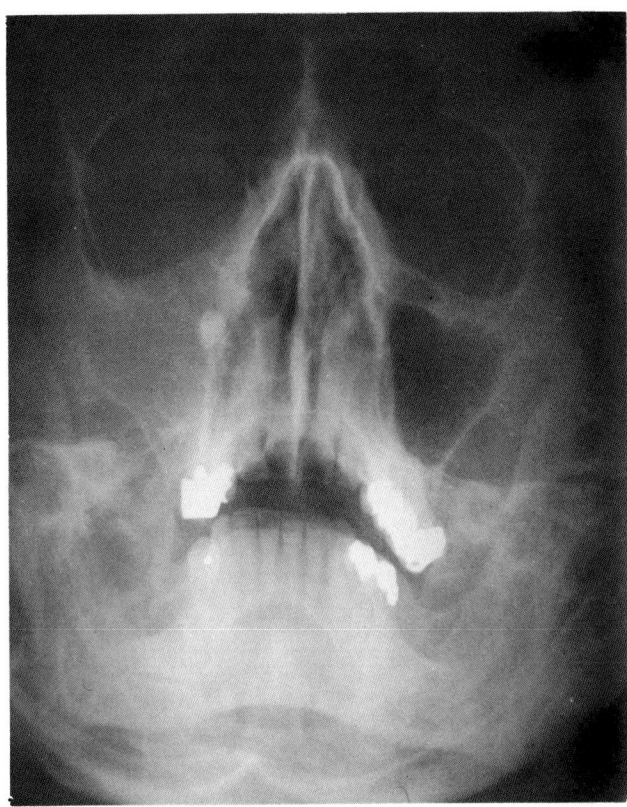

10.23 (top) and 10.24 (bottom) In this example, the root fragment is retained high up on the medial wall of the right antrum, probably blocking its ostium. As a consequence, drainage is prevented and the antrum is infected and fully obscured by radiopaque exudate which demonstrates no fluid level. Note that the other sinuses are normal, confirming again that unilateral sinusitis is often a consequence of dental causes. OM & L

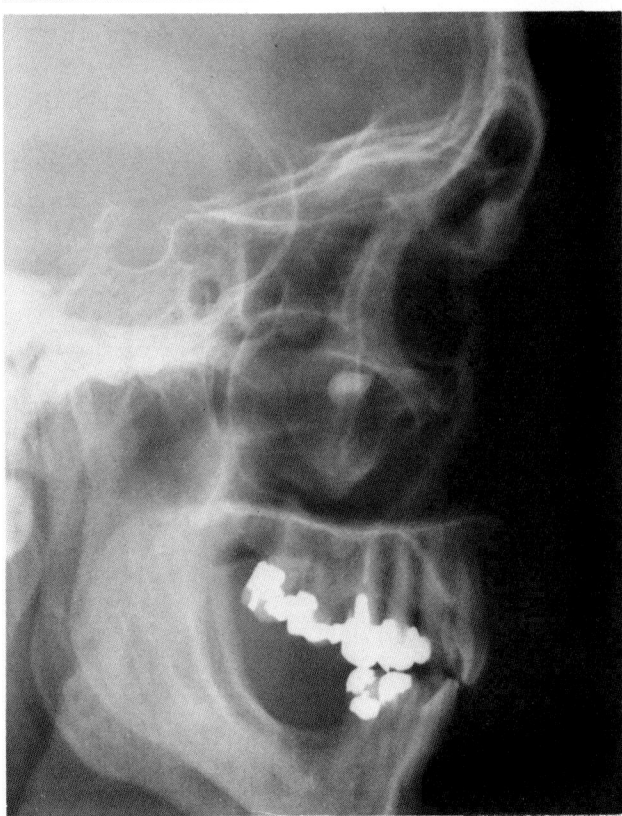

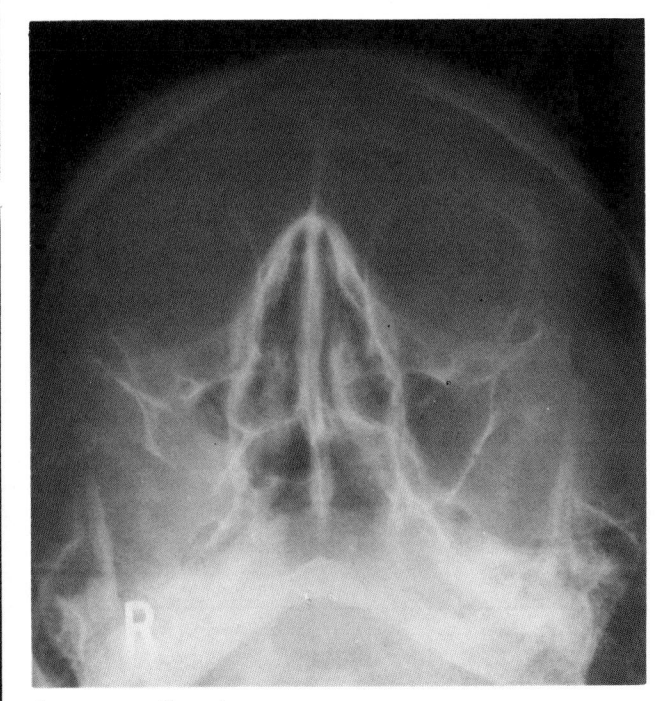

Squamous cell carcinoma
10.25 In the early stages, these tumours which arise from the epithelium lining the antrum, may grow predominantly into its cavity, and thus are frequently of large size before they are detected. In this lesion of the right antrum, the slightly radiopaque tumour mass occupies the inferior and lateral aspects of the antral cavity where it has destroyed the bony walls, and protrudes laterally into the soft tissues. The radiolucent antral air shadow is very much reduced in size, although the infra-orbital margin and foramen remain intact. Note that the foramen ovale is clearly displayed on both sides. OM

10.26 (top), 10.27 (middle) and 10.28 (bottom) This tumour of the left antrum forms a slightly radiopaque shadow extending into the nasal airway and hard palate (arrows), and has destroyed its medial and inferior bony walls which are discontinuous (Fig. 10.26). The destruction of the palate and floor of the antrum is clearly displayed in the panoramic radiograph (Fig. 10.27). Although the soft tissue swelling into the mouth is also shown on this film, it is more clearly demonstrated on the periapical view (Fig. 10.28). The irregular pattern of bone destruction at the margin of the tumour with spikes of bone projecting into the tumour mass, typical of a malignant neoplasm, is clearly demonstrated. Note again the prominent foramen ovale bilaterally. OM, PR & P

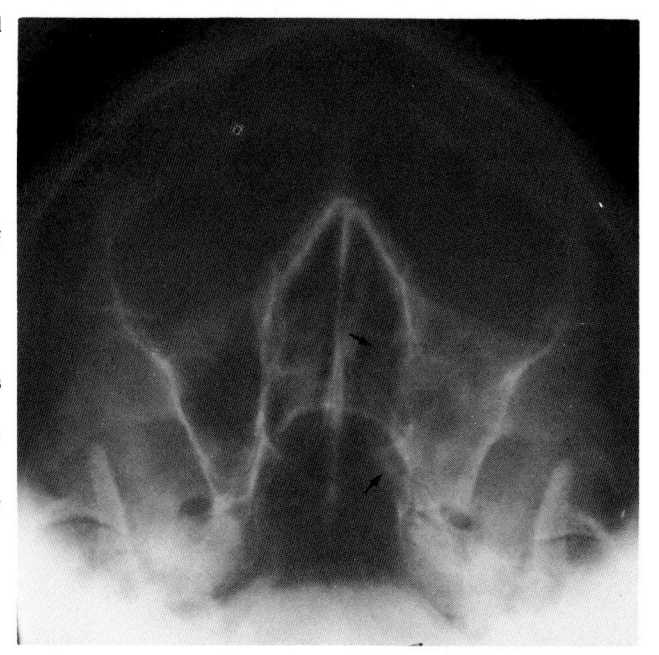

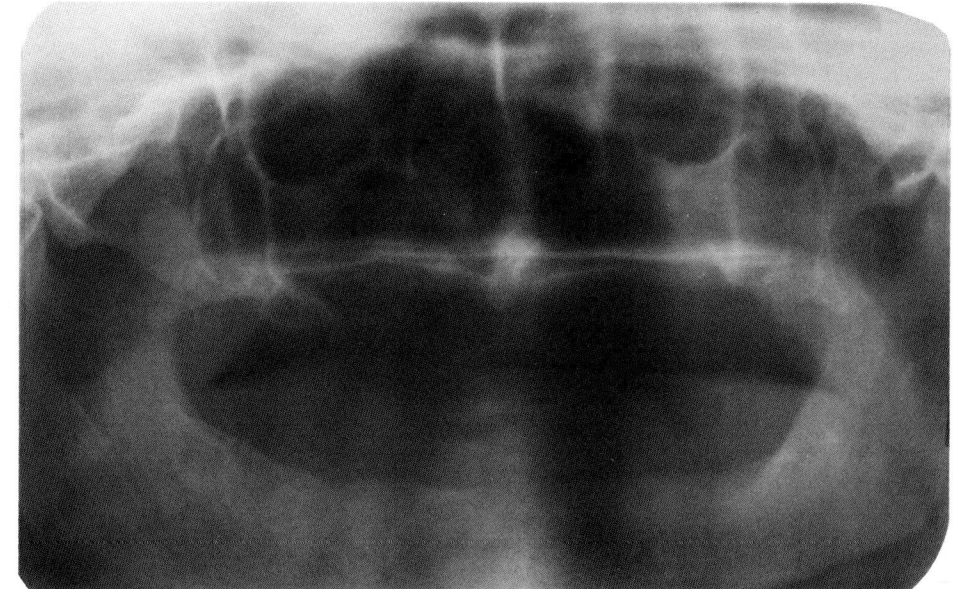

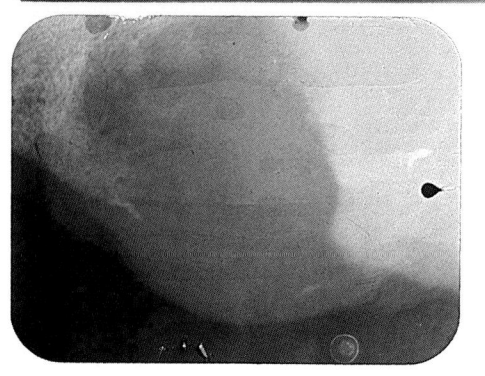

The Maxillary Antrum 237

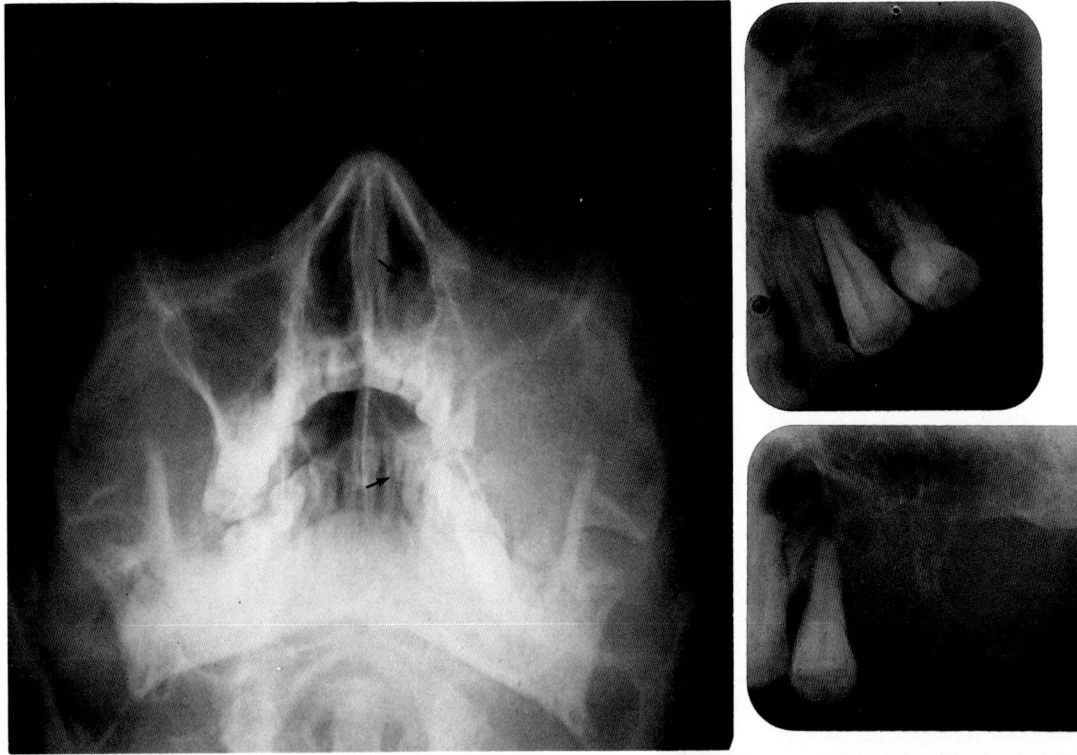

10.29 (above), 10.30 (upper right) and 10.31 (lower right) An advanced neoplasm of the left antrum with almost complete destruction of its medial, inferior and lateral walls. The slightly radiopaque tumour mass is occupying part of the nasal airway (arrow), the oral cavity (arrow) and the infra-temporal fossa (Fig. 10.29). There is thinning of the orbital wall medially and more marked destruction laterally where the outline, including that of the infra-orbital foramen, is indistinct. The intra-oral films (Figs 10.30 and 10.31) show an irregular pattern of bone destruction with patchy areas of radiolucency separated by irregularly arranged bone remnants. There is apical resorption |34 and the periapical areas of increased radiolucency caused by the tumour could be misinterpreted as periapical granulomas. The soft tissue outline overlying the alveolus can just be determined. The greater radiopacity of the bone to the right of the film (Fig. 10.31) is due to superimposition of the shadow of the zygomatic arch, which remains intact. OM & P

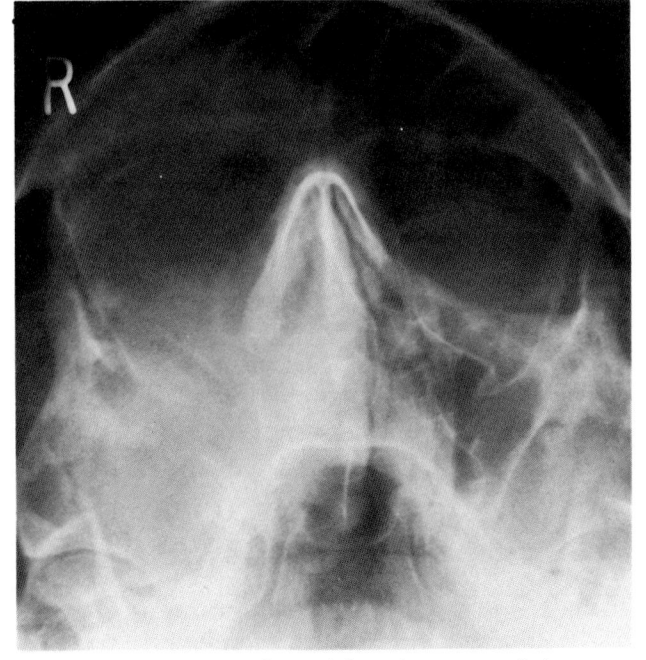

10.32 An extensive neoplasm of the right antrum, all the walls of which have been completely destroyed. The slightly radiopaque mass has spread into the infra-temporal fossa, the lower part of the orbit, and both right and left nasal airways. The nasal septum is discontinuous and displaced to the left, and the left lateral wall of the nasal cavity is partly eroded. OM

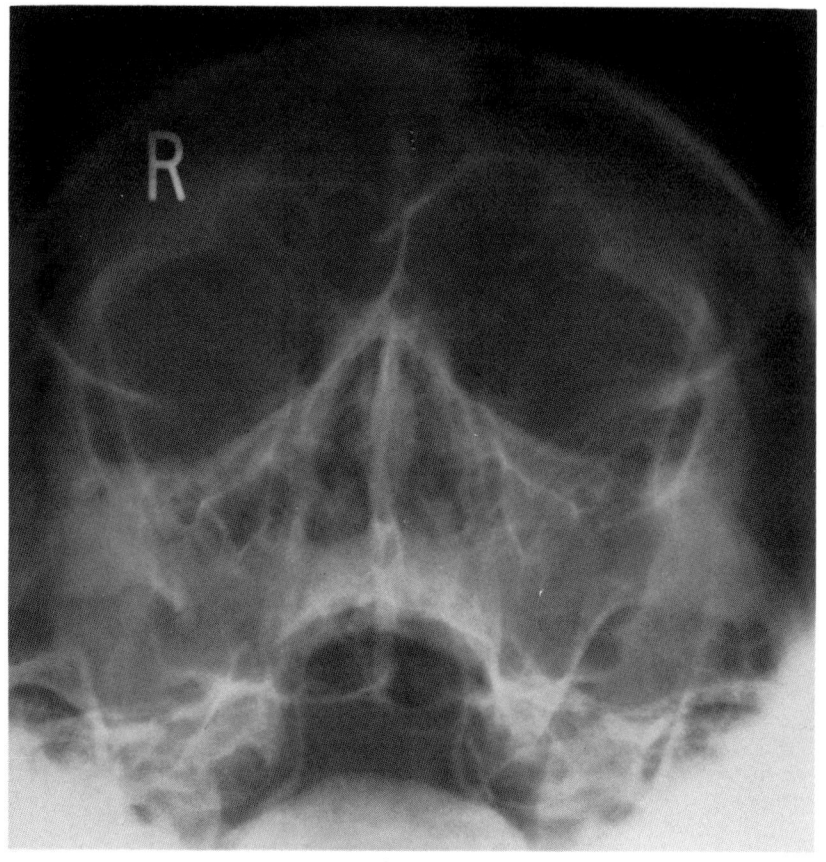

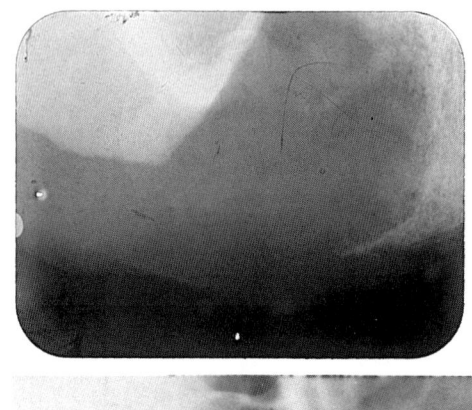

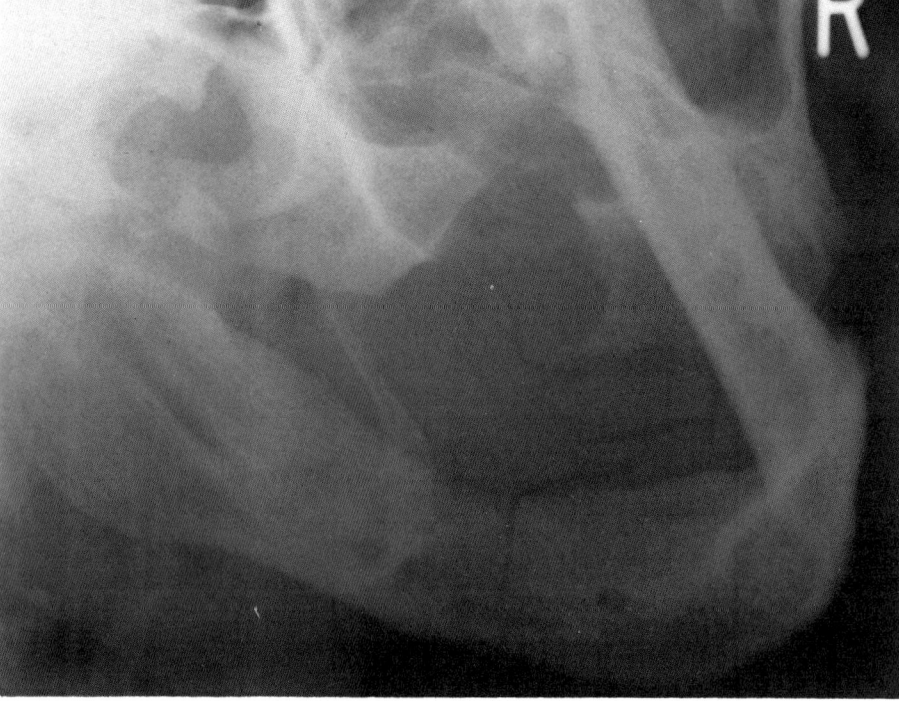

Spindle cell sarcoma 10.33 (top left), 10.34 (left) and 10.35 (above) An undifferentiated sarcoma causing a large radiolucent defect in the right maxillary alveolar process and extending upwards into the antrum (Fig. 10.33). Inferiorly, the bone of the edentulous ridge is completely destroyed and anteriorly the bone margin is shelved and indistinct, exhibiting an irregular pattern of destruction. There is swelling of the overlying soft tissues. The involvement of the antrum is confirmed by the lack of continuity to the cortical lamina demarcating its floor (Fig. 10.34) and the destruction of its lateral wall (Fig. 10.35). P, OLM & OM

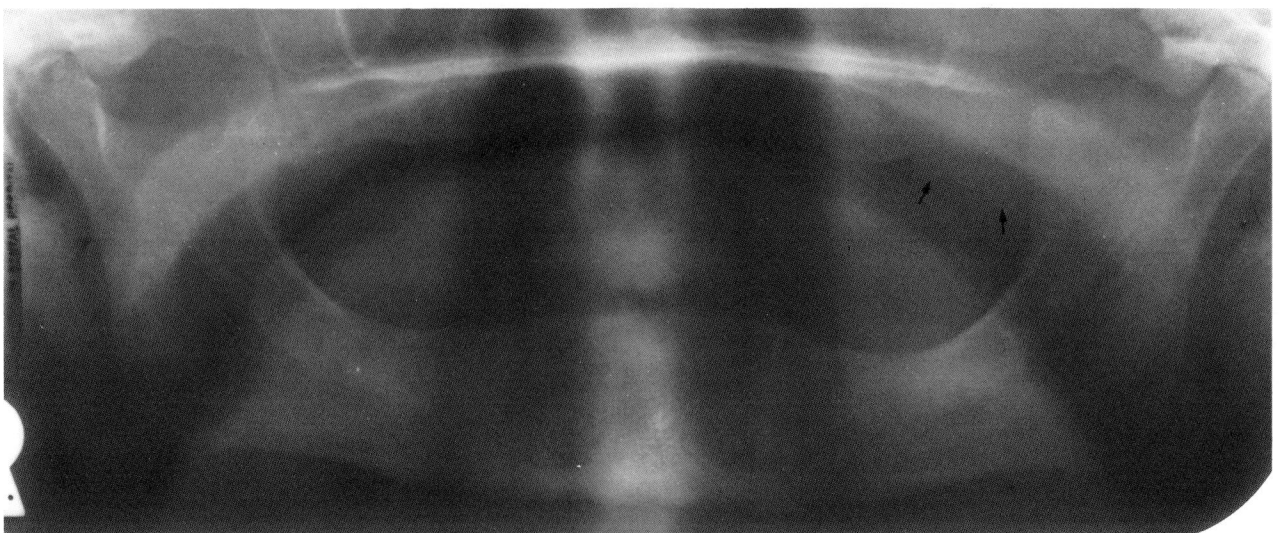

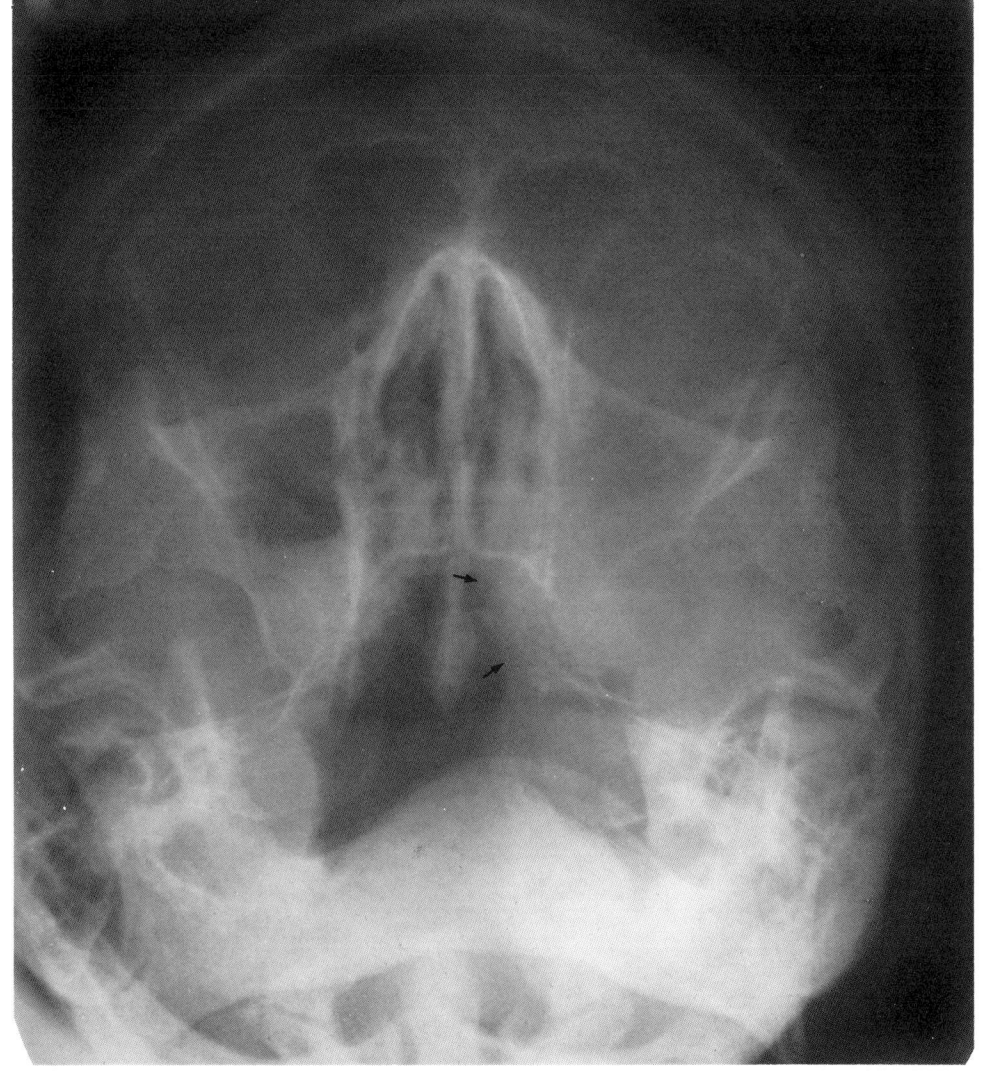

Malignant lymphoma 10.36 (above) and 10.37 (left) A malignant lymphoma of the follicular centre cell type, occupying the entire left antrum, which is opaque. The neoplasm has destroyed the entire lateral wall and the underlying edentulous alveolar ridge, and the superior margin of the antrum is poorly defined medially suggesting that it, too, is involved. The soft tissue tumour mass has caused swelling of the alveolus occlusally (arrows) (Fig. 10.36) and palatally (arrows) (Fig. 10.37). In addition, there is sinusitis of the right antrum which is radiopaque inferiorly with a clearly defined menisciform upper boundary indicating the presence of fluid. Somewhat unusually, the fluid level can also be seen on the panoramic radiograph. PR & OM

Index

A point 3.44
Abscess, acute periapical 5.115–5.117
Abscess, lateral periodontal 6.12, 6.13
Acromegaly 7.205
Adenoma, pleomorphic 7.176–7.178, 9.46, 9.47
Adenomatoid odontogenic tumour 7.147, 7.148
Air cell, mastoid 3.42, 3.48, 3.52, 3.54, 3.56, 3.58
Air gun pellet 9.30, 9.32
Air space, pharyngeal 3.42, 3.60, 7.193
Alveolar crest line 3.3, 3.5, 3.17–3.20, 3.22, 3.36
Alveolus, fracture 7.92, 7.96–7.98
Amalgam fragments 9.14
Amalgam tattoo 9.27
Ameloblastic fibro-odontome 7.52
Ameloblastoma 7.134–7.146
Ameloblastomatoid cyst 7.144–7.146
Amelogenesis imperfecta 5.82
Aneurysm, traumatic 9.44
Aneurysmal bone cyst 7.173, 7.174
Angiogram, carotid 7.56, 9.44
Angle, Frankfort–mandibular plane 3.44
Angle, mandibular incisal 3.44
Angle, mandible 3.39, 3.42, 3.52
Angle, maxillary incisal 3.44
Ankylosis, temporo-mandibular joint 8.17, 8.21–8.23
Ankylosis, tooth 5.65
Anodontia, partial 5.51, 5.66
Antegonial notch 7.9–7.11, 8.18, 8.23
Anterior cranial fossa 3.42, 3.56, 3.58
Anterior ethmoidal sinus 3.48
Anterior midline suture 3.1, 3.9, 3.11, 3.25, 5.152, 7.18
Anterior nasal spine 3.10, 3.11, 3.21, 3.32, 3.35, 3.42, 3.44, 7.15, 7.18, 7.122, 7.131
Antral polyp 10.2, 10.5, 10.8
Antrolith 10.12, 10.13
Antrum, maxillary, cavity 3.12–3.14, 3.16, 3.23, 3.24, 3.26, 3.27, 3.32, 3.34, 3.35, 3.48, 3.50, 3.52, 3.54, 3.56, 3.58
Antrum, maxillary, displaced root 10.17–10.24
Antrum, maxillary, floor 3.12–3.16, 3.22–3.24, 3.26, 3.27, 3.33, 3.42
Antrum, maxillary, squamous cell carcinoma 10.25–10.32
Antrum, maxillary, vascular canals 3.12, 3.14, 3.16, 3.26, 5.123
Antrum, maxillary, wall 3.42
Apicectomy 5.152, 5.154, 5.155
Apron, lead 3.45
Arch, zygomatic 3.39, 3.48, 3.52, 3.54, 3.60, 5.20, 5.65, 7.79, 7.80, 10.18, 10.20, 10.31
Artery, facial 9.44
Artery, maxillary 9.44
Artery, superficial temporal 9.44

Index

Arthritis, rheumatoid 8.16–8.20
Articular eminence, temporo-mandibular joint 3.56, 3.58
Articular fossa, temporo-mandibular joint 3.56, 3.58
Atlas vertebra 3.42, 3.52, 7.31, 7.183
Atrophic mandible 7.119–7.121, 7.184
Attrition 5.81, 5.84, 5.85, 5.119, 5.120, 6.9
Avitaminosis C 6.22
Axis vertebra 7.31
Axis vertebra, odontoid process 3.42, 3.48, 3.50, 3.52

B point 3.44
Basal cell carcinoma 7.187
Benign cementoblastoma 5.96
Bifurcation involvement 6.2, 6.5, 6.10
Bisecting angle technique 2.4, 2.5
Bitewing radiograph 2.7, 3.31
Blade, forceps 5.173
Blow-out fracture 7.128, 7.129
Body, mandible 3.42, 3.48
Body, zygoma 3.42
Bolton plane 3.44
Bolton point 3.44
Buccal cortical plate, mandible 3.36, 3.38
Bone, frontal 3.34, 3.52
Bone, hyoid 3.39, 3.40, 3.42, 3.60, 7.30, 7.31, 7.39, 7.41, 7.53, 7.68, 7.82, 7.111, 7.135, 7.139, 7.141, 7.144, 7.157, 7.166, 7.168, 7.172, 7.192, 9.48, 9.49
Bone, nasal 3.34, 3.42, 3.48, 7.123
Bone, occipital 3.48
Bone, petrous temporal 3.48, 3.54
Bone, Wormian 7.13
Bone, zygomatic 3.48
Bridge, cantilever 9.30
Bridge, fixed/fixed 9.30
Broach, diagnostic 5.140
Buccinator muscle 9.20
Bucket handle deformity 7.118
Bullet 9.33
Bur 5.175

Caffey–Silverman syndrome 7.64
Calcifying epithelial odontogenic tumour 7.151, 7.152
Calcifying odontogenic cyst 7.149, 7.150
Calcinosis 9.50
Calculus, dental 5.100, 5.111, 5.113, 5.124, 6.5–6.7, 6.10, 6.11, 6.21, 7.152, 10.12
Calculus, salivary 9.2–9.20
Canal, external auditory 3.50, 3.52
Canal, Hirschfeld nutrient 3.4, 3.28, 3.29, 7.47
Canal, incisive 3.20
Canal, inferior alveolar 3.7, 3.8, 3.29, 3.30, 3.39, 3.40, 3.42, 3.60, 5.2, 5.6, 5.16–5.19, 5.130, 5.168, 6.16, 7.28, 7.29, 7.37, 7.39, 7.47, 7.66, 7.70, 7.90, 7.91, 7.114, 7.136, 7.152, 7.157, 7.158, 7.185, 7.188, 7.189, 8.6, 8.23
Canal, internal auditory 3.50, 3.52, 3.54
Canal, nasolacrimal 3.32, 3.35, 5.25, 5.26, 5.50, 7.78
Canal, vascular in antral wall 3.12, 3.14, 3.16, 3.26, 5.123
Canine, unerupted 5.23–5.40, 5.51
Carcinoma, basal cell 7.187
Carcinoma, metastatic 7.188–7.191, 8.31
Carcinoma, muco-epidermoid 7.186
Carcinoma, primary intra-osseus 7.185
Carcinoma, squamous cell 7.183, 7.184, 10.25–10.32
Caries, cemental 5.112, 5.113
Caries, cervical 5.110, 5.111
Caries, dental 5.6, 5.10, 5.11, 5.14, 5.15, 5.99–5.114
Caries, fissure 5.99, 5.100, 5.101
Caries, interstitial 5.102–5.109

Caries, irradiation 5.88
Caries, recurrent 5.61, 5.75, 5.89, 5.99, 5.100, 5.114, 5.121, 6.1
Carotid angiogram 7.56, 9.44
Cartilage, thyroid 9.48
Cavernous haemangioma 7.55, 7.56
Cavity, maxillary antrum 3.12–3.14, 3.16, 3.23, 3.24, 3.26, 3.27, 3.32, 3.34, 3.35, 3.50, 3.52, 3.54, 3.56, 3.58, 3.60
Cavity, nasal 3.9, 3.11, 3.12, 3.25, 3.26, 3.32, 3.35, 3.48, 3.60
Cavity, orbital 3.60
Cavity, Stafne's bone 7.63
Cemental caries 5.112, 5.113
Cemental dysplasia, periapical 5.92, 5.93
Cementifying fibroma 5.95
Cementoblastoma, benign 5.96
Cementoma, gigantiform 5.94
Central fibroma 7.168, 7.169
Central giant cell granuloma 7.154–7.156
Central giant cell tumour 7.154–7.158
Central neurilemmoma 7.171, 7.172
Cephalometric radiograph 3.43–3.46
Cervical caries 5.110, 5.111
Cervical radiolucency 3.6, 3.8, 5.73, 5.111, 5.112
Cervical vertebra 3.39, 3.48
Cherubism 7.62
Chondromyxoid fibroma 7.170
Chondrosarcoma 7.194, 7.195
Chronic osteomyelitis 7.66–7.72
Chronic periodontitis 5.10, 5.92, 5.100, 5.113, 5.164, 6.1–6.13, 6.20, 7.63, 7.67, 7.152, 7.203
Cingulum 3.1
Cleft palate 7.1–7.4
Cleido-cranial dysostosis 7.12–7.14
Clivus 3.42, 3.52
Complex composite odontome 5.79, 5.80
Compound composite odontome 5.76, 5.77, 5.78
Compton scatter 2.3
Concha, nasal 10.11
Concrescence 5.89
Condylar hyperplasia 8.3–8.9
Condylar hypoplasia 8.1, 8.2, 10.9
Condyle, dislocation 8.30
Condyle, fracture 7.105, 7.108, 7.109, 8.26–8.29
Condyle, mandible 3.42, 3.48, 3.50, 3.52, 3.54, 3.56, 3.58, 3.60
Contrast medium 7.83, 9.45
Coronoid process, mandible 3.14, 3.15, 3.27, 3.39, 3.42, 3.48, 3.50, 3.52, 3.54, 3.56, 3.58, 3.60, 5.20, 6.11, 6.13, 7.110, 10.18
'Cotton wool' appearance 7.206–7.208, 7.210, 7.211
Crest, internal occipital 3.54
Cribriform plate 3.42
Crista galli 3.50
Cyst, ameloblastomatoid 7.144–7.146
Cyst, aneurysmal bone 7.173, 7.174
Cyst, calcifying odontogenic 7.149, 7.150
Cyst, dental 5.127–5.130, 5.166, 7.77–7.83
Cyst, dentigerous 7.21–7.33
Cyst, globulo-maxillary 7.20
Cyst, haemorrhagic bone 7.175
Cyst, healing 7.84–7.91
Cyst, incisive canal 7.15–7.19
Cyst, lateral periodontal 6.15–6.17
Cyst, mucous of antrum 10.5, 10.9
Cyst, nasopalatine 7.15–7.19
Cyst, odontogenic kerato- 7.34–7.51
Cyst, periapical 5.127–5.130, 5.166
Cyst, primordial 7.35
Cyst, residual 7.77–7.83
Cyst, solitary bone 7.175
Cyst, traumatic bone 7.175

Dens in dente 5.68
Dental calculus 5.100, 5.111, 5.113, 5.124, 6.5–6.7, 6.10, 6.11, 6.21, 7.152, 10.12
Dental caries 5.6, 5.10, 5.11, 5.14, 5.15, 5.18, 5.19, 5.99–5.114
Dental cyst 5.127–5.130, 5.166, 7.77–7.83
Dental development, age 6 3.61
Dental development, age 9 3.62
Dental development, age 12 3.63
Dental development, age 15 3.64
Dental development, age 18 3.65
Denticle 5.76–5.78
Dentigerous cyst 7.21–7.33
Dentinal sclerosis 5.99, 5.109
Dentinogenesis imperfecta 5.83–5.85
Dentinoma 5.97, 5.98
Diagnostic broach 5.140
Diastema 5.40, 5.49, 5.50, 5.66, 5.84, 5.85, 5.152, 6.2, 7.21, 7.22, 7.148
Dilaceration 5.34, 5.42, 5.49, 5.50, 5.56
Dilated odontom 5.69, 5.70
Disease, Hand–Schüller–Christian 7.179–7.181
Disease, Paget's, of bone 7.206–7.211
Disease, Sjogren's 9.23
Disease, Still's 8.16–8.18
Dislocation, mandibular condyle 8.30
Dorsum sellae 3.50, 3.54
Dressing material 5.153, 5.172
Dysostosis, cleido-cranial 7.12–7.14
Dysostosis, mandibulo-facial 7.9–7.11
Dysplasia, ectodermal 5.67
Dysplasia, familial fibrous 7.62
Dysplasia, fibrous 7.57–7.61
Dysplasia, odonto- 5.86
Dysplasia, periapical cemental 5.92, 5.93

Ear-ring 5.28
Ectodermal dysplasia 5.67
Empyema, maxillary antrum 10.2–10.4
Enamel 3.1, 3.2
Enamel hypoplasia 5.81
Enamel pearl 5.75
Enameloma 5.75
Ennis, Y formation 3.12, 3.26
Eosinophilic granuloma 7.182
Epiglottis 7.139, 7.141, 9.47
Epiglottis, mineralised 7.68
Epulis, fibrous 6.18, 6.19
Ethmoidal sinuses 3.50
External auditory canal 3.50, 3.52
External auditory meatus 3.56, 3.58
External oblique ridge 5.172, 6.10, 7.183
Extraction socket 7.92–7.95

Facial artery 9.44
Falx cerebri, mineralisation 7.51, 7.130
Familial fibrous dysplasia 7.62
Fibroma, cementifying 5.95
Fibroma, central 7.168, 7.169
Fibroma, chondromyxoid 7.170
Fibroma, ossifying 7.159–7.163, 7.174
Fibrosarcoma 7.196, 7.197
Fibrous dysplasia 7.57–7.61
Fibrous epulis 6.18, 6.19
Filling, root 5.23, 5.24, 5.122, 6.7, 6.17, 9.30, 9.47
Film holder 3.18, 5.1
First arch syndrome 7.7, 7.8
Fissure caries 5.99–5.101
Fissure, pterygo-maxillary 7.46

Fistula, oro-antral 10.5, 10.16, 10.17
Floor, maxillary antrum 3.12–3.16, 3.22–3.24, 3.26, 3.27, 3.33, 3.42
Floor, nose 3.9–3.12, 3.21, 3.25, 3.26, 3.32, 3.33, 3.35
Fluid level, antrum 7.130, 10.2–10.5, 10.36, 10.37
Foramen, greater palatine 3.52
Foramen, incisive 3.10, 3.11, 3.21, 3.35, 5.117, 7.86
Foramen, infra-orbital 7.44, 7.125
Foramen, lingual 3.3
Foramen magnum 3.52, 3.54
Foramen, mental 3.6, 3.18, 3.19, 3.29, 3.37–3.40, 3.60, 5.171, 6.4, 7.82, 7.91, 7.116, 7.149
Foramen ovale 3.48, 3.52, 10.1, 10.25, 10.26
Foramen, pterygo-palatine 7.46
Foramen rotundum 3.48, 3.50
Foramen spinosum 3.52
Forceps blade 5.173
Foreign body 9.27–9.38, 10.10, 10.11
Fossa, anterior cranial 3.42, 3.56, 3.58
Fossa, glenoid 3.60
Fossa, incisive 3.1, 7.80
Fossa, middle cranial 3.42, 3.52
Fossa, pituitary 3.42
Fossa, retromolar 3.8
Fracture, alveolus 7.92, 7.96–7.98
Fracture, anterior nasal spine 7.122
Fracture, condyle 7.105, 7.108, 7.109, 8.26–8.29
Fracture, fronto-naso-ethmoid complex 7.133
Fracture, genial tubercle 7.99
Fracture, mandible 7.101–7.121
Fracture, maxilla 7.130–7.132
Fracture, maxillary tuberosity 7.100
Fracture, nasal bone 7.123
Fracture, orbital floor 7.128, 7.129
Fracture, pathological 7.156, 7.184
Fracture, root 5.160–5.163, 7.97
Fracture, tooth 5.69, 5.129, 5.157–5.163, 5.166, 9.36, 9.37
Fracture, zygomatic complex 7.124–7.127
Fractured needle 9.39–9.43
Frankfort–mandibular plane angle 3.44
Frankfort plane 3.44
Frontal bone 3.34, 3.52
Frontal process, zygomatic bone 3.50
Frontal sinus 3.42, 3.48, 3.50
Fronto-naso-ethmoid complex, fracture 7.133
30° Fronto-occipital, skull 2.15, 3.53, 3.54
Fronto-zygomatic suture 3.48, 7.127, 7.132

Gardner's sydrome 7.167
Geminated odontome 5.71–5.74
Genial tubercle 3.36–3.38, 7.5, 7.98, 7.99
Ghost teeth 5.86
Gigantiform cementoma 5.94
Gland, parotid 9.14–9.23
Gland, pineal, mineralised 7.197
Gland, submandibular 9.2–9.13
Glass, windscreen 9.34, 9.35
Glenoid fossa 3.60
Globulo-maxillary cyst 7.20
Gnathion 3.44
Gonion 3.44
Gorlin–Goltz syndrome 7.47–7.51
Granuloma, central giant cell 7.154–7.156
Granuloma, eosinophilic 7.182
Granuloma, malignant of maxilla 7.204
Granuloma, periapical 5.118–5.126, 5.131, 5.144–5.148, 5.150–5.151
Greater palatine foramen 3.52
Grid 2.9

244 Index

Groove, meningeal   3.42
Gutta percha point   5.141, 5.142, 5.147, 5.148, 5.150–5.154

Haemangioma, cavernous   7.55, 7.56, 9.1
Haemorrhagic bone cyst   7.175
Hamulus, pterygoid   3.15, 6.13, 10.18
Hand–Schüller–Christian disease   7.179–7.181
Hard palate   3.42, 3.50, 3.60
Healing cyst   7.84–7.91
Hereditary hypophosphataemia   5.177, 5.178
Hirschfeld's nutrient canal   3.4, 3.28, 3.29, 7.47
Histiocytosis X   7.179–7.182
Hyoid bone   3.39, 3.40, 3.42, 3.60, 7.30, 7.31, 7.39, 7.41, 7.53, 7.68, 7.82, 7.111, 7.135, 7.139, 7.141, 7.144, 7.157, 7.166, 7.168, 7.172, 7.192, 9.48, 9.49
Hypercementosis   7.206–7.208
Hyperostosis, infantile cortical   7.64
Hyperparathyroidism   7.212, 7.213
Hyperplasia, condylar   8.3–8.9
Hypertelorism   7.13
Hypodontia   5.13, 5.40, 5.51, 5.66, 5.71, 5.83
Hypophosphataemia, hereditary   5.177, 5.178
Hypoplasia, condylar   8.1, 8.2, 10.9
Hypoplasia, enamel   5.81

Idiopathic resorption   5.133, 5.135–5.137
Incisive canal   3.20
Incisive canal cyst   7.15–7.19
Incisive foramen   3.10, 3.11, 3.21, 3.35, 5.117, 7.86
Incisive fossa   7.80
Incisor tooth   3.1, 3.3, 3.4, 3.9, 3.11
Incisor, unerupted   5.49, 5.50, 5.52, 5.57, 5.58, 5.76, 5.77, 5.80
Infantile cortical hyperostosis   7.64
Inferior alveolar canal   3.7, 3.8, 3.19, 3.29, 3.30, 3.39, 3.40, 3.42, 3.60, 5.2, 5.6, 5.16, 5.17, 5.130, 5.168, 6.16, 7.28, 7.29, 7.37, 7.39, 7.47, 7.66, 7.70, 7.90, 7.91, 7.114, 7.136, 7.152, 7.157, 7.158, 7.185, 7.188, 7.189, 8.6, 8.23
Inferior cortical plate, mandible   3.3, 3.5, 3.7, 3.8, 3.19, 3.28, 3.36, 3.39
Inferior turbinate   3.9, 3.25, 3.50, 3.60
Infrabony pocket   5.118, 6.2, 6.10, 6.11, 6.19
Infraorbital foramen   7.44, 7.125
Infraorbital margin   3.35, 3.48
Internal auditory canal   3.50, 3.52, 3.54
Internal occipital crest   3.54
Interstitial caries   5.102–5.109
Intervertebral space   3.50
Invaginated odontome   5.68–5.70
Inverted tooth   5.22, 5.48, 5.54
Irradiation   5.87, 5.88
Irradiation caries   5.88

Juvenile periodontitis   6.14

Lambdoid suture   3.42, 3.50, 3.54
Lamina dura   3.1, 3.2
Lateral periodontal abscess   6.12, 6.13
Lateral periodontal cyst   6.15–6.17
Lateral skull   2.11, 3.41, 3.42
Lateral wall, orbit   3.42, 3.52
Lead apron   3.45
Le Fort fracture, type II   7.130, 7.131
Le Fort fracture, type III   7.132
Ligament, stylohyoid   7.117, 9.49
Line, alveolar crest   3.3, 3.5, 3.17–3.20, 3.22, 3.36
Line, lip   3.3, 3.4
Linea innominata   3.48, 3.50
Lingual cortical plate, mandible   3.38

Lingual foramen   3.3
Lip line   3.3, 3.4
Lip, soft tissue   3.37, 3.38
Localising plate   5.174
Lower anterior occlusal radiograph   3.36
Lower true occlusal radiograph   3.37, 3.38
Lymph node   7.117, 9.24–9.26
Lymphoma, malignant   7.201, 7.202, 10.36, 10.37

Malignant granuloma of the maxilla   7.204
Malignant lymphoma   7.201, 7.202, 10.36, 10.37
Malignant melanoma   7.203
Mandible, angle   3.39, 3.42, 3.52
Mandible, atrophic   7.117–7.121, 7.184
Mandible, condyle   3.42, 3.48, 3.50, 3.52, 3.54, 3.56, 3.58, 3.60
Mandible, fracture   7.101–7.121
Mandible, oblique lateral radiograph   2.10
Mandible, ramus   3.52
Mandibular incisal angle   3.44
Mandibular plane   3.44
Mandibulo-facial dysostosis   7.9–7.11
Margin, infra-orbital   3.35, 3.48
Margin, supra-orbital   3.48, 3.50
Mastoid air cells   3.42, 3.48, 3.52, 3.54, 3.56, 3.58
Mastoid process   3.50
Material, dressing   5.153, 5.172
Material, impression   9.28, 9.29
Material, root filling   10.10, 10.11
Maxilla, fracture   7.130–7.132
Maxillary artery   9.44
Maxillary incisal angle   3.44
Maxillary plane   3.44
Maxillary sinusitis   10.1–10.7, 10.36, 10.37
Maxillary tuberosity   3.14, 3.15, 3.39
Maxillary tuberosity, fracture   7.100
Meatus, external auditory   3.56, 3.58
Megadontia   5.72
Melanoma, malignant   7.203
Meningeal grooves   3.42
Mental foramen   3.6, 3.29, 3.37–3.40, 3.60, 5.171, 6.4, 7.82, 7.91, 7.116, 7.149
Mental protruberance   3.37
Mental ridge   3.3, 3.4, 3.28, 3.36
Menton   3.44
Mesiodens   5.52, 5.53, 5.55, 5.56, 5.157
Metastatic carcinoma   7.188–7.191, 8.31
Micrognathia   7.7, 7.9–7.11, 8.23
Middle cranial fossa   3.42, 3.52
Middle turbinate bone   3.50
Molar, retained   5.63, 5.64
Molar, submerged   5.65
Molar tooth   3.2, 3.13–3.15
Molar, unerupted   5.1–5.22
Muco-epidermoid carcinoma   7.186
Multiple myelomatosis   7.198–7.200
Myelogram   9.45
Myelomatosis, multiple   7.198–7.200
Mylohyoid muscle   9.9, 9.12
Mylohyoid ridge   3.7, 3.8
Myxoma, odontogenic   7.153

Nasal bone   3.34, 3.42, 3.48
Nasal cavity   3.9, 3.11, 3.12, 3.25, 3.26, 3.32, 3.35, 3.48, 3.60
Nasal concha   10.11
Nasal septum   3.9, 3.11, 3.25, 3.32, 3.34, 3.35, 3.48, 3.50, 3.52, 3.54, 3.60
Nasion   3.44
Nasolacrimal canal   3.32, 3.35, 5.25, 5.26, 5.50, 7.78

Nasopalatine cyst 7.15–7.19
Necrosis, osteoradio- 7.73, 7.74
Necrosis, phosphorus 7.75, 7.76
Needle, fractured 9.39–9.43
Neuro-ectodermal tumour of infancy 7.54
Node, lymph 7.117, 9.24–9.26
Nose, floor 3.9–3.12, 3.21, 3.25, 3.26, 3.32, 3.33, 3.35
Nose, soft tissue 3.25, 3.32
Notch, antegonial 7.9–7.11, 8.18, 8.23
Notch, sigmoid 3.42

Oblique lateral mandible radiograph 2.10, 3.39, 3.40
Oblique ridge 3.7, 3.8, 3.30
Occipital bone 3.48
Occipito-mental radiograph 2.12, 3.47, 3.48
Occiput 3.54
Occlusal plane 3.44
Occlusal trauma 5.63, 5.72, 6.20, 6.21
Occlusion, Class I 3.43
Occlusion, Class II 3.45
Occlusion, Class III 3.46
Odonto-ameloblastoma 7.53
Odontodysplasia 5.86
Odontogenic keratocyst 7.34–7.51
Odontogenic myxoma 7.153
Odontoid process 3.42, 3.48, 3.50, 3.52
Odontome, ameloblastic fibro- 7.52
Odontome, complex composite 5.79, 5.80
Odontome, compound composite 5.76–5.78
Odontome, dilated 5.69, 5.70
Odontome, geminated 5.71–5.74
Odontome, invaginated 5.68–5.70
Onion skin pattern 7.64, 7.65
Orange peel appearance 7.61
Orbit, cavity 3.60
Orbit, lateral wall 3.42, 3.52
Orbital floor, fracture 7.128, 7.129
Orbitale 3.44
Oro-antral fistula 10.5, 10.16, 10.17
Ossifying fibroma 7.159–7.163, 7.174
Osteitis deformans 7.206–7.211
Osteo-arthrosis 8.10–8.15, 9.9
Osteoclastoma 7.157, 7.158
Osteogenic sarcoma 7.192, 7.193
Osteoma 7.164–7.167, 10.6, 10.7
Osteomyelitis, chronic 7.66–7.72
Osteoporosis 7.213
Osteoporosis circumscripta 7.209
Osteoradionecrosis 7.73, 7.74
Osteosclerosis 5.63, 5.123, 5.138, 5.139, 5,172, 7.70, 7.72, 7.101, 7.192, 7.201, 7.202

Paget's disease of bone 7.206–7.211
Palate, cleft 7.1–7.4
Palate, hard 3.42, 3.50, 3.60
Panoramic radiograph 3.59–3.65
Paralleling technique 2.6, 3.17–3.24
Parallax 2.8, 5.23–5.26, 5.32, 5.33, 5.49, 5.50, 5.55, 5.56, 7.16, 7.17, 7.21, 7.22, 7.88, 7.89
Parotid gland 9.14–9.23
Parotid sialogram 3.66, 3.67, 9.18–9.23, 9.46, 9.47
Parotitis, recurrent 9.21, 9.22
Partial anodontia 5.13, 5.40, 5.51, 5.66
Pathological fracture 7.156, 7.184
Pearl, enamel 5.75
Pellet, air gun 9.30–9.32
Periapical abscess, acute 5.115–5.117
Periapical cemental dysplasia 5.92, 5.93

Periapical cyst 5.127–5.130, 5.166
Periapical granuloma 5.118–5.126, 5.131, 5.144–5.148, 5.150, 5.151
Periapical radiograph 3.1–3.20, 3.22, 3.23, 3.25–3.30
Periapical radiolucency 5.10, 5.13, 5.45, 5.64, 5.68, 5.70, 5.109, 5.132, 5.140–5.142, 5.153, 7.58, 7.67, 9.8, 10.10
Periodontitis, chronic 5.10, 5.92, 5.100, 5.113, 5.164, 6.1–6.13, 6.20, 7.63, 7.67, 7.152, 7.203
Periodontitis, juvenile 6.14
Periodontosis 6.14
Periostitis 7.65
Petrous temporal bone 3.48, 3.54
Pharyngeal air space 3.42, 3.60, 7.108, 7.193
Pharyngo-tympanic (Eustachian) tube 3.52
Phlebolith 9.1
Phosphorous necrosis 7.75, 7.76
Photo-electric absorption 2.3
Pineal gland, mineralised 7.197
Pinna 3.60, 7.10, 7.209, 9.49
Pituitary fossa 3.42
Plane, Bolton 3.44
Plane, Frankfort 3.44
Plane, mandibular 3.44
Plane, maxillary 3.44
Plane, occlusal 3.44
Plate, buccal cortical, mandible 3.36, 3.38
Plate, cribriform 3.42
Plate, inferior cortical, mandible 3.3, 3.5, 3.7, 3.8, 3.19, 3.28, 3.36, 3.39
Plate, lingual cortical, mandible 3.38
Plate, localising 5.174
Plate, pterygoid 3.15, 3.42, 5.20, 10.18
Pleomorphic adenoma 7.176–7.178, 9.46, 9.47
Pocket, infrabony 5.118, 6.2, 6.10, 6.11, 6.19
Pogonion 3.44
Point, A 3.44
Point, B 3.44
Point, Bolton 3.44
Point, gutta percha 5.141, 5.142, 5.147, 5.148, 5.150–5.154
Point, silver 5.143, 6.4
Polyp, antral 10.2, 10.5, 10.8
Porion 3.44
Posterior–anterior skull 2.13, 3.49, 3.50
Posterior clinoid process 3.54
Posterior nasal spine 3.44
Potter–Bucky grid 2.9
Premolar, unerupted 5.41–5.48, 5.79
Premolar tooth 3.5, 3.6, 3.12, 3.13
Primary intra-osseous carcinoma 7.185
Primordial cyst 7.35
Process, coronoid 3.14, 3.15, 3.27, 3.39, 3.42, 3.48, 3.50, 3.52, 3.54, 3.56, 3,58, 3.60, 5.20, 6.11, 6.13, 7,110, 10.18
Process, frontal, zygomatic 3.50
Process, mastoid 3.50
Process, maxilla, zygomatic 3.42
Process, odontoid 3.42, 3.48, 3.50, 3.52
Process, posterior clinoid 3.54
Process, styloid 3.60
Process, zygomatic 5.170, 6.3
Process, zygomatic frontal 3.50
Prognathism 7.205
Protruberance, mental 3.37
Pterygoid hamulus 3.15, 6.13, 10.18
Pterygoid plate 3.15, 3.42, 5.20, 10.18
Pterygo-maxillary fissure 7.46
Pterygo-palatine foramen 7.46
Pulp chamber 3.1, 3.2
Pulp sclerosis 5.38, 5.83–5.85, 5.126, 5.133, 5.164–5.166, 5.159

Index

Pulp stone 5.90, 5.91, 5.114

Radiograph, bitewing 2.7, 3.31
Radiograph, cephalometric 3.43–3.46
Radiograph, fronto-occipital 3.53, 3.54
Radiograph, lateral skull 3.41, 3.42
Radiograph, lower anterior occlusal 3.36
Radiograph, lower true occlusal 3.37, 3.38
Radiograph, occipito-mental 3.47, 3.48
Radiograph, oblique lateral mandible 3.39, 3.40
Radiograph, panoramic 3.59–3.65
Radiograph, periapical 3.1–3.20, 3.22, 3.23, 3.25–3.30
Radiograph, postero-anterior 3.49, 3.50
Radiograph, submento-vertex 3.51, 3.52
Radiograph, transcranial of temporo-mandibular joint 3.55–3.58
Radiograph, upper oblique occlusal 3.33
Radiograph, upper standard occlusal 3.32
Radiograph, upper true occlusal 3.35
Radiograph, upper vertex occlusal 3.34
Ramus, mandible 3.52
Reamer 5.141
Recurrent caries 5.61, 5.75, 5.89, 5.99, 5.100, 5.114, 5.121, 6.1
Recurrent parotitis 9.21, 9.22
Residual cyst 7.77–7.83
Resorption, idiopathic 5.133, 5.135–5.137
Resorption, root 5.32–5.36, 5.52, 5.64, 5.65, 5.77, 5.93, 5.96, 5.131–5.138, 5.164, 5.165, 7.23, 7.24, 7.29, 7.42, 7.43, 7.71, 7.101, 7.136, 7.137, 7.147, 7.150, 7.199, 10.30
Retained molar 5.63, 5.64
Retromolar fossa 3.8
Rheumatoid arthritis 8.16–8.20
Rhinolith 10.14, 10.15
Ridge, mental 3.3, 3.4, 3.28, 3.36
Ridge, mylohyoid 3.7, 3.8
Ridge, oblique 3.7, 3.8, 3.19, 3.30, 5.172, 6.10, 7.183
Ring, ear 5.28
Root 5.91, 5.118, 5.123, 5.127, 5.130, 5.167–5.176, 7.58, 7.63, 7.72, 7.73, 7.95, 7.111, 7.205, 9.48, 10.8, 10.12, 10.13, 10.17–10.24
Root canal 3.1, 3.2
Root canal, lateral 5.149
Root canal therapy 5.140–5.155
Root filling 5.23, 5.24, 5.122, 6.7, 6.17, 9.30, 9.47, 10.10
Root fracture 5.160–5.163, 7.97
Root, lateral perforation 5.149–5.151, 6.17
Root resorption 5.32–5.36, 5.52, 5.64, 5.65, 5.77, 5.93, 5.96, 5.131–5.138, 5.164, 5.165, 7.23, 7.24, 7.29, 7.42, 7.43, 7.71, 7.101, 7.136, 7.137, 7.147, 7.150, 7.199, 10.30
Root, zygoma 3.13–3.16, 3.23, 3.24, 3.27, 3.33, 3.60, 5.20, 5.169, 7.93, 7.100

Sarcoma, chondro- 7.194, 7.195
Sarcoma, fibro- 7.196, 7.197
Sarcoma, osteogenic 7.192, 7.193
Sarcoma, spindle cell 10.33–10.35
Scintiscan 9.11
Sclerosis, dentinal 5.99, 5.109
Sclerosis, osteo- 5.63, 5.123, 5.138, 5.139, 5.172, 7.70, 7.72, 7.101, 7.192, 7.201, 7.202
Sclerosis, pulp 5.38, 5.83–5.85, 5.126, 5.133, 5.164–5.166, 5.169
Scurvy 6.22
Sella 3.44
Sella turcica 3.42, 7.205
Septum, nasal 3.9, 3.11, 3.25, 3.32, 3.34, 3.35, 3.48, 3.50, 3.52, 3.54, 3.60
Sequestrum 7.66–7.72, 7.73, 7.75, 7.76
Sialectasis 9.21, 9.22, 9.47
Sialogram, parotid 3.66, 3.67, 9.18–9.23, 9.46, 9.47
Sialogram, submandibular 3.68, 9.10

Sialolithiasis 9.2–9.20
Sigmoid notch 3.42
Silica 9.38
Silver point 5.143, 6.4
Sinus, anterior ethmoidal 3.48
Sinus, ethmoidal 3.50
Sinus, frontal 3.42, 3.48, 3.50
Sinus, sphenoidal 3.42, 3.48, 3.50, 3.52
Sinusitis, maxillary 10.1–10.7, 10.36, 10.37
Sjogren's disease 9.23
Skull, base view 2.14
Skull, 30° fronto-occipital 2.15, 3.53, 3.54
Skull, lateral 2.11, 3.41, 3.42
Skull, occipito-mental 2.12, 3.47, 3.48
Skull, postero-anterior 2.13, 3.49, 3.50
Skull, submento-vertex 2.14, 3.51, 3.52
Skull, Towne's view 2.15
Socket, tooth 5.171, 5.172, 5.175, 7.55, 7.66, 7.68, 7.77, 7.92–7.95, 7.107, 7.110, 7.112, 7.192, 7.195, 7.196, 7.201, 7.202, 7.204, 9.13, 9.14, 10.16, 10.17, 10.20–10.22
Soft tissue, lip 3.37, 3.38
Soft tissue, nose 3.25, 3.32
Solitary bone cyst 7.175
Space, intervertebral 3.50
Space, temporo-mandibular joint 3.54
Sphenoidal sinus 3.42, 3.48, 3.50, 3.52
Spindle cell sarcoma 10.33–10.35
Spine, anterior nasal 3.10, 3.11, 3.21, 3.32, 3.35, 3.42, 3.44, 7.15, 7.18, 7.122, 7.131
Spine, posterior nasal 3.44
Squamous cell carcinoma 7.183, 7.184, 10.25–10.32
Stafne's bone cavity 7.63
Still's disease 8.16–8.18
Stone, pulp 5.90, 5.91, 5.114
Stylohyoid ligament 7.117, 9.49
Styloid process 3.60
Subluxation, tooth 5.156
Submandibular gland 3.68, 9.2–9.13
Submandibular sialogram 3.68, 9.10
Submento-vertex skull 2.14, 3.51, 3.52
Submerged molar 5.65
Sun-ray pattern 7.192
Superficial temporal artery 9.44
Supernumerary tooth 5.52–5.58, 5.157, 5.171, 7.2, 7.3, 7.12, 8.3
Supplemental tooth 5.59–5.62, 7.11
Supra-orbital margin 3.48, 3.50
Suture, anterior midline 3.1, 3.9, 3.11, 3.25, 5.152, 7.18
Suture, fronto-zygomatic 3.48, 7.127, 7.132
Suture, lambdoid 3.42, 3.50, 3.54
Suture, zygomatic-temporal 7.126
Syndrome, Caffey-Silverman 7.64
Syndrome, first arch 7.7, 7.8
Syndrome, Gardner's 7.167
Syndrome, Gorlin–Goltz 7.47–7.51
Syndrome, Treacher–Collins 7.9–7.11
Synovial osteochondromatosis 8.24, 8.25

Tattoo, amalgam 9.27
Taurodontism 5.45, 9.30
Technical error, cone fracture 4.9
Technical error, coning 4.3
Technical error, developer splashing 4.19
Technical error, double exposure 4.10
Technical error, ear-ring artefacts 4.15–4.17
Technical error, electrostatic discharge 4.18
Technical error, film bending 4.4
Technical error, film damage 4.14, 5.17, 7.3
Technical error, film folding 4.5

Index

Technical error, film movement 4.7
Technical error, film reversal 4.6
Technical error, film scratching 4.24
Technical error, fixer splashing 4.20
Technical error, fogging 4.3
Technical error, grid misplacement 4.11
Technical error, image elongation 4.1
Technical error, image foreshortening 4.2
Technical error, incomplete film immersion 4.22
Technical error, metallic foreign body 4.8
Technical error, over development 4.12
Technical error, over fixation 4.23
Technical error, under development 4.13, 4.21
Technique, bisecting angle 2.4, 2.5
Technique, paralleling 2.6
Temporo-mandibular joint, articular eminence 3.56, 3.58
Temporo-mandibular joint, articular fossa 3.56, 3.58
Temporo-mandibular joint space 3.54
Temporo-mandibular joint, transcranial view 2.16, 3.55–3.58
Thompson effect 2.3
Thyroid cartilage 9.48
Tomography 2.17
Tooth fracture 5.69, 5.129, 5.157–5.163, 5.166, 9.36, 9.37
Tooth, ghost 5.86
Tooth, incisor 3.1, 3.3, 3.4, 3.9, 3.11
Tooth, inverted 5.22, 5.48, 5.54
Tooth, molar 3.2, 3.6, 3.8, 3.13–3.15
Tooth, premolar 3.5, 3.6, 3.12, 3.13
Tooth socket 5.171, 5.172, 5.175, 7.55, 7.66, 7.68, 7.77, 7.92–7.95, 7.107, 7.110, 7.112, 7.192, 7,195, 7.196, 7.201, 7.202, 7.204, 9.13, 9.14, 10.16, 10.17, 10.20–10.22
Tooth, subluxation 5.156
Tooth, supernumerary 5.52–5.58, 5.157, 5.171, 7.2, 7.3, 7.12, 8.3
Tooth, supplemental 5.59–5.62, 7.11
Tooth transplantation 5.36–5.38
Tooth transposition 5.51
Torus mandibularis 3.28, 7.5
Torus palatinus 7.6
Towne's view, skull 2.15
Transcranial view, temporo-mandibular joint 2.16, 3.55–3.58
Transplantation, tooth 5.36–5.38
Transposition, tooth 5.51
Trauma, occlusal 5.63, 5.72, 6.20, 6.21
Traumatic aneurysm 9.44
Traumatic bone cyst 7.175

Treacher–Collins syndrome 7.9–7.11
Trifurcation involvement 6.9
Tube, pharyngo-tympanic (Eustachian) 3.52
Tubercle, genial 3.36–3.38, 7.5, 7.98, 7.99
Tuberosity, maxillary 3.14, 3.15, 3.39
Turbinate, inferior 3.9, 3.25, 3.48, 3.50, 3.60
Turbinate, middle 3.50
Tumour, adenomatoid odontogenic 7.147, 7.148
Tumour, calcifying epithelial odontogenic 7.151, 7.152
Tumour, central giant cell 7.154–7.158
Tumour, neuro-ectodermal of infancy 7.54

Unerupted canine 5.23–5.40, 5.51
Unerupted incisor 5.49, 5.50, 5.52, 5.57, 5.58, 5.76, 5.77, 5.80
Unerupted molar 5.1–5.22
Unerupted premolar 5.41–5.48, 5.79
Upper oblique occlusal radiograph 3.33
Upper standard occlusal radiograph 3.32
Upper true occlusal radiograph 3.35
Upper vertex occlusal radiograph 3.34

Vertebra, atlas 3.42, 3.52, 7.31, 7.183
Vertebra, axis 3.42, 3.48, 7.32
Vertebra, cervical 3.39, 3.48
Vitamin D-resistant rickets 5.177, 5.178
Vomer 3.52

Wormian bone 7.13

X-ray 2.1
X-ray tube 2.2

Y formation of Ennis 3.12, 3.26

Zygoma, body 3.42
Zygoma, root 3.13–3.16, 3.23, 3.24, 3.27, 3.33, 3.60, 5.20, 5.169, 7.93, 7.100
Zygomatic arch 3.39, 3.48, 3.52, 3.54, 3.60, 5.20, 5.65, 7.79, 7.80, 10.18, 10.20, 10.31
Zygomatic bone 3.48
Zygomatic bone, frontal process 3.50
Zygomatic complex, fracture 7.124–7.127
Zygomatic process 5.170, 6.3
Zygomatic process, frontal bone 3.50
Zygomatic process, maxilla 3.42
Zygomatico-temporal suture 7.126